Historical and Epidemiological Analyses on the Impact of Infectious Disease on Society

Edward Greenberg
Cigna, USA

A volume in the Advances in Medical Diagnosis, Treatment, and Care (AMDTC) Book Series

IGI Global
PUBLISHER of TIMELY KNOWLEDGE

Published in the United States of America by
IGI Global
Medical Information Science Reference (an imprint of IGI Global)
701 E. Chocolate Avenue
Hershey PA, USA 17033
Tel: 717-533-8845
Fax: 717-533-8661
E-mail: cust@igi-global.com
Web site: http://www.igi-global.com

Library of Congress Cataloging-in-Publication Data

Names: Greenberg, Edward Wertlieb, 1990- author.
Title: Historical and epidemiological analyses on the impact of infectious disease on society / by Edward Wertlieb Greenberg.
Description: Hershey, PA : Information Science Reference, [2022] | Includes bibliographical references and index. | Summary: "This book explores infectious disease from a variety of angles, including the humanities, the social sciences, and medicine and reflects the interaction of knowledge, and of human behavior, with the biology of disease processes"-- Provided by publisher.
Identifiers: LCCN 2021045763 (print) | LCCN 2021045764 (ebook) | ISBN 9781799886891 (hardcover) | ISBN 9781799886891 (paperback) | ISBN 9781799886914 (ebook)
Subjects: LCSH: Communicable diseases--History. | Communicable diseases--Epidemiology. | Communicable diseases--Social aspects.
Classification: LCC RA649 .G74 2022 (print) | LCC RA649 (ebook) | DDC 616.9--dc23/eng/20211103
LC record available at https://lccn.loc.gov/2021045763
LC ebook record available at https://lccn.loc.gov/2021045764

This book is published in the IGI Global book series Advances in Medical Diagnosis, Treatment, and Care (AMDTC) (ISSN: 2475-6628; eISSN: 2475-6636)

British Cataloguing in Publication Data
A Cataloguing in Publication record for this book is available from the British Library.

Advances in Medical Diagnosis, Treatment, and Care (AMDTC) Book Series

ISSN:2475-6628
EISSN:2475-6636

MISSION

Advancements in medicine have prolonged the life expectancy of individuals all over the world. Once life-threatening conditions have become significantly easier to treat and even cure in many cases. Continued research in the medical field will further improve the quality of life, longevity, and wellbeing of individuals.

The **Advances in Medical Diagnosis, Treatment, and Care (AMDTC)** book series seeks to highlight publications on innovative treatment methodologies, diagnosis tools and techniques, and best practices for patient care. Comprised of comprehensive resources aimed to assist professionals in the medical field apply the latest innovations in the identification and management of medical conditions as well as patient care and interaction, the books within the AMDTC series are relevant to the research and practical needs of medical practitioners, researchers, students, and hospital administrators.

COVERAGE

- Alternative Medicine
- Patient Interaction
- Chronic Conditions
- Experimental Medicine
- Emergency Medicine
- Medical Procedures
- Cancer Treatment
- Medical Testing
- Internal Medicine
- Disease Prevention

IGI Global is currently accepting manuscripts for publication within this series. To submit a proposal for a volume in this series, please contact our Acquisition Editors at Acquisitions@igi-global.com or visit: http://www.igi-global.com/publish/.

The Advances in Medical Diagnosis, Treatment, and Care (AMDTC) Book Series (ISSN 2475-6628) is published by IGI Global, 701 E. Chocolate Avenue, Hershey, PA 17033-1240, USA, www.igi-global.com. This series is composed of titles available for purchase individually; each title is edited to be contextually exclusive from any other title within the series. For pricing and ordering information please visit http://www.igi-global.com/book-series/advances-medical-diagnosis-treatment-care/129618. Postmaster: Send all address changes to above address.

Titles in this Series

For a list of additional titles in this series, please visit:
www.igi-global.com/book-series/advances-medical-diagnosis-treatment-care/129618

Handbook of Research on Natural Products and Their Bioactive Compounds as Cancer Therapeutics
Ashok Kumar Pandurangan (B.S. Abdur Rahman Crescent Institute of Science and Technology, India) Suresh Kumar Anandasadagopan (Central Leather Research Institute, India) and Fahad A. Alhumaydhi (Department of Medical Laboratories, College of Applied Medical Sciences, Qassim University, Buraydah, Saudi Aabia)
Medical Information Science Reference • © 2022 • 643pp • H/C (ISBN: 9781799892588) • US $495.00

Exploring the Efficacy and Beneficence of Complementary and Alternative Medicinal Products in Disease Therapy
Etetor Roland Eshiet (Sustainable Energy Environmental and Educational Development (SEEED), USA)
Medical Information Science Reference • © 2022 • 315pp • H/C (ISBN: 9781799841203) • US $295.00

The Pediatric Eye Exam Quick Reference Guide Office and Emergency Room Procedures
Lily Zhu-Tam (Citywide Eye Care Optometry, USA) and Ida Chung (College of Optometry, Western University of Health Sciences, USA)
Medical Information Science Reference • © 2022 • 409pp • H/C (ISBN: 9781799880448) • US $295.00

Medical Atlas of Cornea and External Diseases in Middle Eastern Populations
Anna Hovakimyan (Malayan Ophthalmologic Centre, Armenia)
Medical Information Science Reference • © 2022 • 384pp • H/C (ISBN: 9781799869375) • US $265.00

Using Narrative Writing to Enhance Healing During and After Global Health Crises
Jennifer Lynne Bird (Oxbridge Academy, USA)
Medical Information Science Reference • © 2022 • 241pp • H/C (ISBN: 9781799890515) • US $295.00

IGI Global
PUBLISHER of TIMELY KNOWLEDGE

701 East Chocolate Avenue, Hershey, PA 17033, USA
Tel: 717-533-8845 x100 • Fax: 717-533-8661
E-Mail: cust@igi-global.com • www.igi-global.com

Table of Contents

Preface

TERMINOLOGY AND THE PURPOSE OF THE TEXT

This book is about the context of infectious disease. The causes and effects of any disease are known as its pathology (Funkhouser, 2018). Because so many of those who investigate infectious disease professionally or personally are, for good reason, focused on interactions within the human body, the related field of epidemiology, with its focus on population statistics, vectors, and prevention, may at first glance seem somewhat peripheral to the practice of medicine (Nishi et al., 2016). This distance need not seem the case. In history and political science, a great deal of emphasis is placed on group dynamics, similar to epidemiology. Meanwhile, specific major historical events are often more naturally explained from a broad historical rather than an individual psychological perspective. The purpose of this book is to take the widest possible view of pathology, and investigate the nature of infectious disease in its social and historical context. Biology will be discussed, and is important to the narrative of the book. However, the intent is to discuss outbreaks of disease as the events they are, trying, in the most interdisciplinary way possible, to integrate the norms of pathology with the rich cultural context of epidemiology.

An interdisciplinary project such as this one may require considerable theoretical justification, as it naturally cuts across common disciplinary justifications. As such, much of the subsequent preface will focus on explaining the interdisciplinary approach taken by this book.

THE METAPHYSICS OF DISEASE

Knowledge has a funny way of not fitting neatly into existing categories. The philosopher Martin Heidegger was particularly interested in the distinction between language (which we use to describe reality) and reality itself (Wheeler, 2011; Gale, 2014). While his philosophy is complicated, he ultimately seemed to settle on the idea that the best purpose of philosophy is therapeutic, or to clarify the approaches that are worth pursuing, out of a context where it is sometimes very hard to figure out what other people are talking about, even when they use similar terms. As a practical example--consider an argument between two people where neither can quite understand what the other is even upset at, or why the other is upset. The Heideggerian approach applied to such an interaction would likely consider a key component of conflict resolution to be getting both parties to understand both the concerns of their opposite number, as well as any trivialities that may be unnecessarily inflaming the situation. Maybe the important part of the conversation is not, for example, about how good a hat looks on someone's head, but rather that one party did not check the budget before purchasing the hat.

The whole modern endeavor of science has made an effort to "divide and conquer" the space of potential questions, dividing and dividing down human inquiry into subdomains like the analysis of a particular author, or the behavior of a certain animal. Those who obtain doctoral degrees do so with theses that may address subspecifications even more nuanced. And yet the title "Doctor of Philosophy" clarifies the shared origin of these endeavors, and it is essentially impossible to write any sort of scholarly work that does not owe a great deal to fields outside the thrust of the main topic (math and computers very often being used to conduct analyses, literature embodying the natural state of the writing, and psychology necessarily impacting how the work is received).

The essential and close association of apparently disparate fields is a general theme of this book, which is, naturally, focused on a much more narrow question. That is--how has infectious disease impacted the people who and societies that have naturally formed the backbone of history? It is the hope of the author that through the text, the reader will find new ways of thinking about well-known historical events and processes. Modern historiography arguably defines itself implicitly or explicitly as revolt against the Great Man Theory popularized by Thomas Carlyle (Spector, 2016). That is to say, the idea that certain heroic figures shape the course of destiny has given way to a vision that more fully depicts the roles of individuals in contributing to their society. To give an example of this--if someone is leading a march, moving away from Great Man Theory goes from asking "Why is the leader there?" to "Why is the crowd following?" However, it may be a step further still to say that the environment shapes our world. This goes a step beyond the idea of *subaltern* stories (stories of those considered to have lower social status), and into a space known as "big history."

"Big history" says in effect we are all subalterns (Christian, 1991). What are we subalterns to? The environment itself. Forces like geography, and yes, infectious disease, have had a profound impact on the development of human civilization. Because the impact of infectious disease can in some respects be subtle, before circling onto that topic to stay, it may be useful to see how dramatically geography has impacted human history in a very specific context--human borders.

Borders and countries are a key way children at school are introduced to the natural world. Consider maps and globes, and how often they are colored in bright-but-arbitrary national colors, with the lines between countries potentially as thick as the borders between landmasses and the ocean itself. This, from a certain perspective, is farcical--the land is certainly not composed of monolithic blocks of color--but the implication which may be easy to take for granted is that the human qualification of certain blocks of geography is the most important distinction of that geography. Given regulation of borders, and the different immigration and legal regimes around the world, knowing what country one is in is certainly a very important detail. But the borders themselves have been influenced by geography. France is bounded by the Rhine, the Alps and the Pyrenees. China grew up around two great rivers, the Yellow and the Yangtze. New York State is built around the Hudson River, with a westward extension that follows the Mohawk, and was extended by the Erie Canal. Meanwhile, New York City built up where it was not only because of the site's location at the mouth of the Hudson, but also because of the excellent natural harbor at the location. Other natural harbors that have turned into major places of importance to human civilization include Sydney in Australia and Pearl Harbor in Hawaii. In Africa, Walvis Bay was significant enough that the government of South Africa attempted to hold onto the territory after granting independence to Namibia (Stanley, 1993).

One may object and state that the stories involved in these places (and really, all others) are profoundly human. And this is true. But it is not necessarily an objection. As humans, we must relate to the world around us using the tools that we have at our disposal. Human encounters with the Black Death, with smallpox, with tuberculosis, and with all other diseases are fundamentally mediated through the way in which we perceive them. Disease shaped the human experience, but our understanding of disease has shaped the way disease is defined, considered, and even spread.

The Western concept of a grim reaper, or one of the Four Horsemen of the Apocalypse, is not scientifically tied to disease in any particular way, and yet the association is deeply relevant to engaging with disease. Even when people take pains not to anthropomorphize disease, disease still has what might be deemed anthropomorphic effects. In other words, every effect of disease that is noticeable by humans, or affects humans, is only intelligible by the ways it is notable by humans, or affects humans. This is a tautology, but arguably a very important one, baked into the foundations of medicine. Disease, after all, exists in contrast to a state of health (Scully, 2004). Importantly, disease is not the same as the disease agent. Disease only exists in the context of an organism from a purported baseline. Consider a single viral particle or bacterium entering a human body, and dying, perhaps at the hand of the immune system, without accomplishing anything of note. This is a story of pathogens that can cause disease, certainly. But it is not itself a story of disease *incidence*.

SURVEY OF CHAPTERS

The thought that medicine is fundamentally concerned with deviations from a purported norm, and perhaps only secondarily on the causes of such deviations in their own right, is an invitation to begin to discuss the structure of this book. The first chapter, "Origin Links Between Humans and Infectious Disease Agents," will explore in detail the specific relationship between human beings and the biological and extra-biological causes of infectious disease. To preview just one aspect of this--the fact that a bacterium and a human being seem to share a common evolutionary heritage is not irrelevant to our experience with bacteria, but rather a hint as to the nature of a story that has gone on for billions of years, that we are still experiencing (and interpreting through the lens of concepts like "medicine," and "disease").

The second chapter of the book, "Cultural Explanations of Infectious Disease," will back away from the big historical narration of the first chapter, and engage critically with the range of explanations that have existed surrounding infectious disease. Exploring models for how humans have considered infectious disease is a way of delving into human decision making *in extremis*--how we make sense of catastrophes large and small when we do not necessarily have any immediate insight into their origins.

The third chapter, "Role of Infectious Disease at Pivotal Historical Moments," will shift focus away from any kind of totalizing explanation of infectious disease as a whole, towards descriptions and discussions of significant historical moments that were shaped by the course of infectious disease. It is perhaps common to discuss human history as the annals of human triumph and tragedies, but, in the same way that it may be impossible to discuss the history of any particular region without at least some implication as to its peripheries, it may be impossible to discuss the Columbian exchange that led to the European colonization of the Americas without reference to the infectious disease that hitched rides westward towards immunologically unprepared lands, depopulating and weakening native civilizations just in time for Europeans to take advantage, to conquer, and to exploit. Likewise, it is difficult to explain the complex exchange between Africa and Europe without reference to conditions like malaria, which led to, for example, 1880s mortality rates in Upper Sudan of up to 80% of certain columns of deployed French imperial troops (Cohen, 1983). The Kangxi Emperor, early ruler of the Qing (the last dynasty of China), seems to have been chosen for the throne in part because he had the disease resistance of a smallpox survivor (Zhang, 2002).

In early chapters, the book is concerned with the impressions infectious disease has left on human society, but in the fourth chapter, "The Fight Against Infectious Disease," the book becomes more concerned with the opposite. Humans have done a great deal of work to manage and defeat infectious disease. This story is filled with the travails that come with science in practice. It includes moments of triumph, like the vaccine discoveries of Edward Jenner, and ethical atrocities, like the Tuskegee Syphilis Study, and deserves to be told in its own right.

Chapter 5 is "Quantifying the Lethality of Infectious Disease." Fatality risk, in general, in a fraught concept, with many misconceptions about chances of harm rising in contrast to actual harm. Additionally, even in situations where a disease is clearly highly fatal, there are different ways to think about fatality. Is the most dangerous disease the one that is the least likely for a patient to survive, or is the most dangerous disease one that kills the most people? How do phenomena like environmental sanitation and individual risk factors play into this, since differing "preparedness landscapes" may lead to wildly different disease outcomes in a population? The goal of Chapter 5 is to unpack all of this in as statistically-minded a manner as possible.

The sixth chapter, "Nonlethality in Infectious Disease," goes hand-in-hand with the previous, with an emphasis on describing and analyzing symptoms of infectious disease that do not rise to the level of death. Earth exists in a landscape filled with infectious disease, and anyone who has ever had the common cold, or the flu, has experienced a fragment of the larger narrative presented in so many ways earlier in the book, but it easy enough for so many who get sick to escape relatively unscathed, or at least alive, that the context of nonlethal experiences may seem very much removed from the context of those who lose their lives. This chapter, in keeping with the back half of the book's emphasis on quantifying and contextualizing experiences, aims to bridge the gap between personal memories of infectious disease and the worst infectious disease has to offer.

Chapters 7-11 are effectively case studies, intended to review and reinforce concepts discussed more broadly in the book. Chapter 7, "COVID-19 and Historical Parallels," will cover coronavirus disease 2019 as it is understood to the time of writing, and compare and contrast COVID-19 to prior epidemics. While the coronavirus underlying COVID-19 is not the same as the influenza virus involved in the pandemic starting around 1918, processes surrounding epidemics, including principles surrounding spread, and human response tendencies, have important similarities.

Chapter 8, "Profile: Malaria," will focus on malaria, which John Whitfield, writing for *Nature*, starkly labeled as a disease that "may have killed half of all the people that ever lived" (Whitfield, 2002). This statistic has been criticized directly, and an alternative value of between four to five percent put forward (Pomeroy, 2019). However, it is stubbornly difficult to clearly disprove, in part because humanity evolved in regions of Africa where malaria was endemic (DeMichele, 2016).

Chapter 9, "Profile: Tuberculosis," will focus on a disease once commonly called consumption, which may have killed one in seven people who ever lived (Waters, 2017). Tuberculosis is driven by a bacterial pathogen that largely transmits by air. The disease itself is notable for extended chronic cases featuring long periods of quiescence, where the pathogen is blockaded in granulomas established with the aid of the human immune system. While reactivation is rare, the sheer number of individuals who are infected with this disease worldwide—about two billion people (Babereis et al., 2017)—means that even this rareness is enough to cause an immense human toll. Because of the chronic nature of tuberculosis, those who have weakened immune systems for any reason are at particular risk of an adverse outcome.

Chapter 10, "Profile: Smallpox," will deal with smallpox, a disease which, in addition to playing a critical role in the history of the development of vaccination, also may have killed 300 million people in the 20th century alone, three times the estimated loss in that period from armed conflict (World Health Organization, 2011, pp. 3-21).

Chapter 11, "Profile: Plague," will focus on plague, which as the Black Death may have killed one third of Europe in the wave that began in the 1300s, in addition to uncounted numbers further east (Pamuk, 2007). Plague is less relevant today than in the past because of the use of antibiotics (Anisimov & Amoako, 2006), but the shifting relation of plague with human society, driven by human capacity, should serve as a recapitulation of the central ideas of this book.

In the twelfth and final chapter, "The Relationship Between Vulnerable Populations and the Stigma of Bearing Infectious Disease," the text moves away from biology and history, and instead examines the way infectious disease relates to the common idea of the subaltern. How are those with infectious disease treated? How do they treat themselves? How has cleanliness, and fear of infection, been used to maintain distinctions between social classes? These sorts of questions form the backbone for an investigation of infectious disease that is different from the more top-down style used earlier in the book, but may be no less critical to understanding infectious disease' impact on human society.

This brings a review of book content to a close. From granular details about smallpox and plague, it is time to zoom back out and take stock of the relationship between humanity and infectious disease.

Edward Greenberg
Cigna, USA

REFERENCES

Anisimov, A. P., & Amoako, K. K. (2006). Treatment of plague: Promising alternatives to antibiotics. *Journal of Medical Microbiology*, *55*(11), 1461–1475. doi:10.1099/jmm.0.46697-0 PMID:17030904

Barberis, I., Bragazzi, N. L., Galluzzo, L., & Martini, M. (2017). The history of tuberculosis: From the first historical records to the isolation of Koch's bacillus. *Journal of Preventive Medicine and Hygiene*, *58*(1), E9–E12. PMID:28515626

Christian, D. (1991). The case for "Big History". *Journal of World History*, *2*(2), 223–238. https://www.jstor.org/stable/20078501

Cohen, W. (1983). Malaria and French imperialism. *Journal of African History*, *24*(1), 23–36. doi:10.1017/S0021853700021502

DeMichele. (2016, December 7). *Malaria killed half the people who have ever lived.* Fact / Myth. http://factmyth.com/factoids/malaria-killed-half-the-people-who-have-ever-lived/

Funkhouser, W. K. Jr. (2018). Pathology: The clinical description of human disease. *Molecular Pathology*, 217–229. doi:10.1016/B978-0-12-802761-5.00011-0

Gale, J. (2014). Intersecting heterologies. *European Journal of Psychotherapy & Counselling*, *16*(1), 5–12. doi:10.1080/13642537.2013.879326

Nishi, A., Milner, D. A. Jr, Giovannucci, E. L., Nishihara, R., Tan, A. S., Kawachi, I., & Ogino, S. (2016). Integration of molecular pathology, epidemiology and social science for global precision medicine. *Expert Review of Molecular Diagnostics*, *16*(1), 11–23. doi:10.1586/14737159.2016.1115346 PMID:26636627

Pamuk, Ş. (2007). The Black Death and the origins of the 'Great Divergence' across Europe, 1300–1600. *European Review of Economic History*, *11*(3), 289–317. doi:10.1017/S1361491607002031

Pomeroy, R. (2019, October 3). *Has malaria really killed half of everyone who ever lived?* RealClearScience. https://www.realclearscience.com/blog/2019/10/03/has_malaria_really_killed_half_of_everyone_who_ever_lived.html

Scully, J. L. (2004). What is a disease? *EMBO Reports*, *5*(7), 650–653. doi:10.1038j.embor.7400195 PMID:15229637

Spector, B. A. (2016). Carlyle, Freud, and the great man theory more fully considered. *Leadership*, *12*(2), 250–260. doi:10.1177/1742715015571392

Stanley, W. R. (1993). Southern Africas's Walvis Bay exclave: Apparent tranquility and possible cause for concern. *GeoJournal*, *31*(4), 469–472. doi:10.1007/BF00812804

Waters, D. D. (2017). The rise and fall of tuberculosis and atherosclerosis: First there is a mountain…. *The Canadian Journal of Cardiology*, *33*(3), 295–297. doi:10.1016/j.cjca.2016.11.012 PMID:28081868

Wheeler, M. (2011, October 12). Martin Heidegger. *Stanford Encyclopedia of Philosophy*. https://plato.stanford.edu/archives/fall2020/entries/heidegger/

Whitfield, J. (2002, October 3). Portrait of a serial killer: A round up of the history and biology of the malaria parasite. *Nature*. https://www.nature.com/news/2002/021001/full/news021001-6.html doi:10.1038/news021001-6

World Health Organization. (2011). *Bugs, drugs and smoke: Stories from public health*. World Health Organization. https://www.who.int/about/history/publications/public_health_stories/en/

Zhang, J. (2002). Disease and its impact on politics, diplomacy, and the military: The case of smallpox and the Manchus (1613-1795). *Journal of the History of Medicine and Allied Sciences*, *57*(2), 177–197. doi:10.1093/jhmas/57.2.177 PMID:11995595

Acknowledgment

Many thanks to the following reviewers for their feedback: Jennifer Barnes, Richard Fogarty, Ken Rosenthal, Maureen Straight, Theresa Vaughan, and two anonymous. I would also like to thank the staff at IGI Global for shepherding this book through the publication process. It is my sincere hope that this book is able to contribute to the collection of knowledge about infectious disease.

Chapter 1
Origin Links Between Humans and Infectious Disease Agents

ABSTRACT

This chapter explores in detail the specific relationship between human beings and the biological and extra-biological causes of infectious disease. The fact that a bacterium and a human being seem to share a common evolutionary heritage is not irrelevant to our experience with bacteria, but rather a hint as to the nature of a story that has gone on for billions of years, that we are still experiencing (and interpreting through the lens of concepts like "medicine" and "disease"). From an evolutionary perspective, disease agents and humans share certain foundational characteristics which developed towards the dawn of life, and it is these characteristics that inform on the relationship between diseases and humans today.

EARLY PHYSICS AND EARLY LIFE

The purpose of this chapter is to focus on the shared context of humans and infectious disease agents. Because there is a great deal of difference, the beginning of the narrative is quite early in deep time. The timeline of big history ranges in the billions of years, and is worth exploring in detail. The Big Bang, where the universe exploded in size and complexity from a point, is fixed with reasonable specificity at 13.7 billion years ago (Xu, 2019). Development of the universe then occurred progressively, and initially,

DOI: 10.4018/978-1-7998-8689-1.ch001

with rapid speed--lithium is presumed to have first synthesized within a few minutes of the Big Bang.

Not everything we associate with the modern universe moved nearly so quickly. The first observable star may have formed 30 million years after the Big Bang, and galaxies as massive as our Milky Way seem to have arrived after 400 million years (Naoz et al., 2006). Of course, this still leaves over 13 billion years for the universe to seem somewhat similar to the one we see when we look at the night sky. Somewhat being a key term, as stars exist for an extremely long time. Accretion of Earth's sun is dated to around 4.5 billion years ago (with a birthing process that lasted about one million years); 100 million years after that, the solar system is thought to have been similar to the way it is now (Montmerle et al., 2006).

Despite the enormous timescales involved, our solar system has existed in a recognizable state for a nontrivial fraction of the believed history of the universe. And, perhaps more dramatically, given the focus of this book, it did not take a particularly long fraction of our solar system's history for life to emerge. Earth is thought to have existed in habitable form for 4.3 billion years, and microbes seem to have existed on Earth since at least 3.4 billion years ago (Javaux, 2019). It is a fairly well-known trope in big history to say that humans, and human civilization, have only existed for an eyeblink of the universe. However, if all life on Earth is meaningfully our kin, then the trope is limited. Life existing for around a quarter of the history of the universe does not seem like a particularly narrow pie-slice.

Of course, there is a very important conceit here--what does it mean for the earliest life on Earth to be meaningfully our kin? How similar is a human to a microbe? What is a microbe? One literal answer to that last question is that a microbe is an organism that exists on a scale of approximately 10-6 to 10-4 meters. For comparison, a human hair is about 70 microns wide, with a micron being a unit of 10-6 meters (Sanjuan & Cahill, 2009). However, this literal answer is not particularly satisfying. How does a microbe actually function? How is it linked to humanity in the believed course of the development of life? What is life? These are all questions that get to the heart of this chapter, which is foundationally about the relationship between human beings, and disease-causing organisms which are often microbes.

Let's get started by thinking about life.

MECHANICS OF EVOLUTION

Just as the cosmological history of the universe is a gargantuan topic, so too is the story of life. Life covers everything from the relation of a human being to a tree, a microbe to a tree, and a human being to a microbe, and it does so in a way that, in the framework embraced by modern science, is fundamentally united by the idea of evolution.

Evolution rests on three basic pillars. First, there is some fundamental unit of interest that is distinct from its surroundings. This can be a microbe, a tree, a person, or something else. Second, this fundamental unit of interest has some imperfect ability to reproduce, and create similar, but not exactly-identical versions of itself. (This is a very fancy way of referring to the concept of offspring, or a baby.) Finally, the frequency of this unit of interest, and the way its descendants may split off into different lineages, or disappear entirely, is contingent on how reproduction occurs, or does not occur, in the surrounding environment.

There is a great deal more that can be said about evolution, and its various mechanisms, and patterns, but the above is essentially the core from which can be derived the commentary. Charles Darwin famously built his concept of evolution on the example of birds known as finches, which seemed to be separating into different lineages as evidenced by beak morphology (Podos & Nowicki, 2004). Different beaks were better at achieving success with different food sources, which was tied to all sorts of interesting ways as to how the birds were socializing and arranging themselves in reproductive groups.

While Darwin wrote in the 1800s, there are today four common mechanisms considered to be core to evolution.

1. Natural selection, where organisms with traits more adapted to the environment in which they live are more likely to survive to reproductive age, and pass on those traits to the next generation (Malmquist & Prescott, 2021)
2. Mutation, where copy errors in the genetic sequence of an organism, its DNA (deoxyribonucleic acid), create variation upon which selection can work
3. Genetic drift, where, in small populations, certain traits may leave the gene pool by simple random chance

4. Gene flow, where genes (the inheritable DNA encoding of a trait) may arrive to a population via exogenous factors, such as new members of a compatible species arriving in the area, and reproductively intermixing

Evolution is not necessarily concerned with a tight definition of species. From the perspective of cladistics, a classification methodology for life, lineages continually split (and sometimes merge!) over time, in a naturalistic way (Ridley, 1989). If a population changes so drastically over time that it would no longer be able to interbreed with its far ancestors, according to the cladistic perspective, there is no sharp break, because the individuals that make up the population over time are effectively all individual species. This stands in contrast with the biological species concept, which focuses a boundary line around the idea of ability to successfully breed.

The broader point is that there is explanatory power in seeing life as a giant tree of lineage that traces back from us, through seemingly endless generations, all the way back to a microbial origin about 3.4 billion years ago. What kind of explanatory power? Well, in explaining traits! To start with humans, and trace our tree of ancestry backwards, one can approach the vast number of mammals with four limbs, two eyes, and a head, and consider how, assuming millions of years of development, it is reasonable to imagine those traits only needed to arise once. As a case-in-point, consider the coccyx, or human tailbone (Spinney, 2008). Considered by itself, this protrusion does not have obvious purpose. Considered as a vestigial tail, the end result of a lineage with a tail that shorted and shortened over time, the coccyx is perfectly reasonable.

Hopefully this discussion of humans has framed the evolutionary explanation for how we may relate to a wide variety of other organisms, as well as the basic process by which organisms, instances of life, can relate to each other. Evolutionary toolbox in hand, the narrative will now shift back to the other side of life's lineage on Earth. Its origins. Because it is at the origins of life that some fundamental classifications came into being that are critical to infectious disease.

Relevant to the present narrative, life is intricately tied to reproduction. Above, in the discussion of types of evolution, the concept of the gene was introduced as the *inheritable* DNA encoding of a trait. But there are patterns that fit the schema of evolution that do not involve DNA at all.

What is DNA? What alternatives are there? And how do these alternatives tie to the idea of evolution that has propelled and divided species of life for over three billion years? There are two more fundamental questions. What is life? What did abiogenesis look like?

ABIOGENESIS AND THE DEFINITION OF LIFE

Abiogenesis is the term for the creation of life from nonlife, and thus its explanation is the same as the origin question. Life, on the other hand, is, like evolution, a concept that seems very present-oriented, filled with lots of scholarly debates and terminological quibbling. And so, just as the narrative did with regards to evolution, it is worth looking at a modern definition before returning to Earth's period of abiogenesis over three billion years ago. The reason is to equip the reader with better tools to understand how microbes function, and what sort of entities are similar to them, but distinct.

One reasonable definition of life, from Macklem and Seely (2010), is that life is a "self-contained, self-regulating, self-organizing, self-reproducing, interconnected, open thermodynamic network of component parts which performs work, existing in a complex regime which combines stability and adaptability in the phase transition between order and chaos, as a plant, animal, fungus, or microbe" (p. 330). This seems like rather a lot to unpack, but a lot of the terms in the Maklem-Seely definition are, just as one of their aspects of life, "interconnected."

The first term in the Maklem-Seely definition, "self-contained" refers to the idea of life being distinct from its surroundings. All instances of life have boundaries. It might be a great debate to understand what exactly a human being is, but it is much less controversial to say that a human being, conversationally, is everything at and deeper than the level of the skin. When this boundary breaks down, as with injury, the existence of the individual may be in grave jeopardy. There are interesting quibbles that exist at the edge of "self-contained." For example, how are we supposed to think of the alimentary canal, the tube that runs through us from the mouth to the anus? This canal is external enough to have a vast array of gut microbes contribute to digestive function, while avoiding our bloodborne immune defenses, and yet is critical enough to our continued functioning that it is hard to imagine how humans could exist without it. The idea of "passing gas" is actually a good example of this ambiguity, as flatulence consists significantly of the waste products of gut flora (Quigley, 2006). However, while the concept of mutualism, meaning mutually beneficial dependencies of organisms, is an important one, the alimentary canal should not be so confusing as to lead naturally to tight association between a human being and the air around (human biomagnetism (Zheng et al. 2020), while interesting, will stay in this parenthetical).

The subsequent Maklem-Seely terms are relatively straightforward. "Self-regulating" refers generally to the idea that disruptions from homeostasis, or the organism's normal state, will be addressed by some pressure to restore normality. Consider the immune system itself, or the way breathing rate naturally increases under conditions of exercise, or the phenomenon that produces unpleasant detoxification symptoms when attempting to discontinue a substance of dependence (Diaper et al., 2014; Marhe et al., 2013). "Self-organizing" can be seen as a less defensive parallel to self-regulating--just as a body maintains itself in the face of adversity, it maintains itself regardless. "Self-reproducing" is probably the concept that ties life to evolution the best--life must be able to make copies of itself. Finally, "interconnected" refers to the idea that organisms that are alive have some sense of wholeness--are not randomly scattered parts collected within a border--while the part of the definition starting with "open thermodynamic network" refers broadly to the idea that life remains distinct while engaging in a complicated series of energy exchanges with its environment.

Of this definition, the "self-reproduction" and the "open thermodynamic network" concepts should be the most useful in understanding the origin of life. This is because, fundamentally, life seems to have arisen from entities that were similar, but distinct. What does this mean? The Earth of 3.4 billion or so years ago was filled with chemicals, and was made of chemicals, just like the other planets, and just like the sun. And some of these chemicals, that existed on the surface of the Earth, interacted with each other. Simple chemical reactions are not abiogenesis--there are chemical reactions in stars too. Our sun fuses 600 million metric tons of hydrogen every second, creating 596 tons of helium, and releasing the rest of the mass as energy (Inglis, 2015). However, chemical interactions need not exist on such a gargantuan scale. Not everything in the universe is a stellar factory. Chemicals on Earth were perfectly capable of interacting in more subtle ways. Earth itself is composed of core and mantle and crust, after all, and these layers are made up of elements. And on the surface, likely helped by an aqueous environment (Benner, 2014), certain chemicals in the water came to interact, perhaps not much more than 3.4 billion years ago on geologic timescales, in such a way that was *repetitive and sustainable*.

Consistent active patterns of chemical interaction are not quite the same thing as life, but they are remarkably close. Work on the origin of life done by

Pross and Pascal (2013) uses the phrase dynamic kinetic stability to refer to autocatalytic systems that can sustain themselves. In their framework, dynamic kinetic stability may be *the* critical prerequisite for life, and the authors go so far as to directly assert that Darwinian or evolutionary processes apply to autocatalytic systems. In other words, repetitive and sustainable dynamic kinetic systems that can replicate will succeed and spread in keeping with principles like natural selection. Autocatalytic systems by themselves do not need to have DNA-based genes, a notable departure from the four common mechanisms of evolution discussed above. However, the broader definition of evolution introduced above, which focused on evolution basically as "that which is most sustainable and replicable is more likely to replicate," is still perfectly applicable to an autocatalytic system that has nothing to do with DNA.

So evolution can apply to chemical processes. That sounds very close to being life, without actually being life. Life, applied, is the suggestion (drawing from the Maklem-Seely definition as appropriate) that autocatalytic processes have particular sustainability benefits when they feature self-containment, self-regulation, and self-organization, in addition to the self-reproduction that is the critical link between autocatalysis and evolution. There is a risk, when describing life this way, of being too teleological--there are methods of sustainable catalysis that are quite dramatic, but are not traditionally considered life--but as a way of understanding the fundamental rationale of abiogenesis from a big history viewpoint, the traits of life as being helpful for certain types of chemical stability seems reasonable enough.

With the application of evolutionary concepts to prelife, or nonlife, connecting microbes to trees or people may seem quaint. It is not possible to connect people to stars, or to the Big Bang itself.

What is the purpose of making this connection? Twofold. First, this chapter is still working towards explaining the link between causative agents of infectious disease, and humans, so explaining a potential link between humans and virtually everything else in the universe seems useful as a fundamental. Second, by emphasizing the idea that reproductive systems need not involve DNA, or life, the door opens to discussing autocatalytic systems that may not be considered life, but are very much a part of infectious disease, such as prions or viruses.

The chapter has reached a hinge point. Up until now, the focus was on defining concepts--evolution, life, abiogenesis--that help with the understanding of how humans fit into the grandest possible scope of a big history perspective. This was done at the cost of, for example, describing in practical terms how a microbe could possibly, even with the help of evolution, acquire enough mutations to have its lineage turn into humans. The remainder of the chapter will focus on specific implementations of life, and autocatalytic processes (near-life) that contribute to the landscape of infectious disease, in addition to sketching as much as possible the best available hypotheses for shared lineages among and between the topics of discussion. The terminology discussed above should be a good reference point in understanding the more physical entities that will dominate the rest of this chapter.

REPLICATION

What is required for replication of something like an organism? Near-life can be defined as an entity with replication but missing other of life's definitional components. What did the earliest near-life look like? It may well have been extremely simple. Note that all of the items required for *life*, as defined in the Macklem and Seely definition (self-containing, self-regulating, self-organizing, self-reproducing, etc.) do not strictly include DNA, RNA (ribonucleic acid), or any other physical thing, and near-life may be simpler still. In today's world, the standard "molecular" machine of life, long strings of combined atoms capable of some sort of external function (like catalysis) is the protein. The Central Dogma of molecular biology, which explains much of the functioning of the human body, as well as many, many comparison organisms, states that information in living things is stored in DNA, passes in a sometimes reversible fashion to RNA, and typically, though RNA, finally is implemented in proteins. This dogma, outlined in a published lecture by Francis Crick in 1958 (Morange, 2009), is both extremely valuable and incomplete. The patterns needed to create proteins do not need to be stored in the paired nucleotide language of DNA and RNA for proteins of a given type of spread. The amino acid monomers that are the building blocks of proteins, as well as the nucleotide monomers are the building blocks of DNA and RNA, have been known for decades as being abiotically able to assemble in chains up to 55 monomers long when in the presence of mineral surfaces (Ferris et al., 1996). Montmorillonite works notably well for nucleotide polymerization into polymeric DNA or RNA, while illite and hydroxylapatite does the same sort of work for amino acid assembly into protein strands. Aside from giving more hints as to how science can explain abiogenesis, the importance of replication to life, on multiple levels, also creates the foundation for understanding something that may simultaneous be the embodiment for some of the earliest prelife as on Earth, as well as the causative agent of some of the most terrifying modern infectious disease--the prion.

PRIONS

A prion is a protein with an infective state. Proteins themselves have two basic aspects--the chain sequence of their amino acids, and the folding conformation that allows them to engage in some activity. Importantly, proteins can take on different conformations depending on conditions. Actively infective prions appear to be able to interact with adjacent proteins of the same chain sequence, and refold them into the infective conformer (Linden et al., 2008). The key to prion infections, cellular prion protein (PrP^C), which exists benignly in humans prior to the introduction of an infective conformer, can become extremely dangerous once the infective version starts accumulating in the brain.

The conditions for prions to do their worst are reasonably specific--infectious prion spread is contingent on a Trojan-horse-like protein to already exist in a target. However, prion-style autocatalysis is considered to be a plausible pattern for early prelife to emerge (Lupi et al., 2006). Additionally, prion diseases, despite their dependency on existing PrP^C, progress in a fashion that is uniformly lethal, and exist in externally acquired, hereditary, and sporadically occurring variants (Imran & Mahmood, 2011). In the sporadic variant, the same concept that may have helped organize life's beginnings may today strike down otherwise healthy individuals, and the acquired form of prion disease is no more pleasant. A prominent but now extinct version of externally acquired prion disease, kuru, transmitted through consumption of brain matter by populations in and around the Fore linguistic group of Papua New Guinea, probably originally arose by spontaneous mutation in a single individual (Liberski et al., 2019).

This dualism, that is, the idea that an entity that may have been able to come into being near the dawn of life on Earth may also contribute to infectious disease in our modern age, seems to be no coincidence. Spontaneous prion conformation followed by rapid spread has very different implications when occurring on the aqueous surface of a mineral, versus inside the human body, but the model is essentially identical. Recall the nature of evolution--things that manage to replicate well in a given environment are likely to continue to do so. The fact that one context is a relatively barren Earth, and the other is a body, makes no obvious difference to the specimen that is under Darwinian pressure; it exists in an environment either way. The fact that prion diseases overrun and kill their hosts is both a tragedy and a warning that pressures in the microenvironment can accomplish destruction on a larger level, if left unchecked.

RNA

The next focus is on RNA. The RNA World hypothesis, as first presented by Alex Rich in 1962, suggests that the key molecule in abiogenesis was RNA (Neveu et al., 2013). RNA has properties that allow it to both store genetic information, and conform into forms, or phenotypes, that help catalyze certain reactions. While the genetic aspect of RNA helps allow for reproduction, the catalytic aspect of RNA may help with survivability. This chapter has already discussed how RNA may arise with relative spontaneity with the help of mineral surfaces, and so, a nearly-complete image of RNA as prelife emerges. However, just because this image is coherent does not mean it is correct, or complete; RNA, as the central piece of the Central Dogma, may tie in a more intuitive way to the development of "modern" life than prions do. One way of understanding RNA World (which can be called, both helpfully and confusingly, Lipid-RNA World) is that, in critical stages of abiogenesis, RNA "teamed up" with lipid bubbles to provide sustainability inside the bubble, while the bubble itself provided the inside-outside distinction so critical to the definition of life (Mallik & Kundu, 2012). The short version of the rest of the story would be that, after the lipid-RNA alliance proved fruitful, DNA evolved as an effective information storage system, and proteins evolved as an effective system for expressing phenotypes, creating microbial life, with catalytic activity existing under a lipid cell membrane. Under this framework, RNA, being the center of the original story, hung on in microbes, and larger multicellular life that evolved later. RNA's role was largely as intermediary between more specialized structures.

RNA World, or Lipid-RNA World, has the benefit of being coherent, and of flowing neatly into the Central Dogma that, as stated, is very useful for understanding a critical flow in modern instances of molecular biology. If prion-style proteins had emerged first, then RNA, DNA, and lipid layers in cells would still have to be explained, as would the various complex organelles, such as ribosomes, that exist within cells. Ribosomes, which are made of RNA and protein, and play a critical role in how proteins are manufactured from RNA in modern organisms, may be a particularly difficult challenge to explain under a protein-first abiogenesis hypothesis (Genuth & Barna, 2018; Mallik & Kundu, 2012).

Still worth emphasizing is that RNA World, protein-first synthesis, and all the rest, are competing hypotheses, and an answer to how life arose, via a preponderance of the evidence, is not yet forthcoming (Wulandari et al., 2021). The image of a Lipid-RNA World developing slowly in an aqueous environment near a hydrothermal vent on early Earth, perhaps with the help of some nearby minerals to jumpstart early catalytic processes, is far from fully established. One fascinating alternative framework involves early organic molecules developing complexity as far as viruses, in the atmosphere, before entering the water (Zaritsky et al., 2014).

VIRUSES

WIth reference to something like a virus-first hypothesis of abiogenesis, it is worth examining what a virus is. Viruses are an excellent example of how evolution is not teleological. That is, while viruses are, regardless of when exactly they emerged on Earth, a famous example of a class of structure on the border between life and nonlife (Koonin & Starokadomskyy, 2016), they are also extremely active and competitive with life to the present day. The COVID-19 viral pandemic, ongoing at the time of this writing, is a clear example. Viruses did not need to evolve "up" into plants, animals, or anything else to stay competitive with other entities on Earth. They simply persist, just as microbes do, and prions. What is the structure of a virus?

Viruses contain DNA or RNA, as well as protein, and sometimes have a lipid envelope as their outer layer (Modrow et al., 2013). Their most critical characteristic is their inability to replicate without infecting a living cell and stealing the use of some of the cell's machinery. Viruses do not metabolize materials for energy, as cells do, and they do not contain protein-making ribosomes, either. Their proteins are manufactured in hijacked cellular ribosomes. They are extremely small, and exist on the nanoscale, not the microscale. The small circoviruses can be 16 nm wide, while the large (for a virus) poxviruses can be over 300 nm wide.

From the above description of a virus, it should be clear why viruses did not obviously evolve before microbes. Viral replication *benefits* from microbes and other cell types existing. Viruses are parasites, and take advantage of cellular machinery, without needing to spend the effort to make said machinery. In a basic viral lifecycle, completed virion particles bypass the defenses of a cell, viral replicative compounds, including its DNA or RNA, are injected, and, eventually, the hijacked cell emits new virions out to continue the cycle. A typical method of emission is lysis, which involves the hijacked cell, no longer useful to the virus, now bursting open (Koonin & Starokadomskyy, 2016). However, lysis is not necessary to viral reproduction.

The concept of a mobile element is useful to certain types of viral hijacking strategies--mobile elements are DNA sequences that can inject themselves in a longer genetic code (Frost et al., 2005). The human immunodeficiency virus (HIV), for example, is a retrovirus with a genetic code of RNA that uses the process of reverse transcription to create DNA from RNA as a step towards integrating HIV genes with the target cell (Hu & Hughes, 2012). Still, in keeping with the nature of evolution, there is nothing that requires viral genetic elements to proceed with the construction of virions for external infection, and then lysis of a "hostage parent" cell. Evolution, at its core, circles on the idea that the lineage of successful things tends to stick around, in some form. Traits that might be considered essential to the original design (the ability to trigger lysis, for instance) may become irrelevant, from a cladistics perspective, without a clear break between species.

The point here is to say that viral DNA can survive perfectly well just *staying where it is*, once injected into the genetic code of a living cell. This DNA can then piggyback off of bacterial binary fission, or eukaryotic mitosis (the common style for single-celled microbes, and cells in a multicellular organism, to split, respectively) and be duplicated implicitly just by staying in line with the rest of the DNA while the host cell conducts its process. Lysis is unnecessary for survival of the rogue DNA sequence. Ejection in any form from the host cell is also unnecessary, if the point is merely survival of the viral DNA.

The so-called viral DNA, at this point, does not seem to be behaving much like a virus anymore. But it still bears some evidence of its origin in its construction. Suggesting just how ubiquitous viral DNA "calming down" might have been through the multi-billion year history of life on Earth, fully 44% of the human genome is composed of transposons (a type of mobile element) or transposon-like repetitive elements, though less than 0.05% of these elements are traditionally active (Mills et al., 2007). There are a number of different ways to understand this striking fact about our own bodies. One is that the very blueprints of humanity bear overwhelming scars of past encounters with viruses. Most organisms have methods of suppressing transposon mobility, including methylation of DNA, modification of histones (histones help "wrap up" DNA), and blockading activity by RNA (Wei & Cao, 2016). Another way to think of the existence of these transposons is that the line between infectious behavior, and healthy behavior (as with prions) may be narrow indeed. Because the same biological mechanisms that suppress transposable elements are connected to the general structure of cell regulation, transposable elements contribute to methods of gene expression as phenotypes in a wide variety of modern organisms.

Yet again, topics from the dawn of life help us understand not only the human place in the wider scope of biology, but also the scope of infectious disease. Topics such as viruses and prions also help show how processes that today do not seem particularly infectious between individuals are tied to issues that relate to the concept of infection. Transposable elements that escape suppression are similar in their escape to the dysregulation that occurs in genetically-influenced diseases, like cancer, (Jones & Baylin, 2007; Payer & Burns, 2019). Cancer, which can be roughly understood as dangerously uncontrolled cell growth and metastasis, or mobility (Sarkar et al., 2013), is not traditionally considered an infectious disease at all, but cancer's existence is linked to the idea of infection on a wide variety of levels. The cell regulation that needs to break down for cancer to occur is tied in part to transposons, and then, once cancerous cells are spreading, and not listening to command-and-control signals from a wider organism, the fight becomes one between homeostatic forces intervening on behalf of the larger organism, and the way in which the traits of the cancer assist with, or are irrelevant to, its spread.

A handful more points on viruses before the topic shifts to microbes, and other organisms that are solidly in the category of *life*. First, the success of viruses arguably rivals that of biological life, in terms of the fact that viral life outnumbers life by count, in terms of the fact that viruses maintain a competitive degree of genetic diversity with life, and in terms of the fact that viruses, because of their pared-down nature and high mutation rates, are energy efficient, and can survive and adapt to a vast range of environmental changes (Wasik & Turner, 2013). Second, viruses exist as part of a continuum of relatively-simple infectious entities. Virusoids piggyback off of other viruses to proliferate in the more independent virus' shadow. For example, the hepatitis D virus depends on the presence of hepatitis B, though virusoids are more common with plant viruses (Modrow et al., 2013). Viroids, which also invade plants, are infectious circular RNA that focuses on hijacking only enough cellular tools for its own transcription, without the supplementary protein-creation that is a hallmark of viruses (Di Sero et al., 2014; Modrow et al., 2013).

PHYSICAL NATURE OF LIFE

With a great deal of preliminary work done, attention can now turn to *life*. Life, as it is known on Earth, interacts with its environment through amino acids composed into proteins, and stores replication information as nucleic acids composing into RNA and DNA. This is a simpler definition than Macklem and Seeley but it is relatively coloquial. RNA and DNA molecules are made up of a core structure of the element carbon. Carbon is a critical element not only to life, but to all the other entities that have been leading in this chapter to a discussion of life proper, including protein prions, and the viruses that depend on nucleic acids to propagate their own genome. Carbon has the ability to make four covalent bonds with neighboring atoms, which may or may not be carbon (Petkowski et al., 2020). This flexibility allows for better structural diversity than "competitor" elements, like sulfur and boron.

The fundamentally elemental constraints of life help provide a clearer picture of when and where life originated on Earth. Organic chemistry is defined as chemistry involving carbon. However, nitrogen is an important element for life as well--therefore, life must have originated in a location with plentiful carbon and nitrogen. Above, when describing RNA, two hypotheses for a life origin location were briefly mentioned--the atmosphere, and hydrothermal vents. In the Hadean Eon, the name for the first 550 million years of the Earth's history, a vast range of mineral species, as well as water were already present to serve as potential catalysts, and an environment, for the development of life (Hazen, 2013). Meanwhile, the atmosphere was obviously available, as was UV light (Thomassot et al., 2015), which is valuable as an alternative catalyst to speed up organic reactions (Rimmer & Shorttle, 2019). Rimmer and Shorttle (2019) also propose, as something of an intermediary, surface rather than submarine hydrothermal systems.

It is far from a guarantee that abiogenesis could have occurred in the Hadean Eon (Harrison, 2020). However, the Archean Eon, which began after the Hadean, and continued to 2.5 billion years ago, is a different story (Schopf et al., 2007). The evidence for life that can be gleaned off for rocks from this eon suggests a diverse microbial landscape--regardless of whether life originated in the atmosphere, benthic (seafloor) organic laminae are meaningfully conclusive (Lepot, 2020). As the meteoric bombardment (Grimm & Marchi, 2018), and volcanic activity (Morrison et al, 2018) characteristic of the Hadean began to become less overwhelming, the Archean and its water biomes of microbes suggest an early (if no longer infantile) Earth that, in its most salient aspects, seems like something of a gargantuan petri dish as chemicals over time combined to develop life.

What exactly occurred in this petri dish? The chapter is beyond the point of discussing viruses, prions, and abiogenesis--the focus is now squarely on the organic chemistry of established microbes. And here, strikingly, the narrative of evolution is characterized by the tremendous relevance of infectivity. One way to understand this is to think of one of the important aspects of life--its ability to have a border between itself and the outside world. The critical role a lipid barrier might play in keeping the chemical processes of early life separate from the outside environment has already been discussed, and lipid bilayers are the principle component of cell membranes as we know them today (Qiu et al., 2018). However, the idea of a single layer being all that is needed in cells is too simple. One of the critical aspects of the evolution of early life involved *increasing* the number of relevant layers.

MICROBES

It should be valuable at this point to back up and focus on what entered the petri dish. That is, what the earliest form of Archean life might have looked like. The term 'microbe' should be a valid description, but can be made more specific. Firstly, microbes are not necessarily unicellular. Microbe is a term that refers predominantly to scale, not character. Secondly, microbes may not need be unicellular, but unicelular life is understood to have evolved first (Rainey & De Monte, 2014). That means there is value in imagining the archetypical Archean microbe as unicellular. This imagining may be relatively easy, given the coverage done so far in this chapter. An outer lipid bilayer, plus DNA information storage transcribed at appropriate times into RNA, then translated into protein production--all this has been presented already, and all this is fairly standard for a unicellular organism. The lipid bilayer, here, is at the border of the individual cell, the cell being traditionally accepted as the smallest single unit of life, and the lipid bilayer is also at the border of the larger organism, which, in this case, is just the one cell. However, there are aspects of single-celled life that go beyond the fact of the lipid bilayer as universally present in living cells, as the cell membrane (Karamdad et al., 2015), as well as beyond the Central Dogma of approximately DNA ← → RNA → protein (Crick, 1970) that is commonly accepted as the cornerstone of active life (Koonin, 2012). As stated above, the innovation being given emphasis is the idea of layers.

There are two basic cell types, prokaryotes, and eukaryotes, and prokaryotes. The simpler prokaryotes arose first, though eukaryotes seem to have also evolved in the Archean Eon (Rozanov & Astafieva, 2020). The critical distinction between these two cell types is membrane-bound organelles, which are present in eukaryotes but not prokaryotes (Lynch & Marinov, 2017). What are membrane-bound organelles? Not ribosomes. Those tiny factories, which read RNA and 'print' protein, are ubiquitous in both types of cells. Unique to eukaryotes, rather, are organelles like membrane-inclosed nucleuses for storing genetic material, as well as mitochondria and chloroplasts. The list of available membrane-bound organelles for eukaryotes goes longer than that, but the basic principle is already established. Complexity is not a requirement of evolution, or even a one-way flow, but it is a theme of certain pathways. Eukaryotes rely on a variety of simpler innovations to be able to achieve their framework of organelle "rooms" within a cellular "house."

So eukaryotes seem to have evolved in some manner from prokaryotes, as early as the Archean. This is a deception of what may have happened in that eon's petri dish. The purpose of this evolutionary history lesson is twofold.

First, the discussion here, on the most basic eukaryote, is centered around an organism that appears to be the common ancestor of both some infectious disease-causing organisms, as well as humans ourselves. The point is not that humans descended from the very same microorganisms that exist today, but rather that both share a common evolutionary heritage with tiny older organisms. This overlay, implying certain survival strategy overlaps in categories like reproduction and respiration, is part of the foundation by which humans and disease-causing organisms interact today. More simply, from an evolutionary frame, humans and disease-causing organisms compete because we thrive and reproduce by leveraging the same basic sorts of resources. As eukaryotic humans and the eukaryotic disease-causing organisms share very specific characteristics, the tension between these groups is particularly clear (though there are pathogens that come into conflict with humanity because they share even more basic characteristics, such as simply taking up space–see the section on prions, above).

The second reason for discussing ancient eukaryotes is that a particular infectious process appears critical to creating eukaryotes cells as we know them today. Namely, it is a common hypothesis that both chloroplasts, critical in plants and algae to collect energy from the sun, and mitochondria, critical in how a broader range of eukaryotic cells use a watermill-like process to collect energy from a proton gradient, are both descend from independent species of cells. These pre-chloroplasts and pre-mitochondria, as the hypothesis goes, could be swallowed by early eukaryotic cells, beginning a symbiotic process that extends fruitfully to the present day. Evidence for this hypothesis includes the fact that mitochondria and chloroplasts maintain and replicate with DNA independent of the host cell (Allen, 2015), as well as the fact that both chloroplasts (Cheng et al., 2020) and mitochondria (Thar & Kühl, 2004) bear inner and outer external membranes that are suggestive independent species having been enveloped by a consuming cell some time in the past.

One objection to contrasting the stories of mitochondria and chloroplasts with that of infectious specimens is that the membrane aspect of their morphologies suggests their having been "invited in." This is an interesting point mostly because it sheds light on parasitic mechanisms for cell entrance. Tricking cell membrane barriers into swallowing something they should not be swallowing, is, for example, a common lifecycle event in the behavior of the infectious bacterium *Listeria monocytogenes* (Abuaita & O'Riordan, 2014). For contrast, however, it should be noted that the free-species capture hypothesis is not unchallenged (Harish & Kurland, 2017).

The chapter is now reaching some of its final inflection points. With the arrival of single-celled eukaryotes on the Archean stage, the biggest conceptual hurdle between the microbes discussed so far, and modern species diversity, is probably the dawn of multicellular life. While the two basic subdivisions of prokaryotes are bacteria and archaea (Koonin & Wolf, 2008), both unicellular, and eukaryotes are sometimes unicellular, *all multicellular organisms are eukaryotes* (Combarnous & Nguyen, 2020).

MULTICELLULAR LIFE

When and how did multicellular life originate? Interestingly, the when seems to be the Archean Eon, yet again, in the form of photosynthetic cyanobacterial clusters from around three billion years ago (De Monte & Rainey, 2014). (In an interesting bit of narrative coherence, modern chloroplasts may very well have originated specifically as cyanobacteria (Falcón et al., 2010).) The word mat should be reasonably instructive. One way of understanding the flow of increasing complexity in multicellular evolution goes like this:

First there were individual cells. Because these individual cells often originated from each other, and proliferated in the same environment, they existed near to each other. In certain contexts, there was no particular disadvantage to these cells existing near each other, perhaps matting against an abiotic surface. By doing this, they could use economies of scale to make their environment more friendly. Any process one cell used to "improve" the nearby environment (in accordance with its own definition of fitness) would improve the environment for its neighbors as well, barring any overwhelming issues related to competition for resources. And even in this respect, a mat or cluster of like cells would get some benefit. After all, if there were only so many resources to go around, it would almost definationally be better for a lineage if the resources, regardless of scarcity, went to the lineage. Why give room to any competitor organisms? This sentence should not be understood as if mats of clumps of cells at this stage had a brain, but rather from an evolutionary standpoint, with its tautology: That which is successful, proliferates. Something which can fill a space densely, all other things being equal, has obvious benefits when it comes to proliferation. And that something can perhaps be thought of as a multicellular organism.

At this point, it is worth pointing out an apparent discrepancy. If the origins of multicellular life are in connected cyanobacterial groups, and bacteria are prokaryotes, and all multicellular organisms are eukaryotes, what is going on here? One way of understanding the present conceptual space is that there are legitimate contradictions. Multicellular life at its foundational edges is blurry, and it may be worth revising the statement above to say that *all significantly differentiated multicellular organisms are eukaryotes*. However, this revision may not feel very satisfying. It may be more useful, from the perspective of understanding modern scientific thought on the subject, to say that it is commonly understood that *all multicellular organisms are eukaryotes*, but the precise nature of collectives, such as collectives of individual cells, is a matter for ongoing discussion.

One paper that acknowledges competing definitions of multicellular life, by Niklas and Newman (2013), also provides a useful label for the ambiguous state discussed above--colonial. True multicellularity, arguably, involves more nuanced interactions than mere tight cohabitation. This still leaves the cyanobacteria example in a tight spot, since the question remains of where well-differentiated eukaryotic multicellular organisms came from, if bacterial colonialism is a false start. The answer seems relatively simple, and sheds interesting light on the nature of evolution. Namely, multicellular organisms may have evolved as many as 25 separate times (Grosberg & Strathmann, 2007). Cyanobacterial spreads may have paved the way for others, but eukaryotic multicellularity eventually became respectable. In terms of the key aspect that led multicellularity to be more than simply like cells clustered near each other, Rainey and Kerr (2010) suggest the idea of "cheats," or cells that took advantage of their neighbors and stopped engaging in processes that were maintained by their neighbors. These cells could then specialize, becoming better at a subset of tasks. The idea of gametes, or sex cells (eggs and sperm), is a natural component of this concept--cells that, under specific conditions, are good at being the progenitors of well-coordinated differentiated cells, seem perfectly reasonable under the tenets of evolution.

With clarity now available for complex multicellular life, this chapter is reaching its conclusion. Specialized cell types in a single living organism do not lead immediately to the concept of a fully functional human being, but given that the chapter started with stellar accretion, the path forward seems reasonably clear. The evolution of humans was not, from a biology standpoint, necessary. If various extinction events, such as the oceanic anoxia that existed at the border between the last two of Earth's four geological eons, the Proterozoic and the Phanerozoic (Kimura & Watanabe, 2001) about 543 million years ago (Miller et al., 2005), as well as the famous Chicxulub meteoric impact late in the Phanerozoic in the modern Yucatan, which led to enough temporary environmental damage to destroy the reign of the dinosaurs (Norris, 2020), had not created enough ecological niche carveouts to allow organisms from novel lineages time to awkwardly evolve into filling those gaps, then it is perfectly reasonable to assume humans as we know us would not exist. However, there is evidence for those events, and how the gene pool culls stemming from them contributed to the big history of the earth. Multicellular organisms speciated into animal, plant, protist, and fungi kingdoms, animals grew digestive tracts, animals came out of the water, animals grew land-useful limbs, and then a great deal of evolutionary conservation created the familiar "four limbs and a head" structure we see in so many mammals, amphibians, and reptiles today.

SEPARATION OF DISEASE AGENTS AND HOSTS

Through this process, which occurred over billions of years, the many organisms and entities that created infectious disease co-evolved. Viruses, bacteria, and tiny eukaryotes, to name some of the more obvious culprits, did not go away simply because, for instance, a fish was crawling onto land for the first time. Viruses, bacteria, and other pathogens have their own lineages, which may have diverged from the human lineage back in the Archean Eon, but still were successful enough to propagate down through the many periods and epochs to the present day. They exist in ecological niches, with survival strategies, that are as relevant to their own lives (or near-lives) as ours are to ours. While an important theme of other chapters of this book is the human response to infectious disease, it is valuable to note how similar some of the niche-targeting behaviors of pathogens are to our own patterns. Just as an open wound on a human body might become exploited by infectious bacteria, which take advantage of the opportunity to proliferate on the "wrong" side of our protective skin, so too does human proliferation seem tied to various dramatic disaster events in Earth's history that meaningfully wiped out or damaged our presumptive competition. And, just as a virus or other pathogen might proliferate and optimize for short term success without being concerned for the survival of the host, so too does the current growth of human population and industry seem to be causing extinction of world species at thousands of times the rate that would be present without human interventions (Ceballos et al., 2010).

Despite the ability to make an appalling connection between human beings and pathogens, there is plenty of space for hope. Nearly but not quite nihilistically, just as various infective species have found ways to jump to new hosts after using one up, so too might humanity be so successful at propagating in the face of competition and challenges that we will be able to hop to space, or other planets, and continue our behavior there. Alternatively, we might find new ways of coming to terms with our environment, so to reduce the impact on the environment. Just as humans can take steps to increase the sustainability of the environment, so too can pathogens, at least in the general case, promote the sustainability of *us*. The rhinovirus, for instance, a common pathogen for the common cold, has found a survival strategy that may not be pleasant for its hosts, but is far from lethal. Overcrowding, which promotes a competition for limited resources that would not take place without the proximity (Lowe et al., 2021; Namberger et al., 2019), is a way of thinking about how the significance of competition need not be based on any desire to harm, either on geographic or anatomical scales. This lack of intentionality helps create room for solutions.

Factors in the great divide between humans and the bulk of entities on this planet include our intelligence, as well as our interlinked capacities for tool-use, and ability to network on a global scale. These sorts of benefits to scale are not unlike the benefits that come when a multicellular organism divides the work between its parts, or the mechanism by which the colonies of gut fauna in our digestive tract crowd out microscopic invaders that might otherwise proliferate and do us harm. The difference, of course, is the scale, as vast networking between complex multicellular life builds dramatically on the advantages of specific instances of multicellular life. This level of intentional organization is meaningfully unprecedented in our awareness of big history from the dawn of the universe, and it gives credence to the idea that we as a species might be able to find meaningfully new solutions to old problems. However, as this chapter has indicated, pressures related to infectious disease are all around us, and are tied in many intricate ways to the development of Earth.

REFERENCES

Abuaita, B. H., & O'Riordan, M. X. (2014). Listeria exploits damage and death to spread bad news. *Trends in Microbiology*, *22*(7), 370–371. doi:10.1016/j.tim.2014.06.001 PMID:24934861

Allen, J. F. (2015). Why chloroplasts and mitochondria retain their own genomes and genetic systems: Colocation for redox regulation of gene expression. *Proceedings of the National Academy of Sciences of the United States of America*, *112*(33), 10231–10238. doi:10.1073/pnas.1500012112 PMID:26286985

Benner, S. A. (2014). Paradoxes in the origin of life. *Origins of Life and Evolution of the Biosphere*, *44*(4), 339–343. doi:10.100711084-014-9379-0 PMID:25608919

Ceballos, G., García, A., & Ehrlich, P. R. (2010). The sixth extinction crisis: Loss of animal populations and species. *Journal of Cosmology*, *8*, 1821–1831.

Cheng, Y., Zhang, L., Qi, J., & Zhang, L. (2020). Complete chloroplast genome sequence of Hibiscus cannabinus and comparative analysis of the Malvaceae family. *Frontiers in Genetics*, *11*, 227. doi:10.3389/fgene.2020.00227 PMID:32256523

Combarnous, Y., & Nguyen, T. M. D. (2020). Cell communications among microorganisms, plants, and animals: Origin, evolution, and interplays. *International Journal of Molecular Sciences*, *21*(21), 8052. doi:10.3390/ijms21218052 PMID:33126770

Crick, F. (1970). Central dogma of molecular biology. *Nature*, *227*(5258), 561–563. doi:10.1038/227561a0 PMID:4913914

De Monte, S., & Rainey, P. B. (2014). Nascent multicellular life and the emergence of individuality. *Journal of Biosciences*, *39*(2), 237–248. doi:10.100712038-014-9420-5 PMID:24736157

Di Serio, F., Flores, R., Verhoeven, J. T. J., Li, S. F., Pallás, V., Randles, J. W., Sano, T., Vidalakis, G., & Owens, R. A. (2014). Current status of viroid taxonomy. *Archives of Virology*, *159*(12), 3467–3478. doi:10.100700705-014-2200-6 PMID:25216773

Diaper, A. M., Law, F. D., & Melichar, J. K. (2014). Pharmacological strategies for detoxification. *British Journal of Clinical Pharmacology*, *77*(2), 302–314. doi:10.1111/bcp.12245 PMID:24118014

Falcón, L. I., Magallón, S., & Castillo, A. (2010). Dating the cyanobacterial ancestor of the chloroplast. *The ISME Journal*, *4*(6), 777–783. doi:10.1038/ismej.2010.2 PMID:20200567

Ferris, J. P., Hill, A. R. Jr, Liu, R., & Orgel, L. E. (1996). Synthesis of long prebiotic oligomers on mineral surfaces. *Nature*, *381*(6577), 59–61. doi:10.1038/381059a0 PMID:8609988

Frost, L. S., Leplae, R., Summers, A. O., & Toussaint, A. (2005). Mobile genetic elements: The agents of open source evolution. *Nature Reviews. Microbiology*, *3*(9), 722–732. doi:10.1038/nrmicro1235 PMID:16138100

Genuth, N. R., & Barna, M. (2018). The discovery of ribosome heterogeneity and its implications for gene regulation and organismal life. *Molecular Cell*, *71*(3), 364–374. doi:10.1016/j.molcel.2018.07.018 PMID:30075139

Grimm, R. E., & Marchi, S. (2018). Direct thermal effects of the Hadean bombardment did not limit early subsurface habitability. *Earth and Planetary Science Letters*, *485*, 1–8. doi:10.1016/j.epsl.2017.12.043

Grosberg, R. K., & Strathmann, R. R. (2007). The evolution of multicellularity: A minor major transition? *Annual Review of Ecology, Evolution, and Systematics*, *38*(1), 621–654. doi:10.1146/annurev.ecolsys.36.102403.114735

Harish, A., & Kurland, C. G. (2017). Mitochondria are not captive bacteria. *Journal of Theoretical Biology*, *434*, 88–98. doi:10.1016/j.jtbi.2017.07.011 PMID:28754286

Harrison, T. M. (2020). Could the Hadean Eon Have Been Habitable? In *Hadean Earth*. Springer. doi:10.1007/978-3-030-46687-9_10

Hazen, R. M. (2013). Paleomineralogy of the Hadean Eon: A preliminary species list. *American Journal of Science*, *313*(9), 807–843. doi:10.2475/09.2013.01

Hu, W. S., & Hughes, S. H. (2012). HIV-1 reverse transcription. *Cold Spring Harbor Perspectives in Medicine*, *2*(10), a006882. doi:10.1101/cshperspect.a006882 PMID:23028129

Imran, M., & Mahmood, S. (2011). An overview of human prion diseases. *Virology Journal*, *8*(1), 1–9. doi:10.1186/1743-422X-8-559 PMID:22196171

Inglis, M. (2015). The Sun, Our Nearest Star. In *Astrophysics Is Easy!* Springer. doi:10.1007/978-3-319-11644-0_8

Javaux, E. J. (2019). Challenges in evidencing the earliest traces of life. *Nature*, *572*(7770), 451–460. doi:10.103841586-019-1436-4 PMID:31435057

Jones, P. A., & Baylin, S. B. (2007). The epigenomics of cancer. *Cell*, *128*(4), 683–692. doi:10.1016/j.cell.2007.01.029 PMID:17320506

Karamdad, K., Law, R. V., Seddon, J. M., Brooks, N. J., & Ces, O. (2015). Preparation and mechanical characterisation of giant unilamellar vesicles by a microfluidic method. *Lab on a Chip*, *15*(2), 557–562. doi:10.1039/C4LC01277A PMID:25413588

Kimura, H., & Watanabe, Y. (2001). Oceanic anoxia at the Precambrian-Cambrian boundary. *Geology*, *29*(11), 995–998. doi:10.1130/0091-7613(2001)029<0995:OAATPC>2.0.CO;2

Koonin, E. V. (2012). Does the central dogma still stand? *Biology Direct*, *7*(1), 1–7. doi:10.1186/1745-6150-7-27 PMID:22913395

Koonin, E. V., & Starokadomskyy, P. (2016). Are viruses alive? The replicator paradigm sheds decisive light on an old but misguided question. *Studies in History and Philosophy of Science Part C Studies in History and Philosophy of Biological and Biomedical Sciences*, *59*, 125–134. doi:10.1016/j.shpsc.2016.02.016 PMID:26965225

Koonin, E. V., & Wolf, Y. I. (2008). Genomics of bacteria and archaea: The emerging dynamic view of the prokaryotic world. *Nucleic Acids Research*, *36*(21), 6688–6719. doi:10.1093/nar/gkn668 PMID:18948295

Lepot, K. (2020). Signatures of early microbial life from the Archean (4 to 2.5 Ga) eon. *Earth-Science Reviews*, *209*, 103296. Advance online publication. doi:10.1016/j.earscirev.2020.103296

Liberski, P. P., Gajos, A., Sikorska, B., & Lindenbaum, S. (2019). Kuru, the first human prion disease. *Viruses, 11*(3), 232. doi:10.3390/v11030232 PMID:30866511

Linden, R., Martins, V. R., Prado, M. A., Cammarota, M., Izquierdo, I., & Brentani, R. R. (2008). Physiology of the prion protein. *Physiological Reviews, 88*(2), 673–728. doi:10.1152/physrev.00007.2007 PMID:18391177

Lowe, H., Woodd, S., Lange, I. L., Janjanin, S., Barnett, J., & Graham, W. (2021). Challenges and opportunities for infection prevention and control in hospitals in conflict-affected settings: A qualitative study. *Conflict and Health, 15*(1), 1–10. doi:10.118613031-021-00428-8 PMID:34930364

Lupi, O., Dadalti, P., Cruz, E., & Sanberg, P. R.The Cryopraxis' Task Force for Prion Research. (2006). Are prions related to the emergence of early life? *Medical Hypotheses, 67*(5), 1027–1033. doi:10.1016/j.mehy.2006.04.056 PMID:16814482

Lynch, M., & Marinov, G. K. (2017). Membranes, energetics, and evolution across the prokaryote-eukaryote divide. *elife, 6*. doi:10.7554/eLife.20437

Macklem, P. T., & Seely, A. (2010). Towards a definition of life. *Perspectives in Biology and Medicine, 53*(3), 330–340. doi:10.1353/pbm.0.0167 PMID:20639603

Mallik, S., & Kundu, S. (2012). *The lipid-RNA world.* arXiv preprint arXiv:1211.0413.

Malmquist, S., & Prescott, K. (2021). *1.4 Mechanisms of Evolution.* M. Libraries. https://open.lib.umn.edu/humanbiology/chapter/1-4-mechanisms-of-evolution/

Marhe, R., Waters, A. J., van de Wetering, B. J., & Franken, I. H. (2013). Implicit and explicit drug-related cognitions during detoxification treatment are associated with drug relapse: An ecological momentary assessment study. *Journal of Consulting and Clinical Psychology, 81*(1), 1–12. doi:10.1037/a0030754 PMID:23231572

Miller, K. G., Kominz, M. A., Browning, J. V., Wright, J. D., Mountain, G. S., Katz, M. E., Sugarman, P. J., Cramer, B. S., Christie-Blick, N., & Pekar, S. F. (2005). The Phanerozoic record of global sea-level change. *Science, 310*(5752), 1293–1298. doi:10.1126cience.1116412 PMID:16311326

Mills, R. E., Bennett, E. A., Iskow, R. C., & Devine, S. E. (2007). Which transposable elements are active in the human genome? *Trends in Genetics*, *23*(4), 183–191. doi:10.1016/j.tig.2007.02.006 PMID:17331616

Modrow, S., Falke, D., Truyen, U., & Schätzl, H. (2013). Viruses: Definition, Structure, Classification. *Molecular Virology*, 17–30. doi:10.1007/978-3-642-20718-1_2

Montmerle, T., Augereau, J. C., Chaussidon, M., Gounelle, M., Marty, B., & Morbidelli, A. (2006). 3. Solar System formation and early evolution: The first 100 million years. *Earth, Moon, and Planets*, *98*(1-4), 39–95. doi:10.100711038-006-9087-5

Morange, M. (2009). The Central Dogma of molecular biology. *Resonance*, *14*(3), 236–247. doi:10.100712045-009-0024-6

Morrison, S. M., Runyon, S. E., & Hazen, R. M. (2018). The paleomineralogy of the Hadean Eon revisited. *Life (Chicago, Ill.)*, *8*(4), 64. doi:10.3390/life8040064 PMID:30562935

Namberger, P., Jackisch, S., Schmude, J., & Karl, M. (2019). Overcrowding, overtourism and local level disturbance: How much can Munich handle? *Tourism Planning & Development*, *16*(4), 452–472. doi:10.1080/21568316.2019.1595706

Naoz, S., Noter, S., & Barkana, R. (2006). The first stars in the universe. *Monthly Notices of the Royal Astronomical Society. Letters*, *373*(1), L98–L102. doi:10.1111/j.1745-3933.2006.00251.x

Neveu, M., Kim, H. J., & Benner, S. A. (2013). The "strong" RNA world hypothesis: Fifty years old. *Astrobiology*, *13*(4), 391–403. doi:10.1089/ast.2012.0868 PMID:23551238

Niklas, K. J., & Newman, S. A. (2013). The origins of multicellular organisms. *Evolution & Development*, *15*(1), 41–52. doi:10.1111/ede.12013 PMID:23331916

Norris, R. (2020). Whump, slosh, slosh, slosh—Filling the crater that did in the dinosaurs. *AGU Advances*, *1*(4). doi:10.1029/2020AV000306

Payer, L. M., & Burns, K. H. (2019). Transposable elements in human genetic disease. *Nature Reviews. Genetics*, *20*(12), 760–772. doi:10.103841576-019-0165-8 PMID:31515540

Petkowski, J. J., Bains, W., & Seager, S. (2020). On the Potential of Silicon as a Building Block for Life. *Life (Basel, Switzerland), 10*(6), 84. doi:10.3390/life10060084 PMID:32532048

Podos, J., & Nowicki, S. (2004). Beaks, adaptation, and vocal evolution in Darwin's finches. *Bioscience, 54*(6), 501–510. doi:10.1641/0006-3568(2004)054[0501:BAAVEI]2.0.CO;2

Pross, A., & Pascal, R. (2013). The origin of life: What we know, what we can know and what we will never know. *Open Biology, 3*(3), 120190. doi:10.1098/rsob.120190 PMID:23466673

Qiu, W., Fu, Z., Xu, G. G., Grassucci, R. A., Zhang, Y., Frank, J., Hendrickson, W. A., & Guo, Y. (2018). Structure and activity of lipid bilayer within a membrane-protein transporter. *Proceedings of the National Academy of Sciences of the United States of America, 115*(51), 12985–12990. doi:10.1073/pnas.1812526115 PMID:30509977

Quigley, E. M. (2006). Germs, gas and the gut: The evolving role of the enteric flora in IBS. *The American Journal of Gastroenterology, 101*(2), 334–335. doi:10.1111/j.1572-0241.2006.00445.x PMID:16454839

Rainey, P. B., & De Monte, S. (2014). Resolving conflicts during the evolutionary transition to multicellular life. *Annual Review of Ecology, Evolution, and Systematics, 45*(1), 599–620. doi:10.1146/annurev-ecolsys-120213-091740

Rainey, P. B., & Kerr, B. (2010). Cheats as first propagules: a new hypothesis for the evolution of individuality during the transition from single cells to multicellularity. *BioEssays, 32*(10), 872-880. doi:10.1002/bies.201000039

Ridley, M. (1989). The cladistic solution to the species problem. *Biology & Philosophy, 4*(1), 1–16. doi:10.1007/BF00144036

Rimmer, P. B., & Shorttle, O. (2019). Origin of Life's Building Blocks in Carbon- and Nitrogen-Rich Surface Hydrothermal Vents. *Life (Basel, Switzerland), 9*(1), 12. doi:10.3390/life9010012 PMID:30682803

Rozanov, A. Y., & Astafieva, M. M. (2020). Archean Eukaryotes: A New Outlook. *Paleontological Journal, 54*(1), 1–5. doi:10.1134/S0031030120010086

Sanjuan, E. A., & Cahill, S. S. (2009, February). QFN-based millimeter wave packaging to 80ghz. *2009 IEEE MTT-S International Microwave Workshop Series on Signal Integrity and High-Speed Interconnects*, 9-12. 10.1109/IMWS.2009.4814898

Sarkar, S., Horn, G., Moulton, K., Oza, A., Byler, S., Kokolus, S., & Longacre, M. (2013). Cancer development, progression, and therapy: An epigenetic overview. *International Journal of Molecular Sciences*, *14*(10), 21087–21113. doi:10.3390/ijms141021087 PMID:24152442

Schopf, J. W., Kudryavtsev, A. B., Czaja, A. D., & Tripathi, A. B. (2007). Evidence of Archean life: Stromatolites and microfossils. *Precambrian Research*, *158*(3-4), 141–155. doi:10.1016/j.precamres.2007.04.009

Spinney, L. (2008). Remnants of evolution. *New Scientist*, *198*(2656), 42–45. doi:10.1016/S0262-4079(08)61231-2

Thar, R., & Kühl, M. (2004). Propagation of electromagnetic radiation in mitochondria? *Journal of Theoretical Biology*, *230*(2), 261–270. doi:10.1016/j.jtbi.2004.05.021 PMID:15302557

Thomassot, E., O'Neil, J., Francis, D., Cartigny, P., & Wing, B. A. (2015). Atmospheric record in the Hadean Eon from multiple sulfur isotope measurements in Nuvvuagittuq Greenstone Belt (Nunavik, Quebec). *Proceedings of the National Academy of Sciences of the United States of America*, *112*(3), 707–712. doi:10.1073/pnas.1419681112 PMID:25561552

Wasik, B. R., & Turner, P. E. (2013). On the biological success of viruses. *Annual Review of Microbiology*, *67*(1), 519–541. doi:10.1146/annurev-micro-090110-102833 PMID:23808330

Wei, L., & Cao, X. (2016). The effect of transposable elements on phenotypic variation: Insights from plants to humans. *Science China. Life Sciences*, *59*(1), 24–37. doi:10.100711427-015-4993-2 PMID:26753674

Wulandari, S., Rustaman, N. Y., Widodo, A., & Aryantha, I. (2021). What should be mastered by elementary, junior and senior high school teachers related to theconcept of evolution? *European Online Journal of Natural and Social Sciences*, *10*(1), 9–18.

Xu, K. (2019). A long journey of lithium: From the Big Bang to our smartphones. *Energy & Environmental Materials*, *2*(4), 229–233. doi:10.1002/eem2.12057

Zaritsky, A. R., Grachev, V. I., Vorontsov, Y. P., & Pronin, V. S. (2014). Abiogenesis transition from the atmosphere into the hydrosphere: From vesicles to protocells. *RENSIT*, *6*(2), 221–231. doi:10.17725/RENSITe.0006.201412f.0221

Zheng, W., Su, S., Zhang, G., Bi, X., & Lin, Q. (2020). Vector magnetocardiography measurement with a compact elliptically polarized laser-pumped magnetometer. *Biomedical Optics Express*, *11*(2), 649–659. doi:10.1364/BOE.380314 PMID:32206390

Chapter 2
Cultural Explanations of Infectious Disease

ABSTRACT

This chapter backs away from the big historical narration of the first chapter and engages critically with the range of explanations that have existed surrounding infectious disease. Exploring models for how humans have considered infectious disease is a way of delving into human-decision making in extremis—how humans make sense of catastrophes large and small without necessarily having immediate insight into their origins. Understandings motivate decisions, regardless of how far in advance of the moment of choice those understandings started to form, so this chapter places emphasis on philosophies of knowledge, biological understandings of knowledge, and the way belief relates to knowledge.

INTRODUCTION

The previous chapter attempted to provide a summary of the relationship between infectious disease and the full evolutionary history of our planet. By scouring modern research, a "big history" picture could be patched together, involving the genetic relationship of all life on Earth (along with harder-to-classify entities such as viruses). In this framework, concepts such as evolution, multicellularity, ecological niches, and the prerequisites for life could be discussed as they applied both to humans and our pathogens,

DOI: 10.4018/978-1-7998-8689-1.ch002

shedding light on a complex network of interactions that all fundamentally occur under the constraints of, and the catalyst of, our earthly biosphere.

One problem with the last chapter, that feeds into the content of this one, is that facts are sometimes tricky to assess. Our understanding of the origin of the universe, the origin of life, and the nature of mass extinctions, is ongoing, as is our understanding of virtually every other scientific concept. The information in the previous chapter does reflect the author's best understanding of the current state of scientific literature on the relevant subjects, and, because of the ability of scientific work to make testable predictions, it is quite likely that the bulk of the understandings in the previous chapter are valuable, even if some details will, in years or decades hence, prove not to be valid. However, the very fact that modern science is an *approach* is worth investigating, and investigating deeply. This is not only because scientific thought is not a monolith, and the quest to integrate different approaches is ongoing (understanding the nature of these synthetic attempts is the bent of the biologist E. O. Wilson's work on consilience (Wilson, 1998)), but also because there are modes of human thought that resist integration. There are also modes of human thought that have had extreme impact on past modes of human behavior, even when they are less commonly championed today. One traditional counterpoint to modern allopathic understandings of medicine, for example, is the theorizing on four humors--black bile, yellow bile, phlegm, and blood--that was constructed upon work of the famous Greek physician Hippocrates (460-370 BCE), and remained in vogue in areas influenced by the Hellenic tradition at least until the Renaissance, despite the fact that these humors, when understood as a quartet, seem to only tenuously relate to real biological elements (Neder, 2020).

In essence, the point of this chapter is to take what was for granted in the previous chapter--the value of current scientific understandings about infectious disease--and recontextualize those understandings in a framework that appreciates the world impact of other approaches. As a minimal note to the previous chapter, science, while incredibly valuable, remains in a meaningful amount of flux, and as a much more substantive note, all conceptions of infectious disease, including popular ones that seem invalid, are worth taking seriously, because people have based their lives on the implications of those beliefs.

NATURE OF BELIEF

The question now turns to where to begin an investigation in the breadth of human beliefs about infectious disease. In order to understand where best to start, it is probably worth investigating the nature of belief. Belief, in an Anglophone sense, is understandings an individual might have about themselves and everything around them, but there are interesting and subtle distinctions in how belief can be defined (Schwitzgebel, 2019). The view of *representationalism* is that belief most properly refers to mental models in their most tangible sense. One implication that can be emphasized in representationalist views is that beliefs are only properly about *is*-statements, and not about *oughts*--that is, a desire is not a belief. Representationalism emphasizes the parts of human brains that are most like modern computers. If what Hippocrates thought was yellow bile he other times thought of as black bile, or phlegm, in a way that only misleadingly linked to real world phenomena, then, to representationalism, he was wrong. This description of Hippocrates, however, opens up an issue with representationalism--that is, because an object and a representation can in no usual instance ever be exactly the same thing, the implications of an association may be more coherent than the way brain storage actually matches a thought to some external real phenomenon (Cheruvalath, 2008).

This leads to *dispositionalism* (Schwitzgebel, 2019). In dispositionalism, belief is defined through manifestations of the belief. If Hippocrates goes around discussing the importance of yellow bile and humors, then he believes in yellow bile and humors, and would differ in belief from a modern scientist who would not talk professionally about such things. A basic objection here is how well beliefs actually map to actions. If someone talks enthusiastically about yellow bile, but otherwise engages in tenets consistent with post-Hippocratic understandings of medicine, or if someone is exuberant about yellow bile, or not, depending on whether or not it is raining, then two examples exist of beliefs that are so tangled with other beliefs, or environment conditions, that is extremely difficult to disentangle them. If a single purported belief leads to a variety of behaviors, how can it be a single belief? Practitioners of science and medicine each learned science and medicine to some degree in their own way, in the context of their full set of beliefs, and it is far more likely that two physicians share the same term for a concept than respond identically to that concept. To dispositionalism, belief is shown through behavior.

Next, *interpretationism* attempts to retrench by framing belief as drivers of observable behavior (Schwitzgebel, 2019). That is, if a doctor goes to yellow bile conferences, and tries to publish papers about yellow bile, then the doctor has belief in yellow bile insofar as "believing in that belief" is useful for knowing what kind of diagnoses the doctor might make, or what kind of conferences the doctor might go to in the future. Interpretationism abandons emphasis not only on idealized mental truth states, but also on claims of mental truth states, in favor of the idea that belief predicts.

For some final definitions, *functionalism* frames belief as mental states that are derived from sensory linkages (which seems rather less philosophical than the other approaches), while *eliminativism* asserts that belief as a concept is insufficiently tied to real biology to be useful, and *instrumentalism* makes the compromise that belief is sometimes useful as a shorthand, for, at a minimum, describing what other people call belief (Schwitzgebel, 2019). From all these definitions, it seems the idea of belief is very complicated, which may be problematic when it comes to figuring out what people believe, and how they believe it, on a topic like infectious disease.

BRAIN AND BELIEF

Theorizing may seem somewhat arcane and not instrumental to helping understand actual patterns of thought about infectious disease. However, presenting a variety of ways of understanding belief lends itself naturally to the idea that concepts can be defined flexibly. One detail related to belief that is backed by modern science is that human thought has a strong associative component (Lilienthal et al., 2013). The way human brains actually work is strongly tied to the concept of synaptic plasticity, or adjustments to connections between neurons (Citri & Malenka, 2008). Since perhaps the most foundational physical form of learning involves synaptic plasticity, it stands to reason that one model of human belief with a fair chance of being tied to actual neurochemistry is--humans believe in associations between concepts. The best way of defining a "concept" is probably as intricate as the best way of defining belief, but one way to focus on the biology of important philosophical questions is to put a great deal of emphasis on the fact that neurons, particularly those in the brain, adaptively interlink with each other in ways that are clearly tied to how individuals think and recall (Wang & Cui, 2018). It seems fair to argue that mental associations are not quite the same as executive action, and that human capacity has to work in coordination with task action to accomplish anything (Beaty et al., 2014). However, as all action and thought must flow through an associative net, the impetus to *do* may be most easily understood through the idea of plastic, or dynamic, mental associations. Executive function can thus be addressed as seeming to have a physical origin, likely in the brain's prefrontal region (Xie et al., 2020). Thusly, executive functioning seems to be mediated through the same associative cognitive processes that underlie the neurochemistry of belief and other kinds of thought.

So far, this chapter has addressed the practical necessity of mediating thoughts about infectious disease through a belief structure, as well as philosophical concepts about belief, and an associative model of belief-within-neural-interactions that can complement the abstractions of the philosophical approaches. This train of thought can be made more practical by turning next to one implication of associative thought--the human propensity for pattern recognition. Pattern recognition pervades the breadth of life. In the realms of both tonal and atonal music, predictions as to musical behavior, and adjustments of those predictions, seem to be deeply connected to appreciation of the art form (Mencke et al., 2019). The brain has been characterized as a "prediction machine" (Badcock et al., 2017; Meng et al., 2020). Belief seems very much tied to the nature of how any person can make predictions, while honest explanations are descriptions of perceived associations. In a different work, the next direction of discussion would be to look back on the various philosophical descriptions of belief, and discuss with more detail how this biological framework does or doesn't provide supportive evidence. More useful here is to take the concept of belief-as-association-mediated-prediction and examine how it has interacted with human society. Belief-as-prediction should not be taken for granted, because it characterizes the nature of perhaps every human response ever to infectious disease.

BELIEF WITH INFECTIOUS DISEASE

When perceived, infectious disease must interact with the associative matrix of the human brain, and must necessarily be linked to some prior intuition or experience. The human mind needs a way to understand the things it perceives, because otherwise, in an oddly literal sense, it has no place to put those things. From an evolutionary standpoint, the most useful characterizations of infectious disease are the ones that lead to increased survival of an organism, or fitness, so the most useful early understandings of infectious disease possibly were similar to: "You get sick if you go near the marsh, so try not to go near the marsh if you can help it." This frame, specifically about marshes and their unknown but dangerous character, is present in folk characterizations from Kent and Essex in England dating to around the sixteenth through nineteenth centuries, and reflected specific pragmatic if not epidemiological truisms about malaria (Dobson, 1980). However, a problem with pragmatic truisms is that, without clear causal explanations, they may have difficulty being meshed into the wider range of human cognitive associations. One way of making pragmatic truisms be more recognized is by using stories.

Stories help memory (Smorti & Fioretti, 2016). The existence of fables, and moral "old wives' tales," which may circle on seemingly odd narrations surrounding fairly specific bits of advice (Broom et al., 2014), suggests a sort of "gravitational pull" towards articulating explanations to go with associative beliefs, potentially regardless of any "real" link between the explanation, the phenomenon, and the suggestion. It is unfair and inappropriate to characterize folk belief in a blanket way as attaching poor explanations to potentially-valuable remedies. Language itself is associative (Koerner, 2014), so language that repeatedly brings its users to productive and adaptive conclusions, regardless of how strange it might seem to an outside observer, is epistemologically validated in a very significant way. The danger, specifically, is when explanations for phenomena disassociate with time from the behavior of the phenomena, or are unspecifically applied to apparently similar phenomena, with the link potentially only being validated by associative cognition, rather than in the field. It is not a very large step from "good empirical suggestions that save lives but are framed narratively," to *superstitions*. Both have a narrative aspect.

SUPERSTITION AND THE FOUNDATIONS OF SCIENCE

Superstition, at its root, seems to be about the inappropriate or irresponsible assignment of purpose (Lindeman & Saher, 2007). Each of a pair of events that can be thought of adjacently may have no predictive value on the other, but because they occur together, perhaps trivially or accidentally, a linkage with inordinate emphasis may occur regardless. Here is an example:

"Step on a crack and break your mother's back" seems broadly irrational in the context of sidewalk cracks, but does have the advantage of being a rhyme, dire, and easy to remember. The rhyme is not irrelevant. Poetic structure has a long history of use as memory aid, including in the ancient works of the

Greek Homer (Rubin, 1995, p. 205). Consider a brute implication of belief-as-association. The association can be bizarre in practice, but strengthened by repeated use nonetheless, so long as it is an association. Clearly it is possible to reconsider superstitious thought about the causal link between cracks and backs, but given that much thought is subconscious (Strick et al., 2011), it is eminently plausible that even something as odd as that association can resonate in a person's mind well enough that the association begins to feel true. And once something starts to feel true, it can contribute to actions by making actions feel more obvious. Consider the following anecdote reported by Austin (2002): A mother, asked about the origin of the crack/back saying, hypothesizes that the saying developed to help warn about the danger of loose floorboards. The mother's child, the author, was well aware that stepping on other types of cracks did not seem to be linked to danger, and yet still did not want to do it, out of a sense of filial piety. The power of the rhyme is so strong here that there are multiple attempts to respect its significance. Yet another attempt to do this is in the actual content of Austin's work, which recontextualizes the saying as referring to the street drug crack, in the context that certain zero-tolerance housing policies cause harm to come to families, including mothers, because of drug use among children.

One of the reasons it may be hard to take the crack/back example of powerful superstition seriously is because of the nature of the rest of this text. The exegesis of such a saying in an academic concept may feel less relevant than, say, the exegesis of abiogenesis. However, it is not clear that it should be. The purpose of this chapter, fundamentally, is to point to cultural currents that run besides, or prior to, traditional scientific analysis. Little semi-subconscious rhymes fit that context. Additionally, the broader idea of superstition has been the subject of significant research, particularly in how it interacts with attempts at explaining world problems in the absence of a scientific establishment. The edifice of modern science should not be taken for granted, because it was built atop a wide variety of human efforts at understanding our surroundings, aspirationally, as a more practical way of doing business (Borup et al., 2006). From a learner's perspective, scientific understandings are not priors, and every time an honest student strains to understand a concept, or a scientific idea is misconstrued in popular discourse, the failure is a reminder that modern science is built from, or in reaction to, basic principles.

What basic principles? The anthropologist Sir James George Frazer, in the book *The Golden Bough*, originally published in 1890, put forward two principles of magic, sympathy and contagion (Stewart & Strathern, 2013).

Sympathy relates to the idea that similar things are connected, whereas contagion relates to the idea that things that come into proximity are connected. What is fascinating about these two principles is the ways in which they are and are not tied to the fundamentals of the realm of science. As far as sympathy goes, things that have similar properties are by definition expected to trend in the same way as far as those properties have an effect--any kind of trend line on a graph is built on the idea that quantities can scale towards impacting other quantities. Similarly, contagion is something very similar to the sort of medical history-taking that physicians are trained on. Where someone was, and what sort of physical life they have led, very often has something to do with how they feel or behave. Returning to the malarial example, someone admitting to having spent some time in swamps might be suspected of being more likely to have malaria by both a doctor and a magician, because the way contagion is a concept bridges the realms of superstition and science. Superstition is not trivial. Superstition is often actually predictive, and predictive in ways that are similar to the way science might do things. The key difference, perhaps, between superstition and science, is that science abhors logical leaps, and, at least in the model that stems from the thirteenth century Franscisican and empiricist Roger Bacon (Sidebottom, 2013), must follow directly from experimentation. Going back to the crack/back example, the rhyme might be good enough to create a sympathetic link in a Frazerian context, but may not be good enough in Baconian, because those who repeat the saying do not have clear and direct evidence of a causal link between stepping on a crack, and familial injury. The analogy may be sufficient for one method of investigation, but not the other.

There are some assumptions that have been just introduced that are worth unpacking, because they are not necessarily correct. Superstition and magic are not necessarily synonyms. It seems reasonably clear that superstition is wide enough in its definition to encompass any reasoning that may seem faulty from the perspective of any tradition, as well, as even more appropriately, any reasoning that actually is faulty, but magic means enough different things to people to either squarely fit into that second category, or well and properly escape it. Consider the role of herbal remedies provided by healers (sometimes known as witch doctors) in African traditional medicine--these treatments may at times have poor quality control, but they also have driven pharmacological innovations as worldwide medicine has picked up on chemical efficacies that exist in this space (Ozioma & Chinwe, 2019). Further, a traditional criticism of medicine as practiced within the "modern scientific" tradition is an obsessive focus on treating symptoms at the expense of preventative or holistic approaches (Castanes, 2003; Sun et al., 2013). Consider the fact that primary care physicians in the United States make notably less income in the United States than specialists, and what that says about institutional priorities (Lasser et al., 2008). There is an argument to be made that superstitious logic pervades some structure of the "modern scientific" medical establishment, just as traditional medicine may be built more on empiricism than is obvious to some outside observers.

INTUITION

One way to escape a square-off of "modern scientific" with traditional medicine is to point out that uses of intuition, and more rigorous causal assessment, are both bedrocks of the human experience, cropping up not just in debates between macroscale approaches, but in personal debates as well. In Nobel-Prize-winning economist Daniel Kahneman's book *Thinking, Fast and Slow*, Kahneman purports the utility of thinking of the human mind as engaging in dual tracks, a System 1 and a System 2, wherein System 1 uses the vast array of neurological shortcuts the human mind has available to try to generate decisions quickly, while System 2 is more procedural, and makes measured judgements (2011, pp. 21-62). The theme of Kahneman's book is that both of these strategies are well-used because they have utility in different contexts. These strategies are relevant to this chapter because, insofar as they represent real and accessible decision-making strategies for humans, or ways of levering our neuronal associative matrix, they point out that the challenge in addressing infectious disease properly has at least as much to do with maladaptive decision strategies as traditions. Cultural norms of understanding infectious disease can theoretically spring out of propagated mental models, which can be built on empirical observation of varying degrees of rigor, or even rhyme. Explanation frameworks in human history are at least as ancient as the first time two people ever agreed on something, and can range in rigor from "the marsh is bad" to a sophisticated biochemical understanding of the protozoa that cause malaria. Because sophistication is easiest to achieve when complexity builds atop useful prior complexity, as human civilization proceeded across millenia and archived various findings of real utility, those with the ability to access the knowledge of those before were better able to build out new nuances in understanding. However, there was and is no one pathway, and every step along the way, difficulties in cultural and individual knowledge transmission and acquisition shaped the best understandings of medical minds about infectious disease.

Now that work has been done to explore why diverse understandings of infectious disease exist among, between, and within individuals, cultures, and communities, it is time to explore with specificity what different models can look like. A reasonable place to start is with the divine.

THE DIVINE

Religion, fundamentally, seems to be about coming to grips with the most substantive possible issues, and these issues may relate to group cohesion and survival at least as much as they relate to pursuit of understanding. Religious practices may have started out as journeys into trance-states carried out by hunter-gatherer societies, and from that point developed a framework as to why the trance-states felt special, as well as specialized spaces like temples, specialized practitioners like priests, dogmas, and theology (Dunbar, 2013). Insofar as religion provides meaningful experience, it is outside the bounds of this discussion. Insofar as religion provides meaningful explanations, it is relevant. Religion reaches back to the earliest types of societies, and can be conceptualized as explanatory frameworks that privilege humanlike explanations of cosmic and environmental phenomena (Guthrie, 1996). "Humanlike" is an interesting word. Everything we experience is filtered through some kind of sense perception, and is humanlike in that dimension. It is not obvious, for example, why the electromagnetic spectrum range we think of as visual should be privileged as being more significant, or real, than various ranges we cannot see. Animal sight can range into the ultraviolet and infrared spectrums in ways different than our own vision, and the radiation that our eyes do notice is mediated by the nature of rod and cone cells--not only can sensitivity differ by individual or species, but so too can interpretation, on a very basic, physical level (Kelber & Osorio, 2010). To say that rain falls from a divine being in the sky, or thunderclaps are the gods fighting, or volcanos erupt because of divine rage--all of these concepts can be interpreted with varying degrees of literalness. The idea of the divine presents a helpful interpretative framework with real utility. Stepping outside of religion, providing gender to inanimate objects is baked into the nature of a wide variety of world languages. Tension starts to creep in when the personal explanations of phenomena that religion can offer seem particularly personal, or tied to morality or human behavioral concepts, when alternative explanations are much more impersonal, or seemingly obtuse.

INTRODUCTION TO DIVINE FIGURES AND DISEASE, AND A NARRATIVE OF NERGAL

Across cultures, there have been a wide number of divine figures associated with both causing and curing sickness. Nergal is a Mesopotamian god associated with bringing disease (Trevisanto, 2007). Mami Wata is a divine figure associated with Africa and its overseas diaspora, with special domain over water and healing (Chang, 2016) Sopona is a Yoruba divinity associated with smallpox (Singleton, 1976). Shitala is a Hindu divinity associated with the goddess Durga, and has an association with disease in general and smallpox in particular (Haberman, 2010). Baosheng Dadi is a divine name for a deified Chinese doctor named Wu Tao, who lived in the ninth century (Puett, 2013), and is particularly prominent around Fujian and Taiwan (Li, 2011). The Greeks had the god Apollo, who had medicine as one of his domains, and fathered Asclepius, a mythic doctor who became defied after various adventures (Anselment, 1995, p. 23). The recounting just provided is notably partial, and does not really come close to scratching the surface of the myriad and complex ways that the concept of the divine has been integrated with ideas related to sickness and healing.

To get a better sense of what specific conceptions of divinity can surround disease, Nergal will be explored in additional detail. In the myth text known as *The Marriage of Ereshkigal and Nergal*, with a narrative that dates to at least the fifteenth century BCE. This myth starts with a divine banquet (Mark, 2017). Ereshkigal cannot attend, for Ereshkigal's domain is of the underworld, but Ereshkigal sends her son Namtar in her stead. When Namtar arrives, all the gods rise from their seats to honor Ereshkigal, except for Nergal. Enki, another god, who wanted Ereshkigal to send a proxy, now encourages Namtar to go back to the underworld to tell Ereshkigal of the slight. Ereshkigal is very angry, and demands that Nergal come below, so that Nergal might be killed for his impiety. Nergal is willing enough to head below, but when he finally reaches the place where Namtar and Ereshkigal are waiting for him, he overpowers them both, and threatens to kill Ereshkigal. The tables turned, Ereshkigal now pledges to be Nergal's wife, and to share her power. Nergal, irrepressible, will now spend six months in the underworld, and six months above, continuing to sow strife.

The myth as just presented does not specifically have to do with disease, aside from Nergal's temperament and association with the underworld. However, knowing that Nergal is associated with disease, and knowing that the above narrative is part of Nergal's corpus, there are implications to be made. Namely, the ancient Mesopotamians saw divinity as powerful and dangerous, in intra-divine ways as well as in ways that fell upon humans. There is no sense in the above myth that Nergal has interests beyond his self-interest, and there is even a sense that Enki tried to tame Nergal by setting up a conflict between Nergal and Ereshkigal, only for Nergal to not exactly lose. The gods, in this Mesopotamian context, have characteristics that are reflective of humans (they eat meals; they have conflicts), and the most important departure between those characteristics, and actual human characteristics, is that the potency of the figures have broader implications.

One of the most interesting gaps between the above myth, and human experience, is the discrepancy in Nergal's presence. In the myth, as stated, Nergal acts like, and seems to basically be, a tangible figure with many human characteristics. However, when the Mesopotamians and their neighbors looked for signs of Nergal, what they seemed to find, and recognize as Nergal's work, was much more disembodied phenomena. For example, Nergal was explicitly blamed for what seems to have been a fourteenth century BCE outbreak of tularemia, caused by the bacterial pathogen *Francisella tularensis*, which spread across the Near East, and was even carried into Greek territory by soldiers returning from conflict far from their home (Trevisanto, 2007). This attribution of the pestilence to Nergal did not mean that the world which experienced the outbreak was completely lost as to what to do--the disease potentially did not spread to Egypt because of quarantine measures--but the attribution does help place Nergal in context. Consider the following pattern of thought:

Question: *Why are we getting sick?*
Response: *Because Nergal is acting aggressively, again.*
Question: *How do we know Nergal caused the sickness?*
Response: *Could any besides Nergal cause the sickness?*

Note that this sort of pattern of logic does not exclude the possibility of preventative measures, like quarantine, or maybe offerings of sacrifice. It is simply a basic explication of a linkage between tangible phenomena and the Mesopotamian impression of the divine. One question that hangs over the dialogue above is why anyone would jump to the conclusion that Nergal is responsible for anything, or even that Nergal, such a complex mythic structure, even exists. However, an explication for Nergal's existence, and his linkages, was already touched on above. One way to understand religion, or the divine, is that it is all about attaching meaning and motivation to phenomena that do not obviously have meaning and motivation in a way a human can understand. From such a perspective, the question of why blame for disease jumps to Nergal, a powerful figure, is answered by the very nature of religious tendency in humans. Conversely, stating "Because of invisible organisms" as a component of an answer to the question of "Why are we getting sick?" may be difficult, particularly to individuals from the past who could not look to (then-uninvented) modern allopathic medicine.

SOPONA

The sense of a god's presence behind a disease outbreak was hardly limited to those who lived around Mesopotamia in the second millennium BCE. In order to clarify the way Nergal's relationship to infectious disease may be similar to linkages between infectious disease and other figures, it is worth exploring Sopona, a figure associated with the Yoruba pantheon. Unlike the modern region once known as Mesopotamia, and Europe, where, respectively, Islam and Christianity were the chief religous beneficiaries of displacements of pantheonic beliefs, West Africa, while including many Christians and Muslims, also is home to an active pantheonic Yoruba tradition. From Brazil to Colombia to Cuba, to Benin, to Nigeria (whose southwest is a heartland of the Yoruba people), the Yoruba pantheon may be worshiped in contemporary times by 100 million or more adherents (Emeagwali, 1999). The slave trade, which resulted in a giant African diaspora into the Americas, involving tens of millions of souls, spread traditional African religion into the Americas to no small extent. While it is a matter of debate how closely Yoruban-inspired traditions in the Americas tie to African beliefs (Gordon, 1979; Olanrewaju, 2009), and while it is hard to argue that Sopona is particularly central to the Yoruba pantheon, the fact remains that Sopona is a presence in the Yoruba pantheon (Singleton, 1976). Sopona exists in a meaningfully different context than Nergal, and yet Sopona is surrounded by a story-structure that is similar to Nergal's in interesting ways. Here is a myth about Sopona:

At the divinity Obatala's palace, Sopona wishes to dance (Singleton, 1976). However, Sopona is old, and has a wooden leg, and the other divine figures present think that Sopona is acting ridiculously, so they laugh uproariously. At this affront, Sopona is very angry, and seeks to attack with smallpox. Powerful Obatala intervenes, however, and when the dust settles, Sopona is banished to desolate regions.

This myth has many points of contact with Nergal's. There is a great divine assembly, with an arbiter (in the Yoruba case, Obatala, and in the Mesopotamian case, Enki). Neither Sopona nor Nergal act within the bounds of decorum, though neither Sopona nor Nergal seek violence as their first action. Instead, when the gods and goddesses laugh, in Sopona's case, or, in the Mesopotamian, when Nergal is summoned to the underworld to die, there is an infection moment, and these divine figures of disease are affronted. And then, and only then, does their unusual behavior grow into a furious maelstrom. In the end, Sopona's wrath is blunted by Obatala, and Nergal, while he overwhelms and then joins forces with Ereshkigal, is in turn somewhat blunted by Enki. However, even at the end of the narratives, Sopona and Nergal remain potent, lurking forces. If they can threaten fellow divine figures, it seems obvious that they can also threaten humans with great severity.

Sopona's narratives also offer a clear example of a bridge between the world of the divine and the seemingly mundane world that many humans seem to live in--that of a divine figure in disguise, offering judgment. Consider this tale associated with Sopona:

A young man named Philip, herding goats with some others, encounters an old man (Singleton, 1976). The old man asks for tobacco, but Philip is frightened of the old man, and tries to put off the task on another person present. The old man chastises him, and disappears, and in a matter of days, Philip catches smallpox, and many people in his area die of the same disease.

What may be especially significant about Philip's story is that it takes no particular faith to believe that the events could have happened. People meet strangers all the time, people can be scared of strangers, and calamitous events, such as the transmission of serious infectious disease, can befall people and towns and villages. It is not necessary that Sopona is actually part of the story--it is only context that connects the story to Sopona, a context of belief. However, recall the faith-drive that many humans seem to have, to use a persona to understand events that may not at first glance seem to have a persona. It may not be necessary to make the connection between the smallpox outbreak and the old man, but it may be relatively easy to make the connection, particularly in a region that already tells tales of Sopona.

Since Sopona can be understood both as a divine figure engaging in stories with other divine figures, similar to Nergal, but also as a sort of lurking presence that hides behind very real and unfamiliar faces, the chapter is at an inflection point. There are a vast number of additional myths to tell about infectious disease, but it is probably more useful to delve into ways of considering infectious disease that go beyond the pantheonic divine. Myth-making is not limited to stories of gods and goddesses. Myth-making pervades mundane encounters, and the association between the old man and Sopona is but one example.

SUBTLE MYTHOLOGY

Moving away from religion, and back to superstition--it is a very different sort of myth, but still something of a myth, to think that stepping on a crack can cause some transference of harm. The idea that odd persons, or odd behavior, can lead to dire consequences, may be tied to the principles of sympathy and contagion, and in a narrative way (because sympathy and contagion are all about making associations by any means necessary), but this idea is fantastically pervasive. The idea that the homeless, for example, are diseased, is both common and leads to exclusionary policymaking that may have very little to do with actual danger posed by infectious homeless, and everything to do with perception of threat (Clifford & Piston, 2017). This is like the story of the old man as Sopona, but now no one is asserting that the divine is relevant to the story. The feelings, and desire to *get away* from the other, are simply followed up by support for policies like bans on panhandling or sleeping in public spaces. Social organization in the United States has a way of fighting back against the "horror" of homelessness (with one component of the horror being an association of the homeless with disease) that seems very sophisticated in outcome (with things like ordinances), but may be ultimately rooted in problematic gut instinct.

Consider the natural milieu of human decision-making. The human evolutionary environment. Humans originated in much smaller organizations than we have today, and were concerned with goals more relevant to survival. Civilization is much younger than the human species. In a world with civilization, and the benefits that civilization is capable of bringing–of, for example, using excess wealth to care for even substantially-sized vulnerable populations–the old gut instinct of avoiding dissimilar strangers is still apparently present. Leaving the weak behind to die on their own is almost certainly horrific in any context, but makes more sense in environments with resource constraints, and environments where sophisticated differential diagnoses are not possible, and decisions must be made quickly without time for extensive analysis. The fact that much of human society does not live in such a context, however, may simply be irrelevant, because the proportion of time spent in civilization does not equal the evolutionary impact of the ancestral environment.

A new concept that is useful to understanding the cultural impact of infectious disease, in multiple ways, is known as the founder effect. In the founder effect, a small population that is the progenitors of a larger population, down the line, can have an outside impact on the characteristics of that larger population, regardless of the evolutionary pressures of the new environment. For example, pertaining to the concept of evolutionary niches, a set of birds migrating to an island or other isolated location without large grazers might develop the size and scale useful to become large grazers, like a kind of island elephant. However, because of the characteristics they are starting with, their descendants do not actually become elephants. Instead, they become animals with certain characteristics similar to elephants, but still are recognizably birds. A good example of this sort of phenomenon are the emu of Australia (Phillips et al., 2010). How is the founder effect tied to human belief? The evolutionary idea is that certain patterns of belief that were useful in the human ancestral environment, among the founders or progenitors of the human species, may be problematic today. One central issue here is stigmatizing the other, or strangers, and blaming them for outbreaks of infectious disease regardless of origin.

THE OTHER

At this point, the chapter has discussed the nature of belief, certain religious associations of infectious disease, and certain associations of infectious disease with outgroups, or the "Other." A common point here is the human drive to find an empathetic way, perhaps in terms of awe, and perhaps in terms of disgust, to relate to a topic like infectious disease, which is both important and, at first glance, perhaps, alien. Sometimes infectious disease is even more personal. The idea that Sopona might send smallpox as a punishment is part of a larger constellation of disease-as-punishment concepts. Plague in Early Modern Europe was commonly seen as punishment for sin (Slack, 1988). HIV/AIDS (human immunodeficiency virus/acquired immunodeficiency syndrome) has been seen from certain viewpoints in contemporary times as not much different, with a particular association with homosexuality (Parsons, 2019). The construction of a clinical term, MSM (men who have sex with men), to discuss certain individuals in a health context, (Jeffries IV, et al., 2015), flows into certain restrictions that have been put in place to limit the ability of MSM to donate blood, as well as attendant issues about how ethically or appropriately targeted this policy is when in practice (Galarneau, 2010).

Stigma, as a phenomenon linked to infectious disease, will properly get its own chapter, focusing on ways human psychology comes up with explanations for exclusion. To start to work towards a conclusion in this chapter, the framing will jump back to external explanations for disease and infection, working towards the external explanation that is naturalistic science. This framing is for purposes of utility, and is not meant to imply that the modern conception of science is the obvious endpoint of any line of thinking, or even monolithic--above, the notion was presented that those who "believe" in science can mix that belief with elements from other traditions. However, natural science is extremely popular in the modern world, and its utilities include most of modern allopathic medicine. With the endpoint fixed, the topic for the time being will now move to a basic tenet of holistic medicine, which is sometimes, but far from always, placed in opposition to mainstream medicine, also known as allopathic medicine.

HOLISTIC MEDICINE

Holistic medicine is fundamentally about thinking of the human body as deeply interconnected with itself, and, in a practical sense, the world. This seems a somewhat innocent point that can fit into any open-minded view. However, some of the traditional ways holistic medicine has been quantified fill up these connections with details that are more controversial in some circles. For example, modern academia has labeled a set of traditions and practices in China as traditional Chinese medicine (TCM), and TCM, in turn, is often associated with the category of holistic medicine (Ho, 2006). TCM involves specific practices such as acupuncture, and explanations regarding its practices that are internal to TCM, as opposed to descriptions by outsiders, tend to focus on treatments being motivated by attention to *qi*. What is *qi*? From the teachings of TCM, *qi* is, approximately, the fundamental constituent of the human body, and can be separated into healthy and pathogenic variants (Xu & Zhang, 2020). Treatments like acupuncture (Li et al., 2011), and herbs, that can affect *qi*, have been documented to have real physiological effects (Xu & Zhang, 2020). That these treatments have some kind of effect is not necessarily controversial. What is more controversial to practitioners of allopathic medicine is that the concept of *qi*, and traditional remedies to pathologies derived from an understanding of *qi*, have great credibility among many practitioners at the expense of allopathic approaches (Spence & Li, 2013). What is interesting about this contrast is that it is fundamentally not about a wholesale rejection of allopathic medicine's teachings by TCM practitioners, but rather by a prioritization of traditional texts, and traditional methods of practice. This seems to exactly parallel the attitude of much of allopathic medicine towards TCM (Ho, 2006).

The fact that allopathic medicine, is, in a conventional parlance, "evidence-based" is worth investigating. However, for now, it is important to note that the source of information about *qi* dates back to ancient times, and the body of knowledge about *qi* that has been passed down was not collected using the formal test processes popular in allopathic medicine (Ross, 2009). There are a number of 'life energy' concepts in traditions outside TCM that are similar--*prana* in the Indian-rooted traditions of Ayurveda and and Yoga, *pneuma* among the Ancient Greeks, the Great Spirit in many North American indegenous groups, and the Judeo-Christian concept of breath of life. What binds these concepts together is their sense of unity--that a great variety of symptoms can trace back to shared origins and root causes. This traditional knowledge, which is holistic, has an important aspect at its core that evidence-based medicine seems to have more difficulty with–namely, per the term "holism" itself, that various symptoms caused by infectious diseases and other phenomena really are interrelated.

PLACEBO

Disease progressions involve a wide variety of factors that stretch well beyond the disease itself, from lifestyle elements like diet and exercise, to factors like environment and social network. The placebo effect, which refers to the idea that people can gain some ability to recover from illness because they think they are supposed to recover from illness, is well documented even from a scientific perspective (Moerman & Jonas, 2002). While placebo effectiveness often does not match that of allopathic treatments, and is much more dangerous to rely on in the context of severe and specific diseases--in fact, one general rule for an effective drug is that it is a meaningful better treatment than a placebo like a sugar pill--placebo benefits can often be *competitive* in effect compared to treatment with clear active ingredients, and, by its nature, can create positive side-effects to treatments that otherwise would not have had such side-effects (like mood improvement), if such a treatment is claimed (Moerman & Jonas, 2002). In fact, the placebo effect is so powerful that Jonas (2019) makes the argument that the way the effect is commonly understood is a myth, insofar as belief clearly has a powerful ability to affect real health outcomes. Note that these outcomes can also turn of for ill--individuals who think they are in trouble seem to help make themselves so via the belief (Moerman & Jonas, 2002), in a self-harming sort of manner that contrasts closely with the way stigma can be used to place burdens on others.

HOLISTIC MEDICINE AND ALLOPATHIC MEDICINE

Drawing the discussion of holistic medicine back towards modern allopathic medicine, the evidence-based approach of that latter sort of medicine, which is often narrowly targeted, can be accused of being narrowly focused on superior domain knowledge between well-siloed specialties. In the United States, the "salvaging" of the osteopathic tradition from association with alternative medicine, and the movement of osteopathic doctors into the core ranks of physicians (albeit as physicians with some extra training on certain physical techniques), is an example of how the allopathic tradition can and has taken notes from certain aspects of holism (Esteves et al., 2020). However, just because holism has aspects that point out weaknesses in allopathic medicine, does not mean allopathic medicine rests on a poor foundation. Allopathic medicine has a long history of fighting against quackery, pseudoscience, and miracle cures. The fact that allopathic medicine is firmly attached to experiments, specialization, and the scientific method provides a wide variety of benefits--when allopathic medicine makes a statement, it may be narrow and decontextualized, but it is often rigorously factually correct, which allows for a sort of incrementalism and building of knowledge that has led to remarkable advances in fields like genetics and neuroscience.

The last major turn in this chapter is the birth of modern allopathic medicine itself, out of the troubles of more traditional approaches. Evidence-based reasoning has extensive grounding around the world. Muhammad ibn Musa al-Khwarizmi, who was born in Khiva in 783 in what is now Uzbekistan, did great work in the House of Wisdom in Baghdad, capital of the Abbasid Caliphate, and gave his name to the word "algorithm" (Nabirahni et al.,

2019). Brahmagupta, born in 598 in the Indian region of Rajasthan, is, among other innovations, associated with the discovery of the number zero (Pranesachar, 2012). However, allopathic medicine today has such a strong association with Europe and European immigrants that one problematic name for allopathic medicine is "Western medicine" (Jeffery, 1977). Is Western medicine truly Western? The obvious problem for using this name as a synonym for allopathic, academic, or evidence-based medicine is that, whatever its origins, so-called Western medicine is practiced around the world, and is clearly not purely Western now. Was it ever? Probably not. One possible point at which Western medicine got started was in the 1500s, through the animal dissections of Andreas Vesalius, a doctor from Belgium (Mantri, 2008). However, his work was notable as a threshold because of how it was distinct from the past, particularly the work of the Roman Galen (129-200 CE) (Dunn, 2003).

Galen's work, along with the Greek Hippocrates, dominated medical thinking until the Renaissance, and was built on something like holistic traditions, similar to the traditions described above. Galen developed Hippocrates' system of blood, black bile, yellow bile, and phlegm, which explained illness expression through imbalance of these four humors (Nutton et al., 2005). Galen broke illness causation into three factors--predisposing, exciting, and environmental--and also worked with the idea that contagious illness came from bad air, or miasma (Parvez et al, 2016). Since *qi* can be interpreted as something close to air, the link between holistic traditions outside the West, and holistic traditions inside, seems quite close indeed (Li, 2008). There is also some question of how far apart holism and proto-allopathy were at this point. The idea of bad air itself is not particularly irrational, as, ultimately, many pathogens are airborne, and without microscopy to detect them directly, putting the blame on the air itself may be about as close as one can get to the allopathic idea of a pathogen. An irony is that Galen's anatomical and biological work was, as a whole, so apparently reasonable, and so expansive, that it stayed the cornerstone of medical traditions in his area of the world for around 1400 years, at the expense of independent research (Dunn, 2003). The reason why Vesalius as an anatomist was so innovative was in part because of the way he wanted to find things out for himself, as opposed to read about the human body and sickness by studying the ancient work of Galen.

If the Western tradition, pre-Vesalius, may not have been clearly on the road to allopathy, was anywhere? The easiest answer is the Muslim world. The flourishing of scholarly work in middle east in the time of the early

Abbasid Caliphate does not preclude the accomplishments of other regions and other periods, but is a good example of how tendencies of narrowly-scoped empiricism, in contrast to holism, have emerged in a wide enough way around the world that the contest has arguably been global. Abu-Bakr Mohammad Ibn Zakariya Razi, for example, who flourished in the ninth and tenth centuries, was a major physician who knew enough to be involved in the creation of a separate hospital for the contagiously sick, to set them apart from those with non-transmissible diseases (Parvez et al., 2016).

MEASUREMENT AND FALSIFIABILITY

The key point, as the narrative moves towards the present, is that forces like tradition combine with lack of scientific tools to make it more difficult for experimental research to take place. This sentence is not really scoped to any one particular region or place. It is applicable broadly, even now, and can be seen in boldly pseudoscientific beliefs like homeopathy. One cornerstone of modern homeopathy is the idea of remedy by application of extremely diluted substances--as little as one part in 10^{400}–and even research that embraces the idea that such dilutions contain *something*, and uses advanced microscopy to detect, stops short of connecting the presented evidence of nanoparticles to a mechanism of action (Chikramane, 2010). Compare that situation with physicians in the medieval period following in Galen's tradition. They sincerely believed their great predecessor knew much about human physiology and illness, their line of training paid great homage to his work, and the tools they had at hand did not make it easy to collect clear contraindication to his speculations.

So where did modern science come from? And what defines it? Karl Popper's notion of the key ingredient of science being falsifiability--only asserting things that are possible to be proven wrong--was only articulated in the twentieth century (Olszewski & Sandroni, 2011), and there is even evidence that the human tendency to follow assumptions is so strong that science might be falsifiable in theory, but scientists have great difficulty making this effort in practice (Van Witteloostuijn, 2016). One way of understanding modern science is that it comes from a mixture of rational curiosity and certain advances and spreads of technology that allowed certain chains of thought to be followed fairly deeply towards tentative conclusions. The Italian microscopers Federico Cesi (1585-1630) and Francesco Stelluti (1577-1652) were able to examine bee anatomy, and expound their findings in a manner echoing Vesalius, in part because of their necessary curiosity, and in part because of the tools they had at their disposal (Bardell, 2005). This definition of science has issues, and illuminates how pseudoscience may simply be applying curiosity and complex tools for research objectives that a consensus of scientists deem illegitimate (Gordin, 2017). However, it does point out the cultural aspect of science, which is part of the remit of this chapter. The nineteenth century replacement of miasma by germ theory, which was catalyzed by unsanitary Victorian early industrial conditions, the spread of cholera, and the engineering remit needed to explore both logic and means of sanitation, is a good example of how science in practice is a combination of tools, institutional knowledge, and need (Smeele, 2016). With a little less institutional knowledge, sixteenth century England was more inclined to amalgamate pestilence, rats, miasma, disease, and witches (Cole, 2010).

It would be a mistake to think of history as necessarily tending towards modern science, which has been used as a term of convenience in this chapter for a set of evidence-based practices that did have to be discovered. It is easy to interpret evidence in alignment with an existing belief, or make mistakes of logic, or not be convinced or aware of an important detail, either as a practitioner or as a patient. However, civilizationally, certain evidence about the nature of injury and disease has been collected and used to heal, and the placebo effect tells us that belief has a power of its own to create some recovery regardless.

REFERENCES

Anselment, R. A. (1995). *The realms of Apollo: Literature and healing in seventeenth-century England.* University of Delaware Press.

Austin, R. (2002). Step on a crack, break your mother's back: Poor moms, myths of authority, and drug-related evictions from public housing. *Yale Journal of Law and Feminism*, *14*, 273–289.

Badcock, P. B., Davey, C. G., Whittle, S., Allen, N. B., & Friston, K. J. (2017). The depressed brain: An evolutionary systems theory. *Trends in Cognitive Sciences*, *21*(3), 182–194. doi:10.1016/j.tics.2017.01.005 PMID:28161288

Bardell, D. (2005). The dawn of microscopy. *The American Biology Teacher*, *67*(7), 392–398. doi:10.2307/4451873

Beaty, R. E., Silvia, P. J., Nusbaum, E. C., Jauk, E., & Benedek, M. (2014). The roles of associative and executive processes in creative cognition. *Memory & Cognition, 42*(7), 1186–1197. doi:10.375813421-014-0428-8 PMID:24898118

Borup, M., Brown, N., Konrad, K., & Van Lente, H. (2006). The sociology of expectations in science and technology. *Technology Analysis and Strategic Management, 18*(3-4), 285–298. doi:10.1080/09537320600777002

Broom, A., Meurk, C., Adams, J., & Sibbritt, D. (2014). Networks of knowledge or just old wives' tales?: A diary-based analysis of women's self-care practices and everyday lay expertise. *Health, 18*(4), 335-351. doi:10.1177/1363459313497610

Castanes, M. S. (2003). Major review: The underutilization of vision screening (for amblyopia, optical anomalies and strabismus) among preschool age children. *Binocular Vision & Strabismus Quarterly, 18*(4), 217–232. PMID:14653775

Chang, Y. (2016). Making of Mami Wata: Diasporic Encounter of African, European and Asian Spirits. *Asian Journal of African Studies*, (39), 53–70.

Cheruvalath, R. (2008). The Problem of Phenomenal Consciousness and Connectionist Representationalism. *Acta Philosophica, 17*(1), 135–143.

Chikramane, P. S., Suresh, A. K., Bellare, J. R., & Kane, S. G. (2010). Extreme homeopathic dilutions retain starting materials: A nanoparticulate perspective. *Homeopathy, 99*(4), 231–242. doi:10.1016/j.homp.2010.05.006 PMID:20970092

Citri, A., & Malenka, R. C. (2008). Synaptic plasticity: Multiple forms, functions, and mechanisms. *Neuropsychopharmacology, 33*(1), 18–41. doi:10.1038j.npp.1301559 PMID:17728696

Clifford, S., & Piston, S. (2017). Explaining public support for counterproductive homelessness policy: The role of disgust. *Political Behavior, 39*(2), 503–525. doi:10.100711109-016-9366-4

Cole, L. (2010). Of mice and moisture: Rats, witches, miasma, and early modern theories of contagion. *Journal for Early Modern Cultural Studies, 10*(2), 65–84. https://www.jstor.org/stable/23242141. doi:10.1353/jem.2011.0007

Dobson, M. (1980). "Marsh Fever"—The geography of malaria in England. *Journal of Historical Geography*, *6*(4), 357–389. doi:10.1016/0305-7488(80)90145-0 PMID:11632265

Dunbar, R. I. (2013). The origin of religion as a small-scale phenomenon. In S. Clarke, R. Powell, & J. Savulescu (Eds.), *Religion, intolerance, and conflict: A scientific and conceptual investigation* (pp. 48–66). Oxford University Press. doi:10.1093/acprof:oso/9780199640911.003.0003

Dunn, P. M. (2003). Galen (AD 129–200) of Pergamun: Anatomist and experimental physiologist. *Archives of Disease in Childhood. Fetal and Neonatal Edition*, *88*(5), F441–F443. doi:10.1136/fn.88.5.F441 PMID:12937057

Emeagwali, G. (1999). Editorial: The Yoruba religious system. *Africa Update*, *6*(3). https://web.ccsu.edu/afstudy/supdt99.htm

Esteves, J. E., Zegarra-Parodi, R., van Dun, P., Cerritelli, F., & Vaucher, P. (2020). Models and theoretical frameworks for osteopathic care–a critical view and call for updates and research. *International Journal of Osteopathic Medicine*, *35*, 1–4. doi:10.1016/j.ijosm.2020.01.003

Galarneau, C. (2010). Blood donation, deferral, and discrimination: FDA donor deferral policy for men who have sex with men. *The American Journal of Bioethics*, *10*(2), 29–39. doi:10.1080/15265160903487619 PMID:20131170

Gordin, M. D. (2017). The problem with pseudoscience: Pseudoscience is not the antithesis of professional science but thrives in science's shadow. *EMBO Reports*, *18*(9), 1482–1485. doi:10.15252/embr.201744870 PMID:28794200

Gordon, J. U. (1979). Yoruba cosmology and culture in Brazil: A study of African survivals in the New World. *Journal of Black Studies*, *9*(4), 231–244. doi:10.1177/002193477900900406

Guthrie, S. E. (1996). Religion: What is it? *Journal for the Scientific Study of Religion*, *35*(4), 412–419. doi:10.2307/1386417

Haberman, D. (2010). Faces in the trees. *Journal for the Study of Religion, Nature and Culture*, *4*(2), 173–190. doi:10.1558/jsrnc.v4i2.173

Ho, E. Y. (2006). Behold the power of Qi: The importance of Qi in the discourse of acupuncture. *Research on Language and Social Interaction*, *39*(4), 411–440. doi:10.120715327973rlsi3904_3

Jeffery, R. (1977). Allopathic medicine in India: A case of deprofessionalization? *Social Science & Medicine, 11*(10), 561-573. doi:10.1016/0037-7856(77)90174-3

Jeffries, W. L. IV, Townsend, E. S., Gelaude, D. J., Torrone, E. A., Gasiorowicz, M., & Bertolli, J. (2015). HIV stigma experienced by young men who have sex with men (MSM) living with HIV infection. *AIDS Education and Prevention, 27*(1), 58–71. doi:10.1521/aeap.2015.27.1.58 PMID:25646730

Jonas, W. B. (2019). The myth of the placebo response. *Frontiers in Psychiatry, 10*, 577. doi:10.3389/fpsyt.2019.00577 PMID:31474888

Kahneman, D. (2011). *Thinking, fast and slow*. Macmillan.

Kelber, A., & Osorio, D. (2010). From spectral information to animal colour vision: experiments and concepts. *Proceedings of the Royal Society B: Biological Sciences, 277*(1688), 1617-1625. 10.1098/rspb.2009.2118

Koerner, M. (2014). Beyond Drama: Postdramatic theater in upper level, performance-oriented foreign language, literature and culture courses. *Scenario: A Journal for Performative Teaching, Learning, Research*, 1-16. doi:10.33178/scenario.8.2.1

Lasser, K. E., Woolhandler, S., & Himmelstein, D. U. (2008). Sources of US physician income: The contribution of government payments to the specialist–generalist income gap. *Journal of General Internal Medicine, 23*(9), 1477–1481. doi:10.100711606-008-0660-7 PMID:18592323

Li, C. (2008). A differentiation of the meaning of "qi" on several levels. *Frontiers of Philosophy in China, 3*(2), 194–212. doi:10.100711466-008-0013-y

Li, C. (2011). Folk memory of Baosheng Dadi. *Zhonghua yi shi za zhi, 41*(4), 249-251.

Li, G., Liang, J. M., Li, P. W., Yao, X., Pei, P. Z., Li, W., He, Q.-H., Yang, X., Chan, Q. C. C., Cheung, P. Y. S., Ma, Q. Y., Lam, S. K., Cheng, P. Y. C., & Yang, E. S. (2011). Physiology and cell biology of acupuncture observed in calcium signaling activated by acoustic shear wave. *Pflügers Archiv, 462*(4), 587–597. doi:10.100700424-011-0993-7 PMID:21796340

Lilienthal, L., Tamez, E., Myerson, J., & Hale, S. (2013). Predicting performance on the Raven's Matrices: The roles of associative learning and retrieval efficiency. *Journal of Cognitive Psychology*, *25*(6), 704–716. doi: 10.1080/20445911.2013.791299 PMID:24187609

Lindeman, M., & Saher, M. (2007). Vitalism, purpose and superstition. *British Journal of Psychology*, *98*(1), 33–44. doi:10.1348/000712606X101808 PMID:17319049

Mantri, S. (2008). Holistic medicine and the Western medical tradition. *AMA Journal of Ethics*, *10*(3), 177–180. doi:10.1001/virtualmentor.2008.10.3.mhst1-0803 PMID:23206886

Mark, J. J. (2017, January 17). *Nergal*. https://www.ancient.eu/Nergal/

Mencke, I., Omigie, D., Wald-Fuhrmann, M., & Brattico, E. (2019). Atonal music: Can uncertainty lead to pleasure? *Frontiers in Neuroscience*, *12*, 979. doi:10.3389/fnins.2018.00979 PMID:30670941

Meng, J., Xu, M., Wang, K., Meng, Q., Han, J., Xiao, X., Liu, S., & Ming, D. (2020). Separable EEG Features Induced by Timing Prediction for Active Brain-Computer Interfaces. *Sensors (Basel)*, *20*(12), 3588. doi:10.339020123588 PMID:32630378

Moerman, D. E., & Jonas, W. B. (2002). Deconstructing the placebo effect and finding the meaning response. *Annals of Internal Medicine*, *136*(6), 471. Advance online publication. doi:10.7326/0003-4819-136-6-200203190-00011 PMID:11900500

Nabirahni, D. M., Evans, B. R., & Persaud, A. (2019). Al-Khwarizmi (Algorithm) and the Development of Algebra. *Mathematics Teaching Research Journal*, *11*(1-2), 13–17.

Neder, J. A. (2020). Cardiovascular and pulmonary interactions: Why Galen's misconceptions proved clinically useful for 1,300 years. *Advances in Physiology Education*, *44*(2), 225–231. doi:10.1152/advan.00058.2020 PMID:32412380

Nutton, V. (2005). The fatal embrace: Galen and the history of ancient medicine. *Science in Context*, *18*(1), 111–121. doi:10.1017/S0269889705000384 PMID:16075496

Olanrewaju, J. A. (2009). The relationship between people and supernatural beings in Yoruba traditional culture. *Journal of Adventist Mission Studies*, *5*(2), 41–49.

Olszewski, W., & Sandroni, A. (2011). Falsifiability. *The American Economic Review*, *101*(2), 788–818. doi:10.1257/aer.101.2.788

Ozioma, E. O. J., & Chinwe, O. A. N. (2019). Herbal medicines in African traditional medicine. In P. Builders (Ed.), *Herbal medicine* (pp. 191–214). IntechOpen. doi:10.5772/intechopen.80348

Parsons, S. (2019). Fear of punishment in another world: A follow-up examination of the religious beliefs about HIV/AIDS—a decade of progress? *Journal of Religion and Health*, 1–13. doi:10.100710943-019-00962-z PMID:31863262

Parvez, A., Ahmed, Z., Anwar, N., & Ahmed, K. (2016). Razi's unique approach to Amraz-e-Wabaiya (Infectious Diseases): An overview. *International Journal of Herbal Medicine*, *4*(6), 176–178.

Phillips, M. J., Gibb, G. C., Crimp, E. A., & Penny, D. (2010). Tinamous and moa flock together: Mitochondrial genome sequence analysis reveals independent losses of flight among ratites. *Systematic Biology*, *59*(1), 90–107. doi:10.1093ysbioyp079 PMID:20525622

Pranesachar, C. R. (2012). Brahmagupta, mathematician par excellence. *Resonance*, *17*(3), 247–252. doi:10.100712045-012-0023-x

Puett, M. (2013). Economies of ghosts, gods, and goods: The history and anthropology of Chinese temple networks. In F. Aulino, M. Goheen, & S. J. Tambiah (Eds.), *Radical egalitarianism: Local realities, global relations* (pp. 91–100). Fordham University Press. doi:10.2307/j.ctt1c5cjrj.8

Ross, S. M. (2009). Qigong: An ancient healing tradition. *Holistic Nursing Practice*, *23*(6), 370–371. doi:10.1097/HNP.0b013e3181bf380d PMID:19901612

Rubin, D. C. (1995). *Memory in oral traditions: The cognitive psychology of epic, ballads, and counting-out rhymes*. Oxford University Press.

Schwitzgebel, E. (1348). Belief. *Stanford Encyclopedia of Philosophy*. https://plato.stanford.edu/archives/fall2019/entries/belief/

Sidebottom, E. (2013). Roger Bacon and the beginnings of experimental science in Britain. *Journal of the Royal Society of Medicine, 106*(6), 243–245. doi:10.1177/0141076813488482 PMID:23761584

Singleton, M. (1976). Smallpox in Person: Personification or Personalization (Africa)? *Anthropos, 71*(1/2), 169–179. https://www.jstor.org/stable/40458885

Slack, P. (1988). Responses to plague in early modern Europe: The implications of public health. *Social Research, 55*(3), 433–453. https://www.jstor.org/stable/40970513 PMID:11650270

Smeele, W. (2016). Grounding Miasma, or Anticipating the Germ Theory of Disease in Victorian Cholera Satire. *The Journal of the Midwest Modern Language Association, 49*(2), 15–27. doi:10.1353/mml.2016.0046

Smorti, A., & Fioretti, C. (2016). Why narrating changes memory: A contribution to an integrative model of memory and narrative processes. *Integrative Psychological & Behavioral Science, 50*(2), 296–319. doi:10.100712124-015-9330-6 PMID:26433588

Spence, W., & Li, N. (2013). An exploration of traditional Chinese medicine practitioners' perceptions of evidence based medicine. *Complementary Therapies in Clinical Practice, 19*(2), 63–68. doi:10.1016/j.ctcp.2013.02.003 PMID:23561062

Stewart, P. J., & Strathern, A. (2013). Religion and violence from an anthropological perspective. In M. Juergensmeyer, M. Kitts, & M. Jerryson (Eds.), *The Oxford handbook of religion and violence* (pp. 375–384). Oxford University Press.

Strick, M., Dijksterhuis, A., Bos, M. W., Sjoerdsma, A., Van Baaren, R. B., & Nordgren, L. F. (2011). A meta-analysis on unconscious thought effects. *Social Cognition, 29*(6), 738–762. doi:10.1521oco.2011.29.6.738

Sun, D. Z., Li, S. D., Liu, Y., Zhang, Y., Mei, R., & Yang, M. H. (2013). Differences in the origin of philosophy between Chinese medicine and western medicine: Exploration of the holistic advantages of Chinese medicine. *Chinese Journal of Integrative Medicine, 19*(9), 706–711. doi:10.100711655-013-1435-5 PMID:23975136

Trevisanato, S. I. (2007). The 'Hittite plague', an epidemic of tularemia and the first record of biological warfare. *Medical Hypotheses, 69*(6), 1371–1374. doi:10.1016/j.mehy.2007.03.012 PMID:17499936

Van Witteloostuijn, A. (2016). What happened to Popperian falsification? Publishing neutral and negative findings. *Cross Cultural & Strategic Management*, *23*(3), 481–508. doi:10.1108/CCSM-03-2016-0084

Wang, J. H., & Cui, S. (2018). Associative memory cells and their working principle in the brain. *F1000 Research*, *7*, 108. doi:10.12688/f1000research.13665.1 PMID:29487741

Wilson, E. O. (1998). Consilience among the great branches of learning. *Daedalus*, *127*(1), 131–149. https://www.jstor.org/stable/20027479 PMID:11619830

Xie, S., Wu, D., Yang, J., Luo, J., Chang, C., & Li, H. (2020). An fNIRS examination of executive function in bilingual young children. *The International Journal of Bilingualism*. Advance online publication. doi:10.1177/1367006920952881

Xu, J., & Zhang, Y. (2020). Traditional Chinese medicine treatment of COVID-19. *Complementary Therapies in Clinical Practice*, *39*, 101165. doi:10.1016/j.ctcp.2020.101165 PMID:32379692

Chapter 3
Role of Infectious Disease at Pivotal Historical Moments

ABSTRACT

This chapter shifts focus away from any kind of totalizing explanation of infectious disease as a whole towards descriptions and discussions of significant historical moments that were shaped by the course of infectious disease. It is perhaps common to discuss human history as the annals of human triumph and tragedies, but, in the same way that it may be impossible to discuss the history of any particular region without at least some implication as to its peripheries, it may be impossible to discuss the Columbian exchange that led to the European colonization of the Americas without reference to the infectious disease that hitched rides westward towards immunologically unprepared lands, depopulating and weakening native civilizations just in time for Europeans to take advantage, to conquer, and to exploit. The infectious component of the Columbian exchange is one of the many macro- and micro-events detailed in this chapter.

INTRODUCTION

Infectious disease has shadowed human history. In the first chapter, this point was made in the context of evolutionary history, and in the second, this point was made in terms of the responses humans had to make to the presence of infectious disease. But infectious disease has done more than shape the natural world, and our idea of it. Infectious disease has also shaped more traditional

DOI: 10.4018/978-1-7998-8689-1.ch003

remits of history such as politics and culture. Infectious disease has acted like something of a third wheel. Disease contributed certain historical events in ways that may recontextualize events thought of as conflicts between peoples into deeper-dimensional conflicts that include, as extra players, strange, almost alien species, species with reproductive methods and motives that are hard or shocking to understand. To the author's knowledge, there has never been a major war that involved a major third force consisting of tigers. But there were many conflicts involving warring factions and pathogens.

THE PLAGUE OF ATHENS AND THE PELOPONNESIAN WAR

The first story presented in this chapter involves the Peloponnesian War. This war, which was fought in the fifth century BCE, consisted on a human level of a contest between the Greek *polis* of Athens, the Greek *polis* of Sparta, and their respective allies. The term *polis* can be translated as city-state (Lyttkens, 2006), reflecting the fact that the scale of the Peloponnesian War did not extend much beyond the boundaries of modern Greece. However, to say that Athens and Sparta were simple cities having a small feud would be to misrepresent the context of the conflict. Earlier in the fifth century BCE, many Greek *poleis* had banded together, and had thrown back the invading forces of Persia, which under the Achaemenid dynasty stretched from Anatolia to Egypt to India, and was then one of the dominant powers in the world (Little, 2007). The defeat of Persia left certain powerful Greek *poleis* in a new position to assert their own power, and Athens, a major player, architected itself to the head of a tributary alliance (Jensen, 2010), that had been built to maintain Greek readiness to fight still-powerful Persia (Larsen, 1940). Meanwhile, Sparta, a more land-based *polis*, was less than exuberant about the developing Athenian imperial structure. War broke out, featuring, roughly, Athenian dominance of the sea and Spartan dominance of the land (Nash, 2018). And then, another factor entered the contest:

In the first days of summer the Lacedaemonians [(Spartans)] and their allies, with two-thirds of their forces as before, invaded Attica [(homeland of Athens)], under the command of Archidamus, son of Zeuxidamus, King of Lacedaemon, and sat down and laid waste the country. Not many days after their arrival in Attica the plague first began to show itself among the Athenians. It was said that it had broken out in many places previously in the neighbourhood of Lemnos and elsewhere; but a pestilence of such extent and mortality was nowhere remembered. Neither were the physicians at first of any service, ignorant as they were of the proper way to treat it, but they died themselves the most thickly, as they visited the sick most often; nor did any human art succeed any better. Supplications in the temples, divinations, and so forth were found equally futile, till the overwhelming nature of the disaster at last put a stop to them altogether. (Thucydides, 431 BCE)

There is a great deal of context to be unpacked here. The Spartans invade, and create great upheaval in Attica, and the displacements caused by the invasion seem to create new opportunity for a dangerous sickness to spring up among the people of Athens. The people of Athens, though possessing a powerful military themselves, were unable to combat the disease in any way that Thucydides, the contemporary chronicler of these events, thought to be particularly effective. The doctors of the Athenians tried what treatments they knew, and the people attempted to seek divine aid or guidance, and yet the disease struck anyway, until, Thucydides suggests, many Athenians were given over to despair. It does not seem to be correct to separate the disease outbreak from the war. Thucydides goes on to say:

An aggravation of the existing calamity was the influx from the country into the city, and this was especially felt by the new arrivals. As there were no houses to receive them, they had to be lodged at the hot season of the year in stifling cabins, where the mortality raged without restraint. (Thucydides, 431 BCE)

This description of the nature of the Spartan-induced dislocation clarifies some of the disease causation out of the mere correlation that is explicit in the earlier quote. If nothing else, problems of housing and organizational capacity seemed to create sanitary issues that exacerbated the plague.

The degree to which the Athenians understood the disease is also worth clarifying further. Despite Thucydides stating explicitly that he does not have the capacity to speculate as to the true nature of the disease--"All speculation as to its origin and its causes, if causes can be found adequate to produce so great a disturbance, I leave to other writers...", in his work he does specify that the Athenians knew from experience both that staying away from the ill did help to prevent the diseases, as well as that those who survived the disease acquired some long lasting immunity (431 BCE):

Yet it was with those who had recovered from the disease that the sick and the dying found most compassion. These knew what it was from experience, and had now no fear for themselves; for the same man was never attacked twice-never at least fatally. And such persons not only received the congratulations of others, but themselves also, in the elation of the moment, half entertained the vain hope that they were for the future safe from any disease whatsoever. (Thucydides, 431 BCE).

The human emotional response to the epidemic is relevant to the politics, because it hints not only at the human capacity for compassion, but also at the fact that the outbreak did not stop the war. The Athenians fought for decades after this outbreak, until finally they lost in 404 BCE (Mark, 2020). The great defeat of the Athenian military at Syracuse on the island of Sicily, far afield from Greece, can be seen as critical to their downfall (Russett & Antholis, 1992). However, the plague certainly did not help, at least plausibly figures into the outcome, and certainly has a great deal to do with the *experience* of the war.

What was the disease that rampaged through Athens? The outbreak mentioned in Thucydides' running chronicle cannot be fixed with certainty to a modern diagnosis, despite Thucydides' efforts to describe, at length, the presenting symptoms (Thucydides, 431 BCE). Possible diagnoses for the major outbreak, which likely occurred in 430 BCE, include smallpox, typhus, or bubonic plague (Mark, 2020). The fact that the precise nature of the disease outbreak is unknown reinforces how alien the experience was to the Athenians, who could not really qualify it either. It seems highly plausible that the disease outbreak was just one of a number that occured in the Mediterranean basin and beyond throughout ancient human history, while the reason it is given to us in such detail is merely because the Ancient Greeks were both particularly literate, and situated in the structure of world history such that their civilization had enough of a progenitor relationship to future cultures as to encourage their works to be passed down.

The Plague of Athens, as presented by Thucydides, can be a tool for benchmarking the relevance of infectious disease to world history. Firstly, it has been defined as a pandemic (Cohn, 2012), a term that approximately means a novel disease outbreak, occurring over a wide area (Kelly, 2011). Kelly says that a pandemic need have no particular severity, though, obviously, the pandemics that are most noticeable must be severe in some fashion. Pandemic is an enhancement of the term epidemic, which approximately means a disease outbreak that is greater than anticipated, though, again, an epidemic need require no specific level of severity (Green et al., 2002). The concept of pandemic disease, and epidemics of disease, contrast with the notion of endemic disease, which is typical of a region (Longini Jr. et al., 2002). The fact that spread is not the same as severity is an important invitation to a different way of thinking about the intersection between infectious disease and history. Namely, an infectious disease need not be endemic, or at the expected scale of an epidemic or pandemic, to have a huge impact on history. Endemic, epidemic, and pandemic are all terms that relate to populations. Disease can also affect politics because of how it impacts individuals.

ALEXANDER THE GREAT

Less than a hundred years from the end of the Peloponnesian War, Alexander the Great, a Greek-influenced Macedonian king who, thanks to the work of his father, held the bulk of Greece under his hegemony, decided the time was right to invade Achaemenid Persia. Persian resistance crumbled, and Alexander made it all the way to the edge of India, acquiring the vast Persian Empire almost wholesale. However, in 323 BCE, in Babylon, at the center of his new empire, Alexander died at the age of not quite 33, preventing him from going on to any further accomplishments, and setting up his generals for a power struggle to divide up what Alexander had acquired (Cunha, 2004). Given the abrupt death of such a notable figure, there has been speculation about assassination, possibly involving strychnine poisoning, or even a death that might be associated with a defect of character--alcoholic liver disease. However, such speculation does not engage with a key lesson of the Plague of Athens narrative presented above. That is, infectious disease operates on a logic that is only tenuously connected to human affairs. Just as the easiest way to make a link between the Peloponnesian War and Plague of Athens is that that politics can spread or expose disease, the easiest way to explore the medical aspects of the death of Alexander might be to start with the point that Alexander, by journeying to places far from Macedonia, or Greece, at the head of a military expedition, exposed himself to local endemic diseases. Babylon was, in Alexander's day, a place that experienced significant amounts of malaria and typhoid fever. Given the description of Alexander's death that exists, it is entirely plausible that he simply did not have the adaptive immunity to malaria or typhoid that would likely have available in the bloodstreams of locals exposed to the microscopic pathogens causing those diseases (Doolan et al., 2009; Sarasombath et al., 1987). Thusly, instead of experiencing a sensitizing infection as a child, and then receiving periodic immune system reminders in the form of additional pathogen exposure, Alexander may very well have entered Babylon as a conqueror in the prime of his life, but also as someone whose body simply had not been trained against malaria or typhoid fever when he was a child, and had not faced down a potentially lethal infectious then, when his death would have been tragic, but would have had less geopolitical significance. Since, under this hypothesis, Alexander caught either malaria or typhoid for the first time as an adult, both he and his empire were suddenly in great trouble, from a threat that may have literal similarities to a surprise attack. Accepting this hypothesis for his death, Alexander's end was related to his conquests, and specifically related to him traveling to places with dangers far from what his body was able to expect. The tactics of Darius III of Persia may have been no match for Alexander, but the tactics of malaria, or typhoid, were ones he may have been unable to avoid, even after he settled into Babylon for a time of what might have felt like relative peace.

What is similar about the Plague of Athens and the Alexander narratives is that they both involve a sort of wedge-shaped conflict. On the one side, human versus human war (Athens vs. Sparta, or Alexander vs. his military enemies). On two other sides, human versus pathogen, with the sort of strategies humans could apply to the first category of fighting not available to the others. Neither the causative agent of the Plague of Athens nor the causative agent of Alexander's death could be spotted and isolated, and key tactics people of his day had against the infectious diseases--avoidance, palliative care, and trust in their own bodies/immune systems--were inadequate to the task of defending Alexander.

Given the awkward political vacuum that Alexander's early death left, with powerful generals and an unborn heir, it seems reasonable to believe that if Alexander had survived his brush with death in 323 BCE, the future of world history, possibly inviting a longer-lasting Macedonian empire, would have looked very different (Brunt, 1965).

FEAR OF ILLNESS

So far, this chapter has discussed two instances related to infectious disease that were extremely significant to the Ancient Greek world. What is the best way to look further afield? One reasonable point to make is that *fear* of death, possibly through infectious disease, was a motivating factor that shaped politics in its own right. The first emperor of Qin China, Qin Shi Huang, who lived 259-210 BCE, is famous for not only uniting China after the long decline of the Zhou, but also for being concerned enough with his fate that he may have ingested a mercury elixir that did not provide the intended immortality, but instead cut his life short (Chan, 2014). This way of presenting the death of Qin Shi Huang has a powerful moral component--he was able to unify so many of the lands surrounding the Qin core, but died making a mistake out of fear because he did not know the right way to defeat complex or hidden dangers, like pathogens, that lurked all around him. Regardless of how closely this notorious story matches what actually happened, it provides a meaningful counterpoint to the death of Alexander. Alexander may not have taken pathogens like infectious disease seriously enough. Qin Shi Huang may have been well aware of the danger, but without tutelage on appropriate ways to respond. And, just like Alexander, in his absence, his empire, the Qin Dynasty did not last long without him, though China stayed unified under the Han (Su et al., 2014).

HAMIN MANGHA AND PREHISTORY

There are ways of thinking about infectious disease's impact on world history that go beyond both intervention in recorded wars, and personal challenges for emperors or leaders. Recall one of the key subtexts of the Plague of Athens--it may be famous in large part because it was so well documented by Thucydides. Rolling history back, into points of time documented by archeology, not written records, such that the discussion may more easily be considered one of *prehistory*--mass graves found in housing locations at the site of Hamin Mangha in Inner Mongolia, coupled with evidence of sudden abandonment, suggest that an epidemic roiled the region about five thousand years ago (Yonggang & Ping, 2016). As with the other narratives presented so far, that have better documentation, it is hard to point to a specific cause, but even with the fragmentary evidence available, points of similarity with the Plague of Athens are clear. Just as the Athenians did not know what to do with certain migrants, and so left them in cabins to die, it is entirely possible that people of Hamin Mangha did the best they could before being overwhelmed with plague. The proximity of the bodies to each other, and to housing, suggest both a great tragedy, and one that interacted with social effort.

EPIDEMIC AND ENDEMIC DISEASE

By linking Hamin Mangha to the Plague of Athens, and Alexander to Qin Shi Huang, a structure can be created that will propel the rest of this chapter. One framework that can be constructed about the ways in which infectious disease impacted world history involves two classes. In the first, infectious disease operated on a large scale. In the second, infectious disease attacked, directly or indirectly, individuals whose particular illness would have a disproportionate impact on world history. There is nuance in both of these categories. While small-scale impact can potentially be divided into direct and indirect influence, large-scale infectious disease can be divided further into endemic and epidemic/pandemic phenomena. Both the Plague of Athens and the discovery at Hamin Mangha appear to be epidemics, because the responses and reports tied to their existence do not suggest the Ancient Greeks of two and a half thousand years ago, and the Inner Mongolians of five thousand years ago, expected on a regular basis the calamity that befell them. However, endemic diseases also can have a significant impact on world history.

An example of an important endemic disease is malaria. Malaria, caused by certain types of protozoa (Ndiabamoh, 2020), which are single-celled eukaryotic organisms (Bing, 2021), played a significant role in slowing European colonization of Africa (Shick, 1971). Nevertheless, malaria as an endemic form of resistance has a horrific polar opposite in the experience of the Americas to infectious diseases introduced by Columbus and the Columbian exchange that began in 1492. Before turning to a discussion of that disaster of immunological vulnerability, however, it is worth discussing one more terrible epidemic in the Eastern Hemisphere, which sheds light on more patterns on a huge scale.

PROPAGANDA AND THE BLACK DEATH

A traditional narrative of the Black Death is tied to the intentional spreading of infectious disease. Given the fraught nature of accusing an enemy of biological warfare, it is worth mentioning that certain types of accusations of this sort are likely to be untrue. However, biological warfare is within the bounds of human behavior, and this traditional narrative of biological warfare is associated with how plague, or the Black Death, reached from a port of the Black Sea, throughout the Mediterranean, and beyond (Wheelis, 2002). The following is from the account of Gabriele De' Mussi, a possible eyewitness who described the circumstances surrounding a siege of Caffa, a Genoese outpost in modern Ukraine:

In 1346, in the countries of the East, countless numbers of Tartars and Saracens were struck down by a mysterious illness which brought sudden death. ... Oh God! See how the heathen Tartar races, pouring together from all sides, suddenly invested the city of Caffa and besieged the trapped Christians there for almost three years. There, hemmed in by an immense army, they could hardly draw breath, although food could be shipped in, which offered them some hope. But behold, the whole army was affected by a disease which overran the Tartars and killed thousands upon thousands every day. It was as though arrows were raining down from heaven to strike and crush the Tartars' arrogance. All medical advice and attention was useless; the Tartars died as soon as the signs of disease appeared on their bodies: swellings in the armpit or groin caused by coagulating humours, followed by a putrid fever.

The dying Tartars, stunned and stupefied by the immensity of the disaster brought about by the disease, and realizing that they had no hope of escape, lost interest in the siege. But they ordered corpses to be placed in catapults and lobbed into the city in the hope that the intolerable stench would kill everyone inside. What seemed like mountains of dead were thrown into the city, and the Christians could not hide or flee or escape from them, although they dumped as many of the bodies as they could in the sea. (Wheelis, 2002)

As with the Plague of Athens, this is a conflict that seems to dynamically involve not just two human factions, but also a pathogen. Caffa, a city used as a trading outpost by the then-independent Italian polity of Genoa, existed peacefully under Genoese control at the pleasure of the Golden Horde, a division of the Mongols that controlled the hinterland (Wheelis, 2002). When the Golden Horde came into conflict with Genoa, a siege, or investment, of the city of Genoa began, and, around the same time, the specific disease known as plague began passing through the lands controlled by the Golden Horde. The plague was too much for the Golden Horde to be able to maintain the siege, but they did not seem to want to be the only ones in misery, and so flung the bodies of the dead into Caffa, understanding enough about the spread of disease to think this was a tactic that could inflict special damage. The way Gabriele De' Mussi speculates about the spread of plague--through the stench--is both inappropriate according to modern germ theory, and, because of the limitations of the sense experience in humans of his day (not having access to the implications of equipment like microscopes), is close enough to the truth of invisible pathogens coming through the air (Winderman et al., 2019), or, common to plague, flea-bite, as to clarify how the Golden Horde knew what to do.

Understanding the spread of the Black Death throughout Gabriele De' Mussi's Europe-focused world as the product of ships fleeing plague-infested Caffa may well be overly simplistic. Recall the human inclination to attribute causes for calamity on intentional action. However, disease spread from a point or limited number of points is intrinsic to the exponential growth of contagion. In tandem with travelers or refugees leaving other Mongol centers like Serai and Astrakhan, Caffa seems to have been key in bringing the disease in Europe (Wheelis, 2002). The result when the plague was in Europe--an estimated mortality rate of between 20% and 50% (Gottfried, 2010, p. xvi), is infamous enough to perhaps hide both some of the practical human implications--the economic power of surviving workers rose individually because there were fewer of them, with a plausible positive impact on long-term per capita wealth (Clark, 2016; Voigtländer & Voth, 2013). Another detail that may be hidden by the notoriety of the Black Death in Europe is the impact of the disease on other parts of the world. The Black Death seems to have had roughly comparable effects around the African and Asian rims of the Mediterranean, including Egypt, as well as deep into Asia (Borsch, 2005). The fact that a great deal of Western historiography is built around seeing the Black Death as a European-impacting phenomenon seems to be a limitation of research scope, rather than a detail that has anything to do with the course of the disease.

INFECTIOUS DISEASE IN THE AMERICAS AFTER COLUMBUS

Beginning about a century and a half after the Black Death, the epidemic-driven depopulation of the Americas drove the modern political and demographic state of the modern Western Hemisphere. The Americas were not the only part of the world colonized by Europeans. Africa was too, as was southern and southeastern Asia. However, despite being further away from Europe than Africa, the Americas were mostly controlled by Europe in an earlier period (the sixteenth through eighteenth centuries), than Africa and southern Asia were (the nineteenth century and first half of the twentieth century), as well as for generally a longer period. There are exceptions to this basic frame--the Battle of Plassey in 1757 is a common demarcation for the beginning of British hegemony in India in general and Bengal in particular (Borscheid & Haueter, 2015; Chatterjee, 2019). However, the simple fact that the history of the United States and Canada, even after both countries became independent from Great Britain, is filled with narratives of Native American dispossession at the hands of those with European ancestry, relates starkly with similar narratives from Africa. The country in Africa with arguably the longest-lasting White settlement, South Africa, had a reckoning with the dispossession of Black Africans that came to a head in 1994, with the end of White minority rule. If, in 1991, near the end of White minority rule, Whites in South Africa had been more than the 13.4% of the population they actually were (Treiman et al., 1996), it is reasonable to imagine that the history of the country might have proceeded very differently. In Bolivia, part of the Incan heart of indegenous population concentration when Europeans were entering South America in the sixteenth century, 62% of the population identified as indigenous in the 2001 census (Reyes-García, 2014; Censo, 2001). This seems substantial, but can be understood as a high mark--other countries in South America, particularly the Southern Cone countries of Argentina, Chile, and Uruguay, are far more White, similar to the countries in the far north, Canada and the United States.

With the demographic impact clarified, what was the nature of the infectious-disease-driven depopulation of the Americas? The Columbian exchange as a whole involved plants, peoples, animals, and economic structures, but the infectious disease seems to have overshadowed the rest of it (Crosby Jr., 2003). Modern Mexico, the first major center of Spanish presence in the mainland on the Western Hemisphere, is a reasonably well-documented example (Acuna-Soto et al., 2004). In 1519, when the Spanish arrived, the region is estimated as containing between fifteen and thirty million people. By 1600, the population was down to *two* million. To try to compare this with the hypothesis of Alexander dying in Babylon because of a naive immune system, this is rather as if the diseases of Babylon invaded a land much larger than Greece wholesale, bringing disaster as a vastly larger set of victims tried to cope with the invisible pathogen attack. As with the Plague of Athens, the precise nature or natures of the pathogens that did such horrible damage to the people of the Americas is hard to precisely clarify. Smallpox, measles, and mumps are commonly thought to be key drivers of the catastrophe, along with war and famine--the spread of infectious disease was spread by the affairs of humans, after all. However, more mysteriously, but no less horrifically, outbreaks of hemorrhagic fever called cocoliztli also played a major role. The first outbreak in Mexico of cocoliztli, starting in 1545, killed 80% of the population within three years. The second major outbreak of cocoliztli, which began in 1576, took away 51.36% of the population in 157 districts. Because the Spanish administration was entrenched in the region by that point, there is no invasion-driven lack of records to force demographers to estimate the impact of the outbreak. Census data is straightforward. What is also clear is that cocoliztli was far more dangerous to those of indegenous descent than those of Spanish. Aside from the raw death toll, one of the most horrific aspects of the diseases that took away so much of the population of the Americas in the period starting after the arrival of the Europeans was that the Europeans themselves had immune systems that were sensitized to the infectious diseases they carried with them, while indigenous populations were immunologically naive.

To truly clarify the horror of the demographics in general, and of the situation in Mexico in particular, it is worth moving to a primary source. The Florentine Codex, compiled by the Fransican missionary Fray Bernardino de Sahagún, was something of a life's work, as he arrived in New Spain (the Spanish name for the Mexican colony) in 1529, and labored on the text from 1558 to 1569 (Reeves, 2006). It is notable because of how large sections of the work put the experience of the Nahuatl-speaking indegenous peoples of Mexico in their own words. Many of those words discuss the Spanish conquest from an indegenous perspective, and, because infectious disease was a part of that conquest, the text also discusses outbreak of epidemic.

[Even] before the Spaniards appeared to us, an illness broke out, a sickness of pustules. It began in Tepeilhuitl, and it spread over the people as a great

destruction. Large bumps spread on people; some were entirely covered--on the face, the head, the chest, etc. [The disease] brought great desolation; a great many [people] died from it.

[People] with the illness could not walk, they could only lay in their dwellings and sleeping places. They could not move; they could not stir; they could not change position, nor lie on one side, nor face down, nor on their backs. And when they stirred, they screamed. The pustules that covered people caused great desolation; a great many people died of them, and many just died of hunger; [for] no one took care of others any longer. (de Sahagún, 2020)

One of the most striking parts of this passage is how it ends--the text makes a point of stating that morality seemed to be warped by the disease. The disease discussed here is thought to be smallpox, not cocoliztli (de Sahagún, 2020). However, as part of the cascade of infectious diseases that meet with indegenous populations after arrival of those from across the sea, the above passage seems relevant. Even the multitude of diseases seems relevant. Just as, in times of strife, there might be a variety of different types of human dangers, ranging from armies to robbers, so too do infectious diseases not exist in isolation. The idea of an opportunistic infection, where a vulnerability such as a wound, or a prior present disease, creates space for a new disease to come in, is echoed here in the idea that the ships of the conquistadors had no particular reason to carry only one pathogen. Another important detail is that the impact of the particular epidemic described, as well as others that occured for similar reasons, contributed to the weakening of Amerindian civilizations such that societies imported from the Eastern Hemisphere would drive much of the condition of the West for the next five hundred years.

INFECTIOUS DISEASE AND EMOTIONAL RESPONSES

The combination of infections from similar vectors is also echoed by the combination of directly human and pathogenic vectors mentioned above. In the context of Columbian exchange, illness is combined with great fear on the part of the locals, who feel unable to help each other, as well as by the presence of the Spanish, who both helped to bring the disease. This seems to have been unknowingly to a substantial degree, as germ theory was not common knowledge among the Spanish at the time of their invasion of the Americas. Germ theory took the breadth of the early modern period to be theorized in Europe--Italian physician Girolamo Fracastoro (Hieronymous Fracastorius) had a proposal in 1546, while Viennese doctor Marcus Plenciz had a proposal around 1762 (Opal, 2009). International prominent medical scholars of the Middle Ages were often from the Islamic World, and included Al-Razi (lived 850 to c. 932), who wrote about smallpox and measles, as well as Ibn Sina (980-1037), and Ibn Rushd (1126-1198) (Golzari et al., 2012; Majeed, 2005; Tulchinsky & Varavikova, 2014). (Their works were translated and brought to Christian Europe, and contributed to the world's development of medical knowledge.)

The idea of calamity as often combining dangers from both macroscopic humans and microscopic pathogens is not limited to the horrific events in Mexico and the Americas, either. In the Peloponnesian War description above, issued by Thycidides, there is a quoted segment that seems parallel to the way the passage from the Florentine Codex ends. Namely, Thycidides points out that there was euphoria among those who had overcome the plague of Athens. However, the Plague of Athens also created what might be called euphoria's opposite:

Nor was this [disordered burial rites] the only form of lawless extravagance which owed its origin to the plague. Men now coolly ventured on what they had formerly done in a corner, and not just as they pleased... (Thucydides, 431 BCE)

The Plague of Athens, and the terrors that reached the people of Mexico, were in a cultural sense part of the same continuum. Both the Nahuatl-speaking peoples of the Florentine Codex and then Athenians lost the wars they were fighting, and the fact the ultimate impact on the Americas seems to have been much more significant seems to have been mostly a matter of degree.

INTERCONNECTIVITY AND AWARENESS OF INFECTIOUS DISEASE

The chapter has reached a point where it is worth taking stock of what has been covered. A typology of infectious disease impacts on world history was introduced--impacts on a mass scale (both epidemic and endemic), and impacts through effect on certain persons of particular influence (both directly, and indirectly, through processes such as anxiety). In offering this typology, a number of significant incidents have been discussed, including traditional historiography on the Black Death, the depopulation of the Americas, and, on a smaller scale, the Plague of Athens and the death of Alexander. Additionally, some persistent themes in the impact of infectious disease on world history were also developed. These themes include (1), the way infectious disease can been spread or exacerbated, accidentally, intentionally, or in some in-between level of awareness, by the acts of humans, as well as (2), even with the considerable descriptions or evidence that were left to history of certain waves of infectious disease, descriptions of epidemics that came and went prior to the advent of allopathic medicine are hard to classify. To further explore that second theme, it is worth pointing out that cocoliztli, one of the major illnesses that contributed to the population of the Americas, has recently been associated, through DNA extraction at a cemetery, with the pathogen *Salmonella enterica*, known to cause enteric or typhoid fever, but because the symptoms do not match contemporary occurences of this sickness it seems reasonable that there is more work to be done to get closer to the truth (Vågene et al., 2018; Puente & Calva, 2017). As for the first theme, of the way humans can interact with infectious disease--and spread infectious disease--that topic is worth exploring as a key in its own right.

The culpability of conquistadors and other Europeans of spreading disease into the Americas is a key topic in historiography because of the way a resolution to that issue fits into the narrative of the post-Columbian Americas. If the Europeans largely were observers to, or ignorant of, the horrors their bodies hid, and unleashed, then it is easier to accept some aspects of the old heroic narrative involving certain early colonial immigrants heading to seek fortune in the Americas. However, if some Europeans noticed that they had a horrifying bioweapon at their disposal, and took steps to leverage it--the story then takes another foul turn. One particularly common story in the Americas involves Europeans passing smallpox-contaminated blankets to Native Americans to intentionally decimate them, and while it is certainly possible that certain instances of this terrible behavior were imaginary--recall the human tendency to blame outsiders for misfortunes--there is some documentation of this deed being planned, in writing associated with Jeffery Amherst, a British leader in North America around and after the time of the Seven Years' War (Mayor, 1995).

Worse, there seems to be nothing particularly unique about Jeffery Amherst's behavior, even if it was not widespread. The patterns that happened in the Americas happened in other places. Just as widescale loss of life among the immunologically-vulnerable peoples of the Americas occurred after European contact, so too did widescale loss of life occur among Pacific Islanders in the early modern period when European sailors arrived in that part of the world (Penman et al., 2017). After apparent centuries of not needing innate or adaptive resistance to the diseases common in Eurasia, evolutionary pressures radically shifted in both the Americas and the Pacific, in a way that makes stark just how brutal selection can be--stark enough it is worth reminding the reader that an account of what happened, what *is*, is not close to an ethical account of what should have happened, what *ought* (Greene, 2003).

THE BLACK DEATH IN THE SHADOW OF THE AMERICAS

At this point in the chapter, taking stock again, the narrative has moved through typology, through a recounting of the Black Death, into the horrific demographic shock that the Americas and the Pacific experienced in the early modern age of colonialism, with an emphasis on disease could be conveyed by perilous and even deliberately malicious human activity. There is a coherent way of presenting the Black Death and its effects that seems divorced from the greater history of disease in a way that the infection of the Americas did not, largely because epidemics spreading to the Americas were more effective at wiping out whole civilizations. Is there a better way to connect these vast events, and others like them? The rest of the chapter intends to work towards that goal.

TOWARDS A COHERENT HISTORY OF INFECTIOUS DISEASE: DISPERSAL

Trying to understand the coherent big history of infectious disease on humans and human civilization is a worthwhile pursuit. Having used examples that are accessible to trace major themes in the big history of infectious disease, in a way that is focused more on the concepts than the chronology, the path has been cleared to start back at the beginning, with a new and more connected linear description, and the caveat that this task is limited by the references accessible to the author. The rest of the chapter is in some ways a recapitulation of themes and concepts presented above, but it is a recapitulation that attempts a deeper integration of incidents.

What does a coherent human history interwoven with infectious disease look like? It probably starts in Africa, where humans evolved alongside malaria parasites (Loy et al., 2017). Malaria appears to have been such a shaping force on the human genome. There are a variety of human genetic diseases that appear to have been selected for because some level of the underlying genetics are valuable in malarial resistance. These include blood-related conditions like sickle cell disease (LaMonte et al., 2012), thalassemias (Lell et al., 1999), Glucose-6-phosphate dehydrogenase deficiency, and pyruvate kinase deficiency (López et al., 2010). To give a more precise example, while sickle cell disease is harmful, sickle cell trait, which is a condition that only comes with heterozygous abnormal allele incidence (only inherited from one parent) (Ojodu et al., 2014), provides resistance to malaria (Williams et al., 2005). While the various mechanisms the human body uses internally to fight pathogens, it is a meaningful big history note to point out that our evolution seems to have involved adaptations to fight pathogens, in a way similar to how our lineage evolved bipedalism, binocular vision, and high cognitive capacity for various other substantive reasons.

Regardless, as the ancestral human population spread out of Africa and throughout the world. Modern humans reached the area around the Levant and Europe perhaps 40,000 to 50,000 years ago (Bosch et al., 2015; Richter et al., 2012), then the Americas, via the now-gone Beringia land bridge, perhaps around 20,000 years ago (Vachula et al., 2019). The Pacific islands were settled in an ongoing process that continues through essentially the present with, for example, early signs of settlement in the Marshall Islands dating to about 2,000 years ago (Weisler et al., 2012). Parallel to how a major impact of the human origin in Africa was the spread of genes involved in disease resistance, which in the absence of the disease, are mostly noticed for their negative exacerbations, a major impact of the spread of people all around the world is that various groups far from Eurasia were cut off from close proximity to Eurasian trade, interactions, and disease exposure. The horrors experienced by the Amerindians and Pacific Islanders when Europeans developed the technology needed to establish a direct global colonial and trade network have their origins in the isolation created by the different form of adventuring that the earliest Amerindians and Pacific Islanders took to reach those regions. There is an irony that, just as the sacrifices made by migrants in prehistoric and near-prehistoric times were greater than those of moderns insofar as it would be more difficult to turn back around, another sacrifice made by those migrants to the far reaches of the world was the impact of lack of interaction with major human population densities would have on their genetics, their adaptive immunities, and the fate of many of their descendants. An important point here is that it did not have to turn out the way it did--it is possible, for example, that a dire pathogen might have evolved in the Americas, and the Amerindians might have developed resistance, only for hapless European explorers to bring the disease back to Europe. There is evidence Americas-to-Europe pathogen transfer happened to some degree--one potential candidate is the agent behind syphilis (Harper et al., 2011). However, a problem with assuming that the ultimate horrors inflicted on the Amerindians, Pacific Islanders, and other people who spent centuries developing in relatively isolated locations, were ultimately arbitrary, is that, just as the networks of trade and interconnection that helped Eurasians obtain the goods of their ancient civilizations were larger than that of isolated peoples, so too was their connection to the full lineage of pathogens that coevolved with humans. Malaria, for example, was present in swampy regions of Italy back in the days of Ancient Rome (Sallares, 2002), and was also recognized as occurring around 4,000 years back in Ancient China (Yin et al., 2014). Meanwhile, severe strains of malaria appear to have been absent from the Americas, perhaps cleared away by the period of cold climate conditions the travelers eastward across Beringia had to endure, until the arrival of post-Columbian travel networks (Rodreigues et al., 2018).

Two principles--coevolution and isolation--seem at the heart of understanding key interactions between human history and infectious disease. The two basic ways a disease can strike a large population--through being consistent within certain climatological boundaries, like malaria, or by emerging and decimating through available hosts, like plague, are also tied to these two principles. In ecology, there is a pattern where a predator might overhunt a prey item, causing a prey population crash, followed by a predator population crash, and this pattern analogizes fairly well to the relationship between pandemics and epidemics, or humans. The idea translates as a dangerous disease introduced to a new area for the first time in a while, running rampant, running out of available hosts, and then dying back to reservoirs where it can "await" an opportunity to try again later. Because plague can lurk in rats, for example, rats can act as a reservoir for the pathogen behind the Black Death (Tollenaere et al., 2010). One of the key implications between consistent versus sporadic disease is that it is the shock of the new state of affairs that changes a population's experience, rather than raw harm or mortality. What this means is that, despite malaria's enormous impact on the human experience, the greatest historical impact of it and similar diseases was on long-term population characteristics, as well as migrants to new climes. Meanwhile, a disease more in the pandemic mode, like plague, exerted its impact on populations, and on history, in reasonably short shocks. Endemic diseases find better natural equilibrium with their hosts, through coevolution. Diseases more well-known as epidemics still engage in coevolution, and even may become suddenly virulent because of a genome shift allowing the underlying pathogen to effectively target humans. However, diseases of this class do not by definition exist in close proximity to their ultimate targets for long.

There is a risk at this part of the narrative of falling back into typology at the expense of exploring history. The epidemic/endemic distinction is a typology. However, it is also a framework that can be used to fit in major epidemics and endemic phenomena that are clearly presented by history, and, additionally, it is a framework that helps clarify what is missing. Various epidemics and endemic incidents almost certainly harmed early populations that could not record, going "under the radar" of history. As chronology advances more towards the present, more incidents and phenomena are available to assess, and there is a risk of believing that the most important incidents happened most recently merely because of the documentation. The value of the epidemic/endemic distinction being presented here is to highlight the critical importance of the lacunae as the narrative progresses, and point out that the story told is closer to that which is seen through windows of varying levels of cleanliness, rather than something intrinsically comprehensive. The issue of gaps in the historical record is relevant beyond infectious disease--documentation on a wide variety of historical incidents of past civilizations is lost, missing, or difficult to access via current scholarship. For example, the Indus Valley Script, which promises to contain the records of a widespread ancient civilization, is resistant to being deciphered (Daggumati & Revesz, 2021), and the use of oral tradition in many parts of the world is a barrier to integrating the awareness many people have of their past with text-based formal scholarship (Lebaka, 2019; Cruikshank, 1994). This reinforces the importance of lacunae.

TOWARDS A COHERENT HISTORY OF INFECTIOUS DISEASE: EPIDEMICS

As far as the narrative itself, one way to proceed is to highlight certain epidemics that stood out above the 'noise' of history, as well as the way regionalities associated with disease shaped certain patterns. Ancient Rome experienced three well-known major epidemics. The first, the Antonine Plague, or the Plague of Galen, struck heavily in the eastern part of the Roman Empire from 165 to 189 CE (Zaviyeh & Golshani, 2020). This disease, thought to be smallpox, shaped the environment where the physician Galen honed came to prominence. The second, the Cyprian Plague, from 251 to 270 CE, is harder to diagnose, and with various potential culprits being smallpox, measles, plague, or a viral hemorrhagic fever (Kearns, 2018). In both the cases of the Plague of Galen and the Plague of Cyprian, the diseases are named after famous authors who wrote about the epidemics, with a major lesson here being reinforcement that part of the reason these epidemics are so famous is because of the way they were culturally transmitted. Meanwhile, a major epidemic was present in China from 217-218 CE may have killed half the population of certain regions, but is also difficult to clarify because it must be limited through the lens of surviving local writings of that period, which include Jian'an poetry (Tian, 2020, p.4-15; Williams, 2015). The third major epidemic of the Roman period, or perhaps early Byzantine period, is the Plague of Justianian, identified as truly plague, which began 541-544 CE and progressed in shocks through the eighth century, is easier to tie to a specific political context--the Emperor Justinian was looking to restore the west to the Roman Empire, but was interrupted by an epidemic disease that he had, and survived, but, in four years, perhaps 20% to 25% of the people in his area of the world did not (Findlay & Lundahl, 2017). The ultimate mortality for the Plague of Justinian, in its outbreaks over the next century and a half, may have reached half the affected population, similar to the epidemic of the Jian'an period.

The above description is something of a summary of famous epidemics in the late ancient period of world history, but, unfortunately, is difficult to take as a broad accounting of worldwide epidemics in that period, let alone a representative portrayal of the impact of infectious disease. Frankly, the English-language literature of the 217-218 epidemic in China, being relatively lacking when explored through tools like Google Scholar, is a reasonable example of the larger issue. Even further, while there is at least some clear literature of the above epidemics because they differed so far from the norm, endemic diseases by definition do not draw the same type of ecumenical attention. And, going beyond that, the reason the above recounting started with the late ancient period, and not outbreaks like a thirteenth century BCE tularemia outbreak in Mesopotamia and the Eastern Mediterranean (Trevisanto,

2007), or Hamin Mangha (Yonggang & Ping, 2016), is that the records of the more distance past are necessarily more fragmentary.

In that case, what of forwards? Granting that illnesses that affected specific individuals in late antiquity affected the course of history as well, possibly including, in 117 CE, the powerful Roman Emperor Trajan (Zaviyeh & Golshani, 2020), it may be appropriate to skip forward to a clear epidemic that presented not long after the later shocks of the Plague of Justinian--the smallpox epidemic in Japan that began in 735 CE (Suzuki, 2011). The arrival of smallpox in Japan at this point likely was the first introduction in recorded history, because not only did about a third of the population die in the initial outbreak, but the history of Japan, going forwards, includes smallpox outbreaks with smaller and smaller intervals, until, by the Tokugawa Period that started in the 1600s, smallpox was essentially endemic, predominantly affecting children, who would have to gain immunity from surviving it.

There are a couple takeaways from Japan's experience that tie into the larger world experience with infectious disease. First, in comparing the islands of Japan with more remote Pacific islands, Japan can be seen as a sort of semi-periphery: far enough away from the mainland to be forced to endure great shock when smallpox was introduced, yet close enough that the horrible sensitization happened early enough in Japan's history for the country to be able to treat with Eurasians on a more even basis moving forwards. A Japan that, upon the arrival of Commodore Perry (a nineteenth century United States navy man who worked to "open" Japan to Western influence), was soon after stricken with smallpox, measles, or something like cocoliztli, while interloping Westerners were not, is likely a Japan that would have had a very different experience in the modern era. The second point to make here returns to the epidemic/endemic divide. How could smallpox in Japan, by becoming more prevalent, perhaps fade into the background? One argument is that, with saturation, the number of new cases in Japan, even if they mostly were associated with children, were minimal enough to allow the Japanese to effect useful palliative care, rather than experience their health apparatuses be overwhelmed. Another argument speaks more broadly to the limitations of this chapter in dealing with endemic diseases--horrific incidents that are common simply are less memorable and less disruptive to existing societal structures.

Moving forwards chronologically, a great divide in a world history that focuses on infectious disease is likely the outbreak of plague known as the Black Death. Because this specific pandemic was treated separately above, the brief discussion here will focus on important contexts of the Black Death, rather than its experience. First, how much weight of what was known in Europe as the Black Death fell on Eastern Asia, or sub-Saharan Africa, is unclear. Sussman (2011) has made a firm argument that the major polities in India and China in the mid-1300s, at the time of the initial outbreak of the Black Death (the Delhi Sultanate, and the Mongol-led Yuan Dynasty, respectively) were not subject to the sort of ruptures experienced by Europe, the Mediterranean, and the Middle East. Green (2015), meanwhile, has a different emphasis, pointing out the impact of the plague on lands surrounding the Indian Ocean, including East Africa. Regardless, the impact of plague was substantial. Quite aside from the fact the term "plague," which can be used in a literary fashion to describe a broad range of ailments, is in a restrictive sense linked with the gram-negative bacillus (rod-shaped bacterium) *Yersinia pestis* (Forrester et al., 2017) associated with the Black Death and similar outbreaks like the Plague of Justinian, there is also the fact that plague outbreaks that started with the Black Death persisted around the Mediterranean and Europe for hundreds of years after, in what is called the Second Plague Pandemic (Spyrou, 2019). Unlike the First Plague Pandemic, associated with the Plague of Justinian, and its aftershocks, this Second Plague Pandemic occurred in a world that was increasingly accessible to literacy. Mobile type, a printing technique that allowed for fast creation of texts by application of preformed letters, became prominent throughout Eurasia around the late medieval period, in Song China, Korea, and finally Europe (Gunaratne, 2001; Poon, 1973), created new opportunity for a more thorough documentation of epidemics and other experiences. This may have helped various subsidiary outbreaks of plague have their own identities. For example, the outbreak of plague that reached Naples, Italy, in 1656, via Spain, via Algiers, killed around 1,250,000 people in the whole Kingdom of Italy (Scasciamacchia et al., 2012).

In any event, the fact of Black Death aftershocks should not detract from the horrors inflicted on the Americas about a century and a half after the Black Death struck Europe. That the Second Plague Pandemic struck Europe at the same time that smallpox and other diseases were striking the Americas is important, as is the fact that outsiders could capitalize on what was happening in the Americas, while outsiders could not do the same to Europe. While it is too simple to assert a "Eurasian immunity" to certain common diseases, through genetics or childhood exposure, that people of regions peripheral to the world population concentrations did not possess, this idea does have some value when expanded to be thought of as more of a rule of thumb in the context of a gradient. Europeans had difficulty entering Africa and staying healthy, due in part to malaria and other tropical diseases prevalent in certain areas Europeans wished to enter, while many Native Americans had difficulty merely maintaining in their homelands, because the nature of climates and transportation of persons and diseases meant that diseases found in Europe could migrate to the Americas just as Europeans could.

TOWARDS A COHERENT HISTORY OF INFECTIOUS DISEASE: COLLECTIVE ACTION

The early modern period that can be said to start with Columbus involved more patterns than the spread of epidemics peripherally, of course. Aside from the "revenge" of the Americas that might have come into Europe in the form of less-overwhelmingly-destructive but still unpleasant syphilis, disease in general was able to become continuous and endemic in new ways through increased global connectivity. Smallpox, for example, spread for over two thousand years of human history, branching into variants, like isolates in West Africa, or the more phenotypically mild alastrim/variola minor from the Americas, as it became endemic in different contexts (Li et al., 2007).

One particularly notable example of smallpox's spread, involving leadership, is the Manchu experience with smallpox. The Manchu, a people from north, beyond the Great Wall, managed to conquer China in the seventeenth century, establishing the last dynasty, the Qing, which prevailed in China until the upheaval that led to the People's Republic in the twentieth century. The Manchu, starting from a geographic and epidemiological position vaguely similar to the Japanese from centuries earlier, had leadership not unaware of the dangers of smallpox, and leadership that also knew that, because they had come from a less-exposed part of the world, and now were attempting to rule over the more-populated Chinese heartland, they were at a brand new risk from infectious disease (Zhang, 2002). There is copious evidence that the Manchu really were preoccupied with smallpox. Their records mention concern with the disease, repeatedly, and there seems to have been a government agency devoted to reducing harm from this vector, established in 1622 or sooner, that lasted for more than two centuries, and is without precedent in other Chinese dynasties. The fact that the Manchu were able to mitigate the impact of smallpox enough to successfully rule China should not serve as an argument against the significance of the disease. The Shunzhi Emperor, under whose rule Manchu authority in China was consolidated, died in 1661 after much consternation over the disease, and did indeed die to smallpox, but the decree he promulgated just prior to his death, that future emperors must have already survived smallpox, led to the long-reigned Kangxi Emperor succeeding him.

In other words, the Manchu, a semi-peripheral people to the world's Eurasian population core were able, with care, to manage to battle their way into the heartland of Eurasian population concentrations, and make their authority work despite hostile epidemics, by leveraging a superior state planning apparatus. This success opens a new theme in the remainder of an infectious-disease-focused world history--that of the ability of powerful political organizations to have new exposures to infectious disease, but be able to manage the effects. Despite advances in state planning in the early modern world (Headrick, 1981), disease management is not purely a modern concept--the Roman Empire certainly survived its various epidemics after all--but the ability of early modern polities to break into remarkably new climes, and stay there, is a topic that leads naturally to concepts like sanitization, germ theory, pharmaceuticals, and allopathic medicine that could be harnessed by state governments and other leaders to put certain infectious diseases behind the human experience in a meaningful way. To dwell too much on the nineteenth-century response to various cases of infectious disease is to tell the story of a fight that is beyond the present chapter's scope (but will be presented later). For now, it may be enough to mention that, while the British Empire's exploitation and development of India in the nineteenth century, particularly involving the creation of railroads, created new opportunities for an infectious disease native to India, cholera, to spread throughout the subcontinent, and beyond, the impetus that this Imperial-spread disease implied to find solutions helped drive innovation in sanitation and public health (Klein, 1994).

However, the idea of global interconnectedness and innovation being necessarily able to undo negative effects of interconnection on the world is overly teleological. Invasive species, including pathogens, can wreak havoc on populations that cannot be easily undone. Consider, for example, the likely introduction of yellow fever into the Carribean region from Africa, having been brought to the region by the slave trade (Bryant et al., 2007). One implication of yellow fever settling endemically in the region of modern Haiti is that, after the slaves revolted, and the French tried to restore control in 1802, yellow fever hollowed the nearly 30,000-strong reconquest force to a shell, setting the course for Haiti to achieve independence, and, by weakening French influence in the Americas, created the prerequisites for Napoleon to be willing to sell the French claim to Louisiana to the United States (Marr & Cathey, 2013).

The story of Haiti's birth, and the way it is coupled to the ground being laid for the United States' western expansion, is fairly representative of the complexities of the interconnections between emerging modernity and infectious disease. Without yellow fever being brought to Haiti to be present in 1802, the history of the world might be very different, just as, without slavery and other explotations, the world would look very different. The use of slavery in the Americas was itself tied to the labor demand that was clearly linked to population issues in the Americas, which was itself clearly linked to the epidemic-driven depopulation of the Americas. Some facts cannot be undone. The story of infectious disease and modernity is not primarily the story of modern medicine and technology rising to meet the challenges of pathogens that met people who traveled to new climes, and that hitchhiked on ships to colonize new territories with disease, or to meet disease. Malaria led to, for example, 1880s mortality rates in the region the French saw as Upper Sudan of up to 80% of certain units of deployed French imperial troops (Cohen, 1983), and there is nothing particularly progressive about that level of mortality, or the displacement that comes from military maneuverings. Rather, the story of infectious disease and modernity seems to be the story of an attempted response, starting with simply understanding that disease resistance is largely acquired and not purely based on heredity (Curtin, 1990). The twentieth-century spread of human immunodeficiency virus/acquired immunodeficiency syndrome (HIV/AIDS) into a global epidemic, with around 36 million HIV cases at the dawn of the twenty-first century (Piot et al., 2001), is an example of another disease spread from remote climes around the world with the help of effective transport, which is being met by the development and deployment of costly antiretroviral therapies and effort at international cooperation (Schwartländer et al., 2011). The response to coronavirus disease 2019 (COVID-19), which is also modern, is ongoing, and will be explored in more detail in a later chapter.

In summary: Human diseases spread across the globe with humans. Disease deepens the horrors of conflict like war by taking advantage of displacement and vulnerable immune systems, and benefits from human global transportation. However, disease ultimately might be reduced or tamed by human tools like science.

REFERENCES

Acuna-Soto, R., Stahle, D. W., Therrell, M. D., Griffin, R. D., & Cleaveland, M. K. (2004). When half of the population died: The epidemic of hemorrhagic fevers of 1576 in Mexico. *FEMS Microbiology Letters*, *240*(1), 1–5. doi:10.1016/j.femsle.2004.09.011 PMID:15500972

Borsch, S. J. (2005). *The Black Death in Egypt and England: A comparative study*. University of Texas Press.

Borscheid, P., & Haueter, N. V. (2015). Institutional transfer: The beginnings of insurance in Southeast Asia. *Business History Review*, *89*(2), 207–228. doi:10.1017/S0007680515000331

Bosch, M. D., Mannino, M. A., Prendergast, A. L., O'Connell, T. C., Demarchi, B., Taylor, S. M., Niven, L., van der Plicht, J., & Hublin, J. J. (2015). New chronology for Ksâr 'Akil (Lebanon) supports Levantine route of modern human dispersal into Europe. *Proceedings of the National Academy of Sciences of the United States of America*, *112*(25), 7683–7688. doi:10.1073/pnas.1501529112 PMID:26034284

Brunt, P. A. (1965). The aims of Alexander. *Greece & Rome, 12*(2), 205-215. https://www.jstor.org/stable/642316

Bryant, J. E., Holmes, E. C., & Barrett, A. D. (2007). Out of Africa: A molecular perspective on the introduction of yellow fever virus into the Americas. *PLoS Pathogens*, *3*(5), e75. doi:10.1371/journal.ppat.0030075 PMID:17511518

Censo, I. (2001). *Censo Ind¡gena del Oriente, Chaco, y Amazon¡a. Secretaria de Asuntos Étnicos, de G'nero y Generacionales*. Ministerio de Desarrollo Humano.

Chan, J. C. (2014). Environmental injury to the kidney: Interstitial nephritis. *Hong Kong Journal of Nephrology*, *16*(2), 23–28. doi:10.1016/j.hkjn.2014.09.001

Chatterjee, B. (2019). Old Calcutta Vignettes: 1757-1815. *International Journal Of All Research Writings*, *1*(11), 76–79.

Clark, G. (2016). Microbes and markets: Was the Black Death an economic revolution? *Journal of Demographic Economics*, *82*(2), 139–165. doi:10.1017/dem.2016.6

Cohen, W. (1983). Malaria and French imperialism. *Journal of African History, 24*(1), 23–36. doi:10.1017/S0021853700021502

Cohn, S. K. (2012). Pandemics: Waves of disease, waves of hate from the Plague of Athens to AIDS. *Historical Research, 85*(230), 535–555. doi:10.1111/j.1468-2281.2012.00603.x PMID:25960572

Crosby, A. W. Jr. (2003). *The Columbian exchange: Biological and cultural consequences of 1492, 30th anniversary edition*. Praeger.

Cruikshank, J. (1994). Oral tradition and oral history: Reviewing some issues. *The Canadian Historical Review, 75*(3), 403–418. https://www.muse.jhu.edu/article/574633

Cunha, B. A. (2004). The death of Alexander the Great: Malaria or typhoid fever? *Infectious Disease Clinics of North America, 18*(1), 53–63. doi:10.1016/S0891-5520(03)00090-4 PMID:15081504

Curtin, P. (1990). The end of the "White Man's Grave"? Nineteenth-century mortality in West Africa. *The Journal of Interdisciplinary History, 21*(1), 63–88. doi:10.2307/204918

Daggumati, S., & Revesz, P. Z. (2021). A method of identifying allographs in undeciphered scripts and its application to the Indus Valley Script. *Humanities and Social Sciences Communications, 8*(1), 1–11. doi:10.105741599-021-00713-0

de Sahagún, B. (2020). *Plague Strikes Tenochtitlan* (N. Fitch, Trans.).https://www.historians.org/teaching-and-learning/teaching-resources-for-historians/teaching-and-learning-in-the-digital-age/the-history-of-the-americas/the-conquest-of-mexico/florentine-codex/plague-strikes-tenochtitlan

Doolan, D. L., Dobaño, C., & Baird, J. K. (2009). Acquired immunity to malaria. *Clinical Microbiology Reviews, 22*(1), 13–36. doi:10.1128/CMR.00025-08 PMID:19136431

Findlay, R., & Lundahl, M. (2017). Demographic shocks and the factor proportions model: from the plague of Justinian to the Black Death. In *The Economics of the Frontier* (pp. 125–172). Palgrave Macmillan. doi:10.1057/978-1-137-60237-4_5

Forrester, J. D., Apangu, T., Griffith, K., Acayo, S., Yockey, B., Kaggwa, J., Kugeler, K. J., Schriefer, M., Sexton, C., Ben Beard, C., Candini, G., Abaru, J., Candia, B., Okoth, J. F., Apio, H., Nolex, L., Ezama, G., Okello, R., Atiku, L., ... Mead, P. S. (2017). Patterns of Human Plague in Uganda, 2008-2016. *Emerging Infectious Diseases*, *23*(9), 1517–1521. doi:10.3201/eid2309.170789 PMID:28820134

Golzari, S. E., Mirinejad, M. M., Kazemi, A., Khalili, M., & Ghabili, K. (2012). Avenzoar (1092–1162 AD) and Averroes (1126–1198 AD): Andalusian Muslim Physicians. *World Journal of Surgery*, *36*(10), 2537–2537. doi:10.100700268-012-1711-0 PMID:22767264

Gottfried, R. S. (2010). *Black Death*. Simon and Schuster.

Green, M. H. (2015). Taking "pandemic" seriously: Making the Black Death global. *The Medieval Globe, 1*(1), 27-61. https://www.muse.jhu.edu/article/758495

Green, M. S., Swartz, T., Mayshar, E., Lev, B., Leventhal, A., Slater, P. E., & Shemer, J. (2002). When is an epidemic an epidemic? *The Israel Medical Association Journal: IMAJ*, *4*(1), 3–6. PMID:11802306

Greene, J. (2003). From neural 'is' to moral 'ought': What are the moral implications of neuroscientific moral psychology? *Nature Reviews. Neuroscience*, *4*(10), 846–850. doi:10.1038/nrn1224 PMID:14523384

Gunaratne, S. A. (2001). Paper, printing and the printing press: A horizontally integrative macrohistory analysis. *Gazette (Leiden, Netherlands)*, *63*(6), 459–479. doi:10.1177/0016549201063006001

Harper, K. N., Zuckerman, M. K., Harper, M. L., Kingston, J. D., & Armelagos, G. J. (2011). The origin and antiquity of syphilis revisited: An Appraisal of Old World pre-Columbian evidence for treponemal infection. *American Journal of Physical Anthropology*, *146*(S53), 99–133. doi:10.1002/ajpa.21613 PMID:22101689

Headrick, D. R. (1981). *The tools of empire: Technology and European imperialism in the nineteenth century* (1st ed.). Oxford University Press.

Jensen, S. R. (2010). *Rethinking Athenian imperialism: Sub-hegemony in the Delian League* (Doctoral dissertation). Rutgers University-Graduate School-New Brunswick.

Kearns, A. L. (2018). *A plague in a crisis: Differential diagnosis of the Cyprian Plague and its effects on the Roman Empire in the third century CE*. The University of Arizona.

Kelly, H. (2011). The classical definition of a pandemic is not elusive. *Bulletin of the World Health Organization*, *89*(7), 540–541. doi:10.2471/BLT.11.088815 PMID:21734771

Klein, I. (1994). Imperialism, ecology and disease: Cholera in India, 1850-1950. *The Indian Economic and Social History Review*, *31*(4), 491–518. doi:10.1177/001946469403100403

LaMonte, G., Philip, N., Reardon, J., Lacsina, J. R., Majoros, W., Chapman, L., Thornburg, C. D., Telen, M. J., Ohler, U., Nicchitta, C. V., Haystead, T., & Chi, J. T. (2012). Translocation of sickle cell erythrocyte microRNAs into Plasmodium falciparum inhibits parasite translation and contributes to malaria resistance. *Cell Host & Microbe*, *12*(2), 187–199. doi:10.1016/j.chom.2012.06.007 PMID:22901539

Larsen, J. A. O. (1940). The constitution and original purpose of the Delian League. *Harvard Studies in Classical Philology*, *51*, 175–213. doi:10.2307/310927

Lebaka, M. E. (2019). Misconceptions about Indigenous African music and culture: The case of Indigenous Bapedi music, oral tradition and culture. *European Journal of Soil Science*, *2*(2), 18–30. doi:10.26417/ejss-2019.v2i2-61

Lell, B., May, J., Schmidt-Ott, R. J., Lehman, L. G., Luckner, D., Greve, B., Matousek, P., Schmid, D., Herbich, K., Mockenhaupt, F. P., Meyer, C. G., Bienzle, U., & Kremsner, P. G. (1999). The role of red blood cell polymorphisms in resistance and susceptibility to malaria. *Clinical Infectious Diseases*, *28*(4), 794–799. doi:10.1086/515193 PMID:10825041

Li, Y., Carroll, D. S., Gardner, S. N., Walsh, M. C., Vitalis, E. A., & Damon, I. K. (2007). On the origin of smallpox: Correlating variola phylogenics with historical smallpox records. *Proceedings of the National Academy of Sciences of the United States of America*, *104*(40), 15787–15792. doi:10.1073/pnas.0609268104 PMID:17901212

Little, R. (2007). The Greek City-States in the Fifth Century BCE: Persia and the Balance of Power. In S. J. Kaufman, R. Little, & W. C. Wohlforth (Eds.), *The balance of power in world history* (pp. 47–70). Palgrave Macmillan. doi:10.1057/9780230591684_3

Liu, B., Wang, Q., He, Y., & He, P. (2021). Research progress on immune regulation of medical protozoa-related proteins. *Chinese Journal of Parasitology and Parasitic Diseases*, *39*(1), 112–119. doi:10.12140/j.issn.1000-7423.2021.01.017

Longini, I. M. Jr, Yunus, M., Zaman, K., Siddique, A. K., Sack, R. B., & Nizam, A. (2002). Epidemic and endemic cholera trends over a 33-year period in Bangladesh. *The Journal of Infectious Diseases*, *186*(2), 246–251. doi:10.1086/341206 PMID:12134262

López, C., Saravia, C., Gomez, A., Hoebeke, J., & Patarroyo, M. A. (2010). Mechanisms of genetically-based resistance to malaria. *Gene*, *467*(1-2), 1–12. doi:10.1016/j.gene.2010.07.008 PMID:20655368

Loy, D. E., Liu, W., Li, Y., Learn, G. H., Plenderleith, L. J., Sundararaman, S. A., Sharp, P. M., & Hahn, B. H. (2017). Out of Africa: Origins and evolution of the human malaria parasites Plasmodium falciparum and Plasmodium vivax. *International Journal for Parasitology*, *47*(2-3), 87–97. doi:10.1016/j.ijpara.2016.05.008 PMID:27381764

Lyttkens, C. H. (2006). Reflections on the origins of the polis. *Constitutional Political Economy*, *17*(1), 31–48. doi:10.100710602-006-6792-z

Majeed, A. (2005). How Islam changed medicine. *BMJ (Clinical Research Ed.)*, *331*(7531), 1486–1487. doi:10.1136/bmj.331.7531.1486 PMID:16373721

Mark, J. J. (2020, April 1). *Thucydides on the Plague of Athens: Text & Commentary*. https://www.ancient.eu/article/1535/thucydides-on-the-plague-of-athens-text--commentar/

Marr, J. S., & Cathey, J. T. (2013). The 1802 Saint-Domingue yellow fever epidemic and the Louisiana purchase. *Journal of Public Health Management and Practice*, *19*(1), 77–82. doi:10.1097/PHH.0b013e318252eea8 PMID:23169407

Mayor, A. (1995). The Nessus shirt in the new world: Smallpox blankets in history and legend. *Journal of American Folklore*, *108*(427), 54–77. doi:10.2307/541734

Nash, J. (2018). Sea power in the Peloponnesian war. *Naval War College Review*, *71*(1), 119–139. https://www.jstor.org/stable/26398094

Ndiabamoh, C. O. M. C., Ekali, G. L., Esemu, L., Lloyd, Y. M., Djontu, J. C., Mbacham, W., Bigoga, J., Taylor, D. W., & Leke, R. G. F. (2020). The immunoglobulin G antibody response to malaria merozoite antigens in asymptomatic children co-infected with malaria and intestinal parasites. *PLoS One*, *15*(11), e0242012. doi:10.1371/journal.pone.0242012 PMID:33170876

Ojodu, J., Hulihan, M. M., Pope, S. N., & Grant, A. M., & Centers for Disease Control and Prevention (CDC). (2014). Incidence of sickle cell trait—United States, 2010. *MMWR. Morbidity and Mortality Weekly Report*, *63*(49), 1155–1158. PMID:25503918

Opal, S. M. (2009). A Brief history of microbiology and immunology. *Vaccines. Biography*, 31–56. doi:10.1007/978-1-4419-1108-7_3

Penman, B. S., Gupta, S., & Shanks, G. D. (2017). Rapid mortality transition of Pacific Islands in the 19th century. *Epidemiology and Infection*, *145*(1), 1–11. doi:10.1017/S0950268816001989 PMID:27609550

Piot, P., Bartos, M., Ghys, P. D., Walker, N., & Schwartländer, B. (2001). The global impact of HIV/AIDS. *Nature*, *410*(6831), 968–973. doi:10.1038/35073639 PMID:11309626

Poon, M. S. (1973). The Printer's Colophon in Sung China, 960-1279. *The Library Quarterly*, *43*(1), 39–52. doi:10.1086/620094

Puente, J. L., & Calva, E. (2017). The One Health Concept—The Aztec empire and beyond. *Pathogens and Disease*, *75*(6). Advance online publication. doi:10.1093/femspd/ftx062 PMID:28605517

Reeves, H. M. (2006). Sahagún's "Florentine Codex", a little known Aztecan natural history of the Valley of Mexico. *Archives of Natural History*, *33*(2), 302–321. doi:10.3366/anh.2006.33.2.302 PMID:19845064

Reyes-García, V., Paneque-Gálvez, J., Bottazzi, P., Luz, A. C., Gueze, M., Macía, M. J., Orta-Martínez, M., & Pacheco, P. (2014). Indigenous land reconfiguration and fragmented institutions: A historical political ecology of Tsimane' lands (Bolivian Amazon). *Journal of Rural Studies*, *34*, 282–291. doi:10.1016/j.jrurstud.2014.02.007

Richter, J., Hauck, T., Vogelsang, R., Widlok, T., Le Tensorer, J. M., & Schmid, P. (2012). "Contextual areas" of early Homo sapiens and their significance for human dispersal from Africa into Eurasia between 200 ka and 70 ka. *Quaternary International*, *274*, 5–24. doi:10.1016/j.quaint.2012.04.017

Rodrigues, P. T., Valdivia, H. O., de Oliveira, T. C., Alves, J. M. P., Duarte, A. M. R., Cerutti-Junior, C., Buery, J. C., Brito, C. F. A., de Souza, J. C. Jr, Hirano, Z. M. B., Bueno, M. G., Catão-Dias, J. L., Malafronte, R. S., Ladeia-Andrade, S., Mita, T., Santamaria, A. M., Calzada, J. E., Tantular, I. S., Kawamoto, F., ... Ferreira, M. U. (2018). Human migration and the spread of malaria parasites to the New World. *Scientific Reports*, *8*(1), 1–13. doi:10.103841598-018-19554-0 PMID:29386521

Russett, B., & Antholis, W. (1992). Do democracies fight each other? Evidence from the Peloponnesian war. *Journal of Peace Research*, *29*(4), 415–434. doi:10.1177/0022343392029004005

Sallares, R. (2002). *Malaria and Rome: a history of malaria in ancient Italy*. Oxford University Press on Demand. doi:10.1093/acprof:oso/9780199248506.001.0001

Sarasombath, S., Banchuin, N., Sukosol, T., Rungpitarangsi, B., & Manasatit, S. (1987). Systemic and intestinal immunities after natural typhoid infection. *Journal of Clinical Microbiology*, *25*(6), 1088–1093. doi:10.1128/jcm.25.6.1088-1093.1987 PMID:2439536

Scasciamacchia, S., Serrecchia, L., Giangrossi, L., Garofolo, G., Balestrucci, A., Sammartino, G., & Fasanella, A. (2012). Plague epidemic in the Kingdom of Naples, 1656-1658. *Emerging Infectious Diseases*, *18*(1), 186–188. doi:10.3201/eid1801.110597 PMID:22260781

Schwartländer, B., Stover, J., Hallett, T., Atun, R., Avila, C., Gouws, E., Bartos, M., Ghys, P. D., Opuni, M., Barr, D., Alsallaq, R., Bollinger, L., de Freitas, M., Garnett, G., Holmes, C., Legins, K., Pillay, Y., Stanciole, A. E., McClure, C., ... Padian, N.Investment Framework Study Group. (2011). Towards an improved investment approach for an effective response to HIV/AIDS. *Lancet*, *377*(9782), 2031–2041. doi:10.1016/S0140-6736(11)60702-2 PMID:21641026

Shick, T. W. (1971). A Quantitative Analysis of Liberian Colonization from 1820 to 1843 with Special Reference to Mortality. *Journal of African History*, *12*(1), 45–59. doi:10.1017/S0021853700000062 PMID:11632218

Spyrou, M. A., Keller, M., Tukhbatova, R. I., Scheib, C. L., Nelson, E. A., Valtueña, A. A., ... Krause, J. (2019). Phylogeography of the Second Plague Pandemic revealed through analysis of historical Yersinia pestis genomes. *Nature Communications*, *10*(1), 1–13. doi:10.103841467-019-12154-0 PMID:31578321

Su, Y., Fang, X., & Yin, J. (2014). Impact of climate change on fluctuations of grain harvests in China from the Western Han Dynasty to the Five Dynasties (206 BC–960 AD). *Science China. Earth Sciences*, *57*(7), 1701–1712. doi:10.100711430-013-4795-y

Sussman, G. D. (2011). Was the Black Death in India and China? *Bulletin of the History of Medicine*, *85*(3), 319–355. doi:10.1353/bhm.2011.0054 PMID:22080795

Suzuki, A. (2011). Smallpox and the epidemiological heritage of Modern Japan: Towards a total history. *Medical History*, *55*(3), 313–318. doi:10.1017/S0025727300005329 PMID:21792253

Thucydides. (431 BCE). *The history of the Peloponnesian war: The second book* (R. Crawley, Trans.). http://classics.mit.edu/Thucydides/pelopwar.2.second.html

Tian, X. (2020). *The Halberd at Red Cliff: Jian'an and the Three Kingdoms*. Brill.

Tollenaere, C., Rahalison, L., Ranjalahy, M., Duplantier, J. M., Rahelinirina, S., Telfer, S., & Brouat, C. (2010). Susceptibility to Yersinia pestis experimental infection in wild Rattus rattus, reservoir of plague in Madagascar. *EcoHealth*, *7*(2), 242–247. doi:10.100710393-010-0312-3 PMID:20443044

Treiman, D. J., McKeever, M., & Fodor, E. (1996). Racial differences in occupational status and income in South Africa, 1880 and 1881. *Demography*, *33*(1), 111–132. doi:10.2307/2061717 PMID:8690135

Trevisanato, S. I. (2007). The 'Hittite plague', an epidemic of tularemia and the first record of biological warfare. *Medical Hypotheses*, *69*(6), 1371–1374. doi:10.1016/j.mehy.2007.03.012 PMID:17499936

Tulchinsky, T. H., & Varavikova, E. A. (2014). A History of Public Health. *The New Public Health*, 1–42. doi:10.1016/B978-0-12-415766-8.00001-X

Vachula, R. S., Huang, Y., Longo, W. M., Dee, S. G., Daniels, W. C., & Russell, J. M. (2019). Evidence of Ice Age humans in eastern Beringia suggests early migration to North America. *Quaternary Science Reviews*, *205*, 35–44. doi:10.1016/j.quascirev.2018.12.003

Vågene, Å. J., Herbig, A., Campana, M. G., García, N. M. R., Warinner, C., Sabin, S., ... Krause, J. (2018). Salmonella enterica genomes from victims of a major sixteenth-century epidemic in Mexico. *Nature Ecology & Evolution*, *2*(3), 520–528. doi:10.103841559-017-0446-6 PMID:29335577

Voigtländer, N., & Voth, H. J. (2013). The three horsemen of riches: Plague, war, and urbanization in early modern Europe. *The Review of Economic Studies*, *80*(2), 774–811. doi:10.1093/restud/rds034

Weisler, M. I., Yamano, H., & Hua, Q. (2012). A multidisciplinary approach for dating human colonization of Pacific atolls. *Journal of Island & Coastal Archaeology*, *7*(1), 102–125. doi:10.1080/15564894.2011.616923

Wheelis, M. (2002). Biological Warfare at the 1346 Siege of Caffa. *Emerging Infectious Diseases*, *8*(9), 971–975. doi:10.3201/eid0809.010536 PMID:12194776

Williams, N. M. (2015). Echoing through the Rafters: The Afterlife of Jian'an. In Imitations of the Self: Jiang Yan and Chinese Poetics (pp. 105-144). Brill.

Williams, T. N., Mwangi, T. W., Roberts, D. J., Alexander, N. D., Weatherall, D. J., Wambua, S., Kortok, M., Snow, R. W., & Marsh, K. (2005). An immune basis for malaria protection by the sickle cell trait. *PLoS Medicine*, *2*(5), e128. doi:10.1371/journal.pmed.0020128 PMID:15916466

Winderman, E., Mejia, R., & Rogers, B. (2019). " All smell is disease": Miasma, sensory rhetoric, and the sanitary-bacteriologic of visceral public health. *Rhetoric of Health & Medicine, 2*(2), 115-146. https://www.muse.jhu.edu/article/729140

Yin, J. H., Zhou, S. S., Xia, Z. G., Wang, R. B., Qian, Y. J., Yang, W. Z., & Zhou, X. N. (2014). Historical patterns of malaria transmission in China. *Advances in Parasitology*, *86*, 1–19. doi:10.1016/B978-0-12-800869-0.00001-9 PMID:25476879

Yonggang, Z., & Ping, J. (2016). Investigation on the Mass Graves Found in House Foundations at the Hamin Mangha Site, Inner Mongolia: Exploration and Reflection on Prehistoric Catastrophic Events. Archaeology and Cultural Relics, 5.

Zaviyeh, S. F. S. A., & Golshani, S. A. (2020). Recognition of the Outbreak of Deadly Diseases of the Antonine or Galen Era in the Second Century AD (96-192 AD). *Medical History*, *11*(41), 81–92. doi:10.22037/med%20 hist%20j.v11i41.30020

Zhang, J. (2002). Disease and its impact on politics, diplomacy, and the military: The case of smallpox and the Manchus (1613-1795). *Journal of the History of Medicine and Allied Sciences*, *57*(2), 177–197. doi:10.1093/ jhmas/57.2.177 PMID:11995595

Chapter 4
The Fight Against Infectious Disease

ABSTRACT

While infectious disease has left strong impressions on human society, this chapter is concerned with the impression human society has left on disease. Humans have done a great deal of work to manage and defeat infectious disease. This story is filled with all the travails that come with science in practice. It includes moments of triumph, like the discovery of vaccination, and ethical atrocities, like the Tuskegee Syphilis Study, which deserves to be explained in its own right. Other major topics include sanitation, grappling with information about transmission and epidemiology, the discovery of microorganisms, and the role of accidents in medical research.

INTRODUCTION

Thus far, infectious disease has been presented as connected to the science and narratives of human evolution and civilization, but the major effects of this connection have been explored insofar as they pertain to humans. Humans split from infectious disease pathogens, according to the evolutionary model. Humans have grappled to understand infectious disease, through culture, faith, and science. Humans have been influenced by infectious disease at key historical moments, and it is not hard to argue that, at a bare minimum, the demographics and politics of the Western Hemisphere would be wildly different had infectious disease not come along with the Columbian exchange,

DOI: 10.4018/978-1-7998-8689-1.ch004

and destroying a vast portion of the native population at exactly the time outsiders were ready to enter and press their own claims. On a more narrow scale, humans have stigmatized each other for bearing infectious disease, placing burdens on top of burdens. However, humans have also impacted the pathogens of infectious disease a great deal, as well. Humans have responded to unpleasantness, and danger, with a vast array of practical strategies, defenses, and attacks, that have, for example, eradicated smallpox outside of scientific facilities in Russia and the United States (MacIntyre, 2020; Meyer et al., 2020). Aside from such deliberate tactics, our own bodies offer up a vast array of defenses to tame and control infectious disease. This chapter will focus on deliberate social, scientific, and political interventions against infectious disease, and save the body's strategies for handling infectious disease for later in the book.

SANITATION

Where to begin? Inoculations, vaccinations, and antibiotics became especially important tools into the modern era, but the fight against infectious disease did not begin in the modern era. Sanitation, a key technique in preventing harmful microbes from getting close to our bodies, has been widely practiced throughout human history. Between about 2,185 years before the anchor date of radiocarbon dating, 1950, and 965 years before that anchor, the Maya used a filtration system at Tikal, wherein crystalline zeolite and fine grains of quartz removed microorganisms and toxins from their drinking water (Tankersley et al., 2020). Full sanitation and systems go back further than that. At Mohenjo-Daro, a major site of the Indus Valley Civilization that flourished between around four thousand and five thousand years ago, full bathrooms have been unearthed from dig sites (Kalbermatten, 1991). Mohenjo-Daro has been characterized as a place where nearly every habitation included a flushable latrine connected to the city's sewer system (Scobie, 1986). Storm sewers existed in Ancient Greece, four thousand years ago (Angelakis & Spyridakis, 2010). A sanitation system has value beyond infectious disease, but is certainly relevant to controlling the spread of such, and sanitation systems, at least in some regions of the world, date back to truly old times when written records were scarce, absent, or spotty. While the human experience has never been consistent, sanitation systems seem to have existed in various places, and in many places, since meaningfully early on in the world's development of cities. Further, these systems existed before humans acquired the sort of modern scientific evidence about pathogen-driven disease spread that lets people in the current era point to specific culprits of ill health. It was enough, it seems, for people in ancient times to understand stochastically, through patterns of incidents, that keeping clean was a good way of avoiding certain types of misfortunes.

UNDERSTANDING TRANSMISSION

So if it may be said that the earliest collective response to disease involved engaging in behaviors known to keep disease at bay, and one of the early ways this was done was through urban hygiene, there still seems to be a missing piece–directly leveraging evidence and theory to model infectious disease transmission so that infectious disease could be more effectively targeted and fought. The idea that infectious disease is largely caused by tiny pathogens actually seems to have been a moderately intuitive idea for some individuals even in ancient times, and early models of infectious disease did incorporate this idea to various degrees. The Roman-era physician Galen, whose thoughts dominated so much of the discourse of European medicine until the early modern period, had a concept of contamination that involved 'seeds' of fever (Nutton, 1983). The concept of miasma, or bad air, common around the world, while presented earlier in this book with its misapprehensions relative to allopathic medicine emphasized, is itself not terribly far away from the reality of the situation, given that airborne pathogens, when miasma theory first developed, were too small to see.

In other words, the "tiny bad particle" idea, a valuable first step in understanding infectious disease from an allopathic perspective, and helpful in coming up with coherent models of spread, is a fairly ancient idea to go hand-in-hand with ancient principles of sanitation. Why, then, did it apparently take so long to develop other ideas useful to the modern practice of allopathic medicine, including concepts like vaccination? Technology-driven accessibility seems like a key culprit. Without high levels of information sharing, the same useful assumptions can be built up and lost, time and time again, without doing much to add to humanity's collective knowledge. Paying deep honor to the works from renowned ancient medical authors like Hippocrates and Galen, works which did have much to offer, was a limited substitute to the sort of learning that seems able to take place with formal research structures, and information sharing in an empirical mindset.

HIPPOCRATES AND BAGHDAD

To really point out just how ready ancient doctors might have been to develop modern-seeming concepts about infectious disease had the right information-sharing systems been in place, consider how many seemingly-modern concepts actually began with Hippocrates. Hippocrates, who, among his many deeds, was involved in combating the same fifth century BCE plague outbreak described by Thucydides, was so able to give accurate clinical conditions of the condition he called "typhos" that there is a clear link between this "typhos" and the modern typhoid fever caused by *Salmonella enterica Typhi* (Yapijakis, 2009). Hippocrates also carefully described tuberculosis, malaria, and tetanus (Pappas et al., 2008). Modern medical words coined by Hippocrates include cancer, coma, diagnosis, paralysis, panic, sepsis, symptom, therapy, and trauma (Kleisiaris et al., 2014). His careful evidence-based practice and attention to ethics are so well regarded to this day that the idea of a Hippocratic Oath to protect is one of the cornerstones of what it means to be a modern physician. In light of all this contribution to world knowledge, what is interesting about Hippocrates being considered the father of modern medicine is the gap between his work and the timing of so many of the major innovations that came after him (Pappas et al., 2008). Why did it take so long between some of the basic elements of allopathic medicine being laid down, and the creation of a "full" antibiotic/antiseptic/vaccine/genetic-research system? The "information sharing" hypothesis may be persuasive when examined by the facts, but it also may not feel convincing.

In any event, the potentially-arbitrary gap between the framework that Hippocrates laid down, and the modern system that embraces him, did not prevent the man himself from being innovative. There is even legend that he directly intervened in Athens at the time of the plague, and used techniques like burning the air to reduce impurities (Yapijakis, 2009). Regardless of the veracity there, the idea that such a technique could be associated with him seems appropriately thematic, given that heat can, in the right context, sterilize environments (Abrham et al., 2020). Further, Hippocrates as someone who was talented and capable of disseminating knowledge did not exist completely alone, even if he was deprived of certain tools that would exist in a modern context. One common example about how the struggle to establish tools and institutions of scientific research went beyond Europe is in the role the Islamic world played in storing and building upon ancient knowledge during the medieval period. Particularly famous scholars like Ibn Sina contributed their own thoughts to the nature of medicine and the spread of infectious disease, which he thought involved "traces" in the air (Tschanz, 2003). Muhammad ibn Zakaryia Al-Razi (c. 841-926), who worked as a hospital director in Baghdad, emphasized the collaborative aspect of medicine. The work that these and other scholars of the Islamic world produced eventually filtered back to Europe, as texts and knowledge continued to be shared and discussed.

However, the global spread of medical knowledge prior to the explosion of scientific literature that came into its own around the modern era is difficult to describe as other than sporadic, given the way texts or knowledge that was disseminated regularly had significant gaps and required re-learning (Šimunić, 2018). Another contributor to this pattern was the significant, potentially excessive, respect for the institutional knowledge that did exist (Pasipoularides, 2014). However, a simplification like "the medieval world only believed in Galen" is too much (Nutton, 2005).

QUARANTINE

From the above foundation, the ability to progress in the fight against infectious disease lurked. Due to how transmission of records work, it is easiest to point to an explosion of new developments in the fight against infectious disease once the timeline reaches the early modern period, but time itself is not so familiar with arbitrary barriers. One significant innovation that came earlier emerges clearly from the mists of history in association with the Black Death--quarantine. Quarantine is distinct from isolation because of its use as a precautionary measure, rather than a measure applied to someone who is more certainly sick. Quarantine as word seems to tie to 1377 in then-Venetian Ragusa, now known as Dubrovnik, when in 1377 the rector decided to impose an isolation period for travelers--thirty days for those on ship, and forty days for those coming by land (Gensini et al., 2004; Tognotti, 2013). Note the way the root of the word "quarantine" connects to the Romantic language root for the word "forty," which in Italian is *quaranta.* The concept of a quarantine spread far from this origin, as Venetians continued the policy through the centuries as plague continued to emerge (Konstantinidou et al., 2009). The idea behind quarantine, however, spread much farther than lands ruled by Venice. Quarantine, for example, occurred in the British Isles (McDonald, 1951). One particularly striking instance of quarantine occurred in the village of Eyam during the 1665 outbreak of plague in Britain (Whittles & Didelot, 2016). The villagers imposed a quarantine upon themselves, and though the plague struck their town terribly, taking 257 lives within 14 months (Whittles & Didelot, 2016), the plague did not seem to gain a new vector, out of the village (Spitale, 2020).

It may seem at first glance unlikely that the Ragusan quarantine was the first time anyone had thought to restrict the motions of people coming from potentially-infected areas, and indeed, this does not seem to have been the case. In Tang China of the ninth century, and earlier, a variety of state responses to epidemic seem to have been employed, including establishing hospitals, isolating infected individuals, and burying the dead (Yu, 2020). Ancient Egypt of the fourteenth century BCE may have avoided a major outbreak of tularemia by quarantine measures (Trevisanato, 2007). These examples of quarantines or quarantine-like instances prior to Ragusa of 1377 are not meant to be a full recounting of such instances, but rather, samples of reasonable measures taken by people in different parts of the world before the advent of global medicine and associated record-keeping. It seems, interestingly, that the very scarcity of information regarding ancient quarantine practices may be less an indication that such practices did not occur, and more an example of the process by which innovation was slow in the ancient era--that with limited information being passed from region to region or generation to generation, the same sort of techniques would have to be discovered again and again. The “correct” way of thinking about the human response to infectious disease prior to the early modern period may not be one that involves radically different doctor’s intuitions than the intuitions of doctors today, but rather that these intuitions had to constantly be rebuilt without the help of access to modern comprehensive research and libraries. This point has been belabored somewhat but seems critical to a reasonable understanding of the early human response to infectious disease.

Quarantine was not the only development in the fight against infectious disease that was pioneered in ancient times. Ancient India, China, and perhaps Africa also seem to have developed the process of inoculation (Boylston, 2012; Edsall, 1964; Normansell, 1996; Ma, 1995; Sheng, 2008). Inoculation, as distinct from vaccination, is a term associated with the process of applying a living pathogen to the body, with the intention of provoking a mild infection and long-term adaptive immune response that will prevent against the dangers of a more virulent infection in the future. Note the stochastic element here. Without knowing the specific microbiology of the adaptive immune response, it seems impossible for ancient physicians to have known exactly why inoculation had a beneficial effect. However, it seems very realistic to imagine that they knew it did work, and, in an environment where infectious disease could be deadly, had some satisfaction in knowing the result, if not the mechanism. Techniques for inoculation could be elaborate. In variolation, a form of inoculation linked to the smallpox virus, liquid or scabs from those with smallpox were collected and applied (Niu, 2020).

VARIOLATION

Variolation was present in the Ottoman Empire in the early eighteenth century, having been brought to the lands of modern Turkey by the Seljuks who entered the area in the eleventh century, who themselves may have picked up the technique from ancient India, Tibet, or other parts of Asia (Dinc & Ulman, 2007). The Ottoman Empire in the eighteenth century was in a state of balance with lands further into Europe, the country's advance further northwest having been halted only a few decades earlier. Thusly, many diplomats and foreigners had interest in the area, and a British ambassador's wife, Lady Mary Wortley Montagu, had keen interest in some of the practices that went on around the Ottoman capital. Namely, variolation. She described what she witnessed thusly:

The small-pox, so fatal, and so general amongst us, is here entirely harmless, by the invention of engrafting, which is the term they give it. There is a set of old women, who make it their business to perform the operation, every autumn, in the month of September, when the great heat is abated. People send to one another to know if any of their family has a mind to have the small-pox; they make parties for this purpose, and when they are met (commonly fifteen or sixteen together) the old woman comes with a nut-shell full of the matter of the best sort of small-pox, and asks what vein you please to have opened. She immediately rips open that you offer to her, with a large needle (which gives you no more pain than a common scratch) and puts into the vein as much matter as can lie upon the head of her needle, and after that, binds up the little wound with a hollow bit of shell, and in this manner opens four or five veins. (Montagu, 1717)

What is fascinating about this passage is how it shows in a very specific way how Westerners learned from another culture. There will be a danger, as the chapter progresses, and many of the seminal moments are associated with Europe, of thinking that Europe was necessarily essential to the fight against infectious disease. Europeans certainly contributed a great deal. However,

Europeans contributed as part of global society, and the Lady Mary Wortley Montagu passage shows one specific example of knowledge transfer flowing west--her writing was a watershed moment in introducing the practice of variolation to Britain (Dinc & Ulman, 2007). Work done by Lady Montagu helped introduce the practice of inoculation into Europe, where it served as a new substrate which physicians could use to treat and innovate.

The practice of variolation spread across the Atlantic Ocean. In 1721, around Boston, at the time of a smallpox epidemic, variolation was practiced to try to reduce harm (Dinc & Ulman, 2007). As the decades passed, and the British colonies on the Atlantic seaboard came to agitate for independence, smallpox was so relevant to even the political situation that George Washington made the effort to inoculate the Continental Army (Drew, 2015), placing United States soldiers on a more even footing with the British.

VACCINATION

The next step in this chapter reaches what is perhaps the pivotal moment in the history of the fight against infectious disease--vaccination itself. Vaccination involves preparing the body to resist an infectious disease without going so far as to introduce virulent particles of the actual disease. What was the mechanism by which vaccination worked? One way to answer this question is by presenting Edward Jenner, a pioneer credited in traditional historiography as the key figure in presenting vaccination to the world, in his own words:

The more accurately to observe the progress of the infection I selected a healthy boy, about eight years old, for the purpose of inoculation for the cow-pox. The matter was taken from a sore on the hand of a dairymaid..., who was infected by her master's cows, and it was inserted, on the 14th of May, 1796, into the arm of the boy by means of two superficial incisions, barely penetrating the cutis, each about half an inch long.

On the seventh day he complained of uneasiness in the axilla, and on the ninth he became a little chilly, lost his appetite, and had a slight headache. During the whole of this day he was perceptibly indisposed, and spent the night with some degree of restlessness, but on the day following he was perfectly well.

The appearance of the incisions in their progress to a state of maturation were much the same as when produced in a similar manner by variolous matter.

The only difference which I perceived was in the state of the limpid fluid arising from the action of the virus, which assumed rather a darker hue, and in that of the efflorescence spreading round the incisions, which had more of an erysipelatous look than we commonly perceive when variolous matter has been made use of in the same manner; but the whole died away (leaving on the inoculated parts scabs and subsequent eschars) without giving me or my patient the least trouble.

In order to ascertain whether the boy, after feeling so slight an affection of the system from the cow--pox virus, was secure from the contagion of the smallpox, he was inoculated the 1st of July following with variolous matter, immediately taken from a pustule. Several slight punctures and incisions were made on both his arms, and the matter was carefully inserted, but no disease followed. The same appearances were observable on the arms as we commonly see when a patient has had variolous matter applied, after having either the cow--pox or smallpox. Several months afterwards he was again inoculated with variolous matter, but no sensible effect was produced on the constitution. (Jenner, 1798)

The above passage is seminal in the history of vaccination, even though it may not have been the first vaccination. For example, a farmer named Benjamin Jestsy may have performed a vaccination in Dorset, England, some 22 years before Jenner's work (Pead, 2003). Regardless, something really did happen around Jenner's place and time that led to a worldwide discovery of vaccination. The word is telling--vaccination comes from the Latin *vacca*, or cow. There are a number of secrets hiding behind Jenner's work, which emphasize that despite Jenner's accomplishment, there were steps yet to be taken to reach current understandings of medical science and ethics.

The first of these hidden aspects is actually reasonably apparent when combining the text of the passage with its context. Namely, the boy who was vaccinated in this case was a test subject. Jenner was experimenting with a child around the age of eight. This is not very consistent with modern norms of medical ethics. From Jenner's perspective, there seem to have been aspects of expediency involved--the child was around, and the child did not seem to have been infected by smallpox previously. There is an argument to be made that the child, being someone at risk for smallpox infection, was in a group urgently needing attention, but it seems reasonable that an adult more cognizant of the risks and benefits could have been involved in the trial. Obviously, the result--the development of the modern field of vaccination-

-seems to have been very clearly a net positive, but is an important asterisk on Jenner's work that this net positive may have been in spite of, rather than because of, certain aspects of his practices. In science, there is no guarantee of specific outcomes, so in important ways, agreements about process are part of the outcome.

The second hidden aspect in the above message is somewhat less obvious. The basic idea behind Jenner's vaccine was to give his subject cowpox, not smallpox, which was much more mild, but was similar enough to smallpox to grant the body lasting immunity to both. The problem is that the modern smallpox vaccine, which theoretically should have a direct line of descent from Jenner's work, is actually made of vaccinia virus, which is another agent entirely, though it has similar properties to cowpox (Damaso, 2018). There are two basic solutions to this mystery. In the first solution, Jenner was not able to correctly identify the vaccine agent he used. In the second, at some point in the history of the smallpox vaccine, a swap was made, but because the essential properties stayed consistent, this swap was not noticed until much later. What is important about this aspect of the smallpox vaccine is how much it emphasizes that so much of the work done in the fight against infectious disease has been contingent and subject to forces that can escape human comprehension. Consider the various theories related to miasma, or bad air, which contained some practical lessons for getting away from hotspots, but still did not model pathogenic particulars perfectly. The situation with Jenner, despite leading to a better outcome, is remarkably similar. Either he was not able to categorize what he was looking at, or, down the line, part of the succession of caretakers of the smallpox vaccine made a mistake in keeping the vaccine isolated, and then compounded this mistake by still not knowing what they were looking at. The fact that the accident was at least a neutral one should not take away from the fact that a significant misapprehension occurred. That the discovery that the vaccine was not made out of what was expected first occurred in 1939 with the immunological assays of Allan Downie says something positive about the progression of science in that era (Esparza et al., 2018). However, the general theme of this story says something about science's limitations, and how they can contextualize the successes.

Another context of Jenner is his location. He was from Britain, and was even variolated as part of the push that Lady Montagu helped set up (Dinc & Ulman, 2007). Britain, being a major center of science in the eighteenth and nineteenth centuries, when much of the groundwork for modern medical practices was laid, contained many figures who were involved pivotally in the fight against infectious disease. However, this is, in part, just one more example of the importance of contextual communication. At the start of the twenty-first century, English was to a meaningful degree the most important language of scholarly discourse (Flowerdew, 1999), and this detail is tied in various ways to the relevance of Great Britain in the development of modern techniques in the fight against infectious disease. On the one hand, it is unreasonable to believe that all of the brightest lights in the fight shone from Great Britain, but on the other, one of the major throughlines of this chapter has been the way in which researchers and physicians are limited by the structure of their relationships with peers, and are constrained by limited access to peer knowledge. The focus in this chapter of individuals from Britain can thus be understood doubly. First, as a limitation in research material available to the author. Second, as a limitation in research material potentially available to people in other parts of the world.

JOHN SNOW AND EPIDEMIOLOGY

In any event, the next major figure to be discussed is the anesthesiologist John Snow, also from Britain, who was very active in laying the basis for modern epidemiology in the middle of the nineteenth century (Oleckno, 2008). The following is an excerpt from his book, *On the Mode of Communication of Cholera*:

On proceeding to the spot, I found that nearly all the deaths had taken place within a short distance of the pump. There were only ten deaths in houses situated decidedly nearer to another street pump. In five of these cases the families of the deceased persons informed me that they always sent to the pump in Broad Street, as they preferred the water to that of the pump which was nearer. In three other cases, the deceased were children who went to school near the pump in Broad Street. Two of them were known to drink the water; and the parents of the third think it probable that it did so. The other two deaths, beyond the district which this pump supplies, represent only the amount of mortality from cholera that was occurring before the irruption took place.

With regard to the deaths occurring in the locality belonging to the pump, there were sixty-one instances in which I was informed that the deceased persons used to drink the pump-water from Broad Street, either constantly, or occasionally. In six instances I could get no information, owing to the death or departure of every one connected with the deceased individuals; and in six cases I was informed that the deceased persons did not drink the pump-water before their illness.

The result of the inquiry then was, that there had been no particular outbreak or increase of cholera, in this part of London, except among the persons who were in the habit of drinking the water of the above-mentioned pump-well. (Snow, 1855)

This is modern epidemiology in an embryonic form. It seems highly unlikely that tracing infections to causes did not occur repeatedly before John Snow performed his analysis. However, his tracing of cholera cases to a specific contaminated pump marks something of a shift of the process into a more permanent collective memory. Cholera, for its part, is an infectious disease that spread around the world in part due to modernity, being lifted out of India and Southeast Asia, and traveling in the nineteenth century through modern lines of interconnection to a wide variety of places, including Britain, home of the government that ruled much of India at that time (Naruszewicz-Lesiuk & Stypułkowska-Misiurewicz, 2017). Its hallmark symptom is severe acute diarrhea, and the disease is caused by the bacterium *Vibrato cholera* (Tulchinsky, 2018). Cholera, in other words, seems to have become a problem because of modernity, and the way modernity can organize and unify, but at the same time measures against cholera could begin to be managed because aspects of the same extractive system that carried cholera further than many people would have wished also managed to extract, and publish, John Snow's insights. The role of communication of information, so much a motif in this chapter, is particularly critical in Snow's interactions.

There are two different implications of Snow's work that are worth exploring for their benefit to the narrative. First, it took a great deal of time for all of the implications of Snow's work to find their way into actual epidemiological practice used on a large scale to track and mitigate the spread of infectious disease (Tulchinsky, 2018). There was resistance against accepting Snow's work as it related to germ theory, which was far from settled science in his day. There is a risk, in this sort of retrospective, to assume that just because Snow's work seems familiar, his context was. Unfortunately, his context was miasma theory, and the inertia of existing understandings. Just because Snow theorized that cholera spread due to contaminated water, did not mean that the people around him could immediately accept what was then a meaningfully novel idea. Miasma might mean, approximately, "bad air," but one of the issues with having only an approximate understanding of disease transmission is that sometimes the right thing to look for in transmission is "bad water."

The second major implication of Snow's work is that while the doctor was able to provide some measure of relief for those in his environs, the release of cholera from its home around the Bay of Bengal spread the disease to parts of the world that did not have the same hints of compensatory science. The story is not--humans overturn a rock they should not, and then work together to fix the aftermath. The story, rather, is that while humans overturn a rock, or, in this case, make the Bay of Bengal a center of shipping, and inadvertently transport contaminated bilge water by ship, those people and places who can receive useful treatments receive them, while those who cannot, and who may be largely unrelated to the processes that spread a given disease in the first place, experience some of the consequences (Tulchinsky, 2018). The interconnection of the world has costs. One of the ways cholera seems to have spread to reach Snow's home in Britain was through bilge water filled with cholera in ships streaming from the Bay of Bengal.

ANTISEPTICS

Again, however, if the theme of this chapter is interconnection, there were many incidents of interconnection that proceeded in the nineteenth century that were beneficial to humankind. One was the antiseptic discoveries associated with Joseph Lister. Lister, another from Great Britain, was extremely interested in the way wounds healed, and leveraged the discoveries of the Frenchman Louis Pasteur to develop the idea and practice of antiseptics (Pitt & Aubin, 2012). Here is a passage from one of Lister's writings that is representative:

My house-surgeon, Mr. Hector Cameron, applied carbolic acid to the whole raw surface, and completed the dressing as if for compound fracture. The hand remained free from pain, redness or swelling, and with the exception of a shallow groove, all the wound consolidated without a drop of matter, so that if it had been a clean cut, it would have been regarded as a good example of primary union. The small granulating surface soon healed, and at present a linear cicatrix alone tells of the injury he has sustained, while his thumb has all its movements and his hand a fine grasp. If the severest forms of contused and lacerated wounds heal thus kindly under the antiseptic treatment, it is obvious that its application to simple incised wounds must be merely a matter of detail. (Lister, 1867)

What may be most interesting about this passage involving Lister is, again, how normal it seems. The patient was treated with an antiseptic, in this case carbolic acid, and an injury was then healed "kindly." This sounds similar to modern treatments, but was cutting-edge at the time, and showcases how sometimes developments occur in spurts. While carbolic acid no longer has pride of place as an antiseptic (carbolic acid has a side effect of living tissue irritation, and inappropriate use can lead to poisoning requiring hospitalization (Gupta et al., 2008)), the principle demonstrated by Lister has endured (Hirsch et al., 2010). Next, here is a passage where Pasteur presents his understanding of the relationship between microorganisms, control, and disease:

It was necessary therefore to attempt to cultivate the septic vibrio either in a vacuum or in the presence of inert gases-such as carbonic acid.

Results justified our attempt; the septic vibrio grew easily in a complete vacuum, and no less easily in the presence of pure carbonic acid.

These results have a necessary corollary. If a fluid containing septic vibrios be exposed to pure air, the vibrios should be killed and all virulence should disappear. This is actually the case. If some drops of septic serum be spread horizontally in a tube and in a very thin layer, the fluid will become absolutely harmless in less than half a day, even if at first it was so virulent as to produce death upon the inoculation of the smallest portion of a drop.

Furthermore all the vibrios, which crowded the liquid as motile threads, are destroyed and disappear. After the action of the air, only fine amorphous granules can be found, unfit for culture as well as for the transmission of any disease whatever. It might be said that the air burned the vibrios.

If it is a terrifying thought that life is at the mercy of the multiplication of these minute bodies, it is a consoling hope that Science will not always remain powerless before such enemies, since for example at the very beginning of the study we find that simple exposure to air is sufficient at times to destroy them. (Pasteur, 1878)

Pasteur in this passage describes how infection can be linked to a specific microorganism. Through careful specimen cultivation, he was able to remove so many of the extraneous factors that confused the thinking of his forebears, and reduced the nature of the germ to a simple cause and effect. His discoveries were contextual--not all cultures of pathogens causing infectious disease die through simple exposure to air. However, they were meaningful and foundational.

MICROORGANISMS, ROBERT KOCH, AND MODERN MEDICINE

Another researcher who was working around the same time was Robert Koch, from Germany, and by looking at Koch's four postulates for whether a microorganism causes a disease, one can see more developments in the fight against infectious disease, including a new organized perspective.

The first criterion is that the microorganism appears only in individuals with disease. (Segre, 2013) The second criterion is that the microorganism can be extracted, and cultured, from samples from an individual with the disease. The third criterion is that spreading the organism to a healthy individual causes the disease. Finally, the fourth criterion is that the organism can be extracted, and cultured, from samples of an individual who has been spread the disease by the experiment suggested in the third criterion.

These postulates are a foundation and not a conclusion. One important context is that disease-causing microorganisms can indeed be found in healthy individuals--not everyone infected with a specific pathogen shows the same symptoms, or any meaningful symptoms at all. While a specific pathogen can be said to have a high likelihood of causing an illness, the link is not perfect. Another issue in the Koch postulates is medical ethics--the postulates themselves are built on the idea that to really understand if a given organism is the cause of a disease, controlled infections must be studied. While in his day there were fewer ways of testing a pathogen's mechanism of action, making this protocol more reasonable, the hint that a pathogen cannot be considered causative without experimental infection has a problematic aspect.

Mirroring the importance of contextualizing the postulates, Koch became famous for more than just the postulates. An army doctor in the Franco-Prussian War, he, among his accomplishments, isolated the anthrax bacillus in 1876 (Blevins & Bronze, 2010).

At this point a narrative has been presented that shows increasing awareness of microorganisms and techniques to combat them, including quarantine, vaccination, sanitation, and antiseptics. Quarantine, one of the least technologically-demanding interventions, has not been supplanted by the others--a well-rounded approach to fighting infectious disease can involve slowing or halting spread at every step of the process. Quarantines were used throughout the nineteenth century, and continue to be used today, though one issue worth analysis whenever they are used is if their burden may fall disproportionately on immigrant communities (Markel, 1999).

ACCIDENTS

The collection of techniques presented above build on each other to some degree--understandings from vaccination are related to understandings about antiseptics, and understandings about quarantine are related to understandings about sanitation. However, as this narrative of techniques against infectious disease builds towards the modern day, one phenomenon worth pointing out is the effects of serendipity. A particularly potent antibacterial drug, penicillin, essentially created the modern concept of antibacterials (Gaynes, 2017). Antiseptics, in contrast, were perfectly good for sterilization but are not in their common use put inside the human body, to reach the pathogen of a disease that had already been contracted. One of the key features of the discovery of penicillin is how truly accidentally it seems to have been found. Reading from discoverer Alexander Fleming's 1945 Nobel speech:

Then in 1928 an accidental contamination of a culture plate by a mould set me off on another track. I was working on a subject having no relation to moulds or antiseptics and if I had been a member of a team engaged on this subject it is likely that I would have had to neglect the accidental happening and work for the team with the result that penicillin would not then have been described and I would not be here today as a Nobel Laureate. But, fortunately for myself – and may be for the world – I was situated so that I could leave my previous line of research work and follow the track which fate hade indicated for me.

I isolated the contaminating mould. It made an antibacterial substance which I christened penicillin. (Fleming, 1945)

To reiterate, what is striking about penicillin, which catalyzed the age of antibiotics, was that it was discovered on accident. Well into the age of scientific discovery, and allopathic medicine, where bacilli could be seen under microscopes, and the link between the agents of cholera and anthrax, and their effects, had been made, Fleming was a physician, microbiologist, and beneficiary from Scotland of the institutional medical knowledge and infectious disease research apparatus available to researchers in Great Britain. Thus placed, Fleming stumbled upon something that let humanity lurch from awareness to impact. The history of the human response to infectious disease began with practical measures made by people with understanding of cause and effect, but who naturally did not have direct understanding of specific microorganisms they could not see. Then tools built up in haphazard and sometimes unintuitive ways, but there is a way to push back against the "randomness" thesis. Namely, just because Fleming was lucky enough to notice the mold did not mean he had sporadic luck in all ways. He had a lab to analyze the interesting substance, which itself was the product of a great deal of scientific discovery that was obtained before him, and passed down.

IMPLEMENTATION

At this point the chapter reaches something of a pivot. Many of the key planks of modern allopathic treatment have already been mentioned, because, as it turns out, many of the key planks of allopathic treatment are at least about a couple centuries old. The various tools mentioned above are accessible and known in different parts of the world in different ways, and one of the key aspects that connects them is skill at implementation. As an example of a quarantine implementation that was particularly successful, in relatively recent times, consider strict border control in the Pacific in the period of the 1918 to 1919 influenza pandemic. Continental Australia, Tasmania, American Samoa, and New Caledonia implemented strict maritime quarantines to leverage their physical isolation, and were rewarded both by delaying the date upon which the disease arrived at their shores, and then, through remarkably low comparative mortality rates (McLeod et al., 2008). Pacific island nations that did not leverage their innate protections suffered horrific amounts of death. As a representative comparison, while American Samoa had a death rate of *0* in 1,000, the area today known as Samoa, which then too was separate politically, had a mortality rate of 220 per 1,000.

Science has, nevertheless, continued to advance in more modern times. Standard vaccine regimes have built up where available--in the United States, the tetanus toxoid, reduced diphtheria toxoid, and acellular pertussis (Tdap) vaccine is relatively standard, as is an influenza shot (Kahn et al., 2018). The post-World War II era brought many promises and perils to the fight against infectious disease. One of the greatest positives came in the shape of the field of genetics--a way to understand not just the structure of biology, but its causes, in such a way that a researcher might be able to read the DNA instructions for building the cells of a physical person, or a physical bacterium. Proceeding from merely appreciating the key role that DNA plays in shaping the phenotypes of life to being able to leverage the coding language of DNA to perform interventions for the sake of health, has been an ongoing process. The human genetic code was not sequenced until 2001 (International Human Genome Sequencing Consortium, 2004), but advances in genetics are continuing to proceed with rapidity, with two major mRNA vaccines being released to combat the 2019 coronavirus pandemic (Noor, 2021), and, prospectively, gene editing being a technology set up to be an increasingly major part of the future (Lino et al., 2018).

The ability to harness facets of infectious disease opens the door for impact more fine-tuned than that of the horrific plague blankets spread to Native Americans. Infectious disease can be weaponized more directly, and released more directly. Alternatively, infectious disease might be harnessed by the world's military-industrial complex by accident, as in a virus escaping a lab. The resistance of Russia and the United States to destroying their last samples of smallpox can be seen as a positive insofar as it opens the door to possible health research (Impelluso & Lentzos, 2017). However, widescale smallpox vaccinations in the United States have desisted, due to the disease being wiped out in the wild via a concerted vaccination campaign (Mandra et al., 2021; Simpson et al., 2020). This desistance in turn has led to the phenomenon where only older individuals may have general vaccination-related protection to a disease with a fatality rate of around 30% (Simptson et al., 2020). Therefore, the continued existence of smallpox samples contains danger. Smallpox vaccination has declined because the sometimes-deadly side effects (serious adverse events on the order of 0.001%, and death on the order of 0.0001%) in the face of effective elimination, no longer seemed worth the benefits (Kemper et al. 2002). Presumably, it would not be prohibitively difficult to start mass distribution of a new smallpox vaccine, should the need arise. However, the modern experience of vaccine rollouts taking many months for the 2019 coronavirus epidemic, purely on the logistics, even discounting the research time, seems to be a hint as to the significant lethality of smallpox in a nightmare scenario (Lee & Chen, 2021). There is more to contemplate in an era where the biology of infectious diseases can be so effectively studied. A smallpox virus, for example, that is sequenced, is a smallpox virus that might be reconstructed regardless of the existence of actual preserved samples. The promise of the most cutting-edge technologies, like mRNA vaccines, is thus a hint of technologies and outcomes that might be worse.

ETHICS, TECHNOLOGY, AND LIMITED INFORMATION

Another great challenge into the modern era involves ethics. The study of infectious disease is a space where a great deal can be on the line, and, consequently, the incentives to collect data by any means are high as well. Into the breach has come a number of ethical standards for modern science, focusing heavily on the concepts of both informed consent and relevance to the subject--a given participant in a study should know what is going on, approve of their participation in that light, and, if there is any chance of harm from the study, have a commensurate chance of benefiting from the results (Brim & Miller, 2013). However, these standards did not emerge out of pure philosophy.

One seminal experiment that is repeatedly referenced in the literature surrounding research ethics was the Tuskegee Syphilis Study. In this experiment, which proceeded over the years of 1932 to 1972, centered in the United States state of Georgia (Thomas & Quinn, 1991), Black individuals with syphilis were recruited and then monitored over long periods of time, while their syphilis went untreated. The callousness of this research clearly connects to some of the principles that were developed in its aftermath--the participants in this study may have agreed to be present, but they certainly were not informed to the study's purpose, and certainly were not benefiting from the process of having syphilis untreated while while suffering for decades. It is not hard to draw a line between the Tuskegee Syphilis Study and some lack of trust for vaccines in the modern day, attitudes which are complicated in parts of the world where successful vaccination campaigns have made the threat of diseases like smallpox and measles much less obvious.

Reinforcing fear of mistreatment may be the complexity. Modern vaccines exist in many different types. These include live-attenuated (a weakened form of the actual pathogen is introduced to the vaccine recipient) and inactivated (a dead form of the actual pathogen is introduced to the vaccine recipient) (Vetter et al., 2018). There are also various other approaches, though approaches prototypically involve showing a piece of the pathogen in question to the human adaptive immune system so that it will be able to respond much more quickly and effectively, in the case of a natural infection, than if it had not been forewarned. In addition to the number of vaccine types, the manner of their operation is not trivial–what may be particularly counterintuitive is just how much vaccines are tied to the normal workings of the adaptive immune system (Yürüyen et al., 2018).

In the context of a human species that struggles to make the best choices in a realm of limited information, the social context of infectious disease is especially important. The idea of a coronavirus disease 2019 (COVID-19) passport, discussed as part of the protective toolkit in the early stages of the outbreak (Brown et al., 2020), and implemented stringently in places like Lithuania (Walkowiak et al., 2021), is not dissimilar to yellow fever passports that help give individuals clear bills of health to travel in Africa (Vanderslott & Marks, 2021), and is also not dissimilar to the various mandated vaccinations that exist in the United States prior to entry into various schools (Paquette, 2021). However, tools combating the spread of infectious disease necessarily exist as social levers on a population that has a combination of interests and incentives. All tools in society's fight against infectious disease are predicated on not only the knowledge to harness them, but also social acceptance in wide segments of the population, which cannot be taken for granted.

REFERENCES

Abraham, J. P., Plourde, B. D., & Cheng, L. (2020). Using heat to kill SARS-CoV-2. *Reviews in Medical Virology*, *30*(5), e2115. doi:10.1002/rmv.2115 PMID:32614102

Angelakis, A. N., & Spyridakis, D. S. (2010). A brief history of water supply and wastewater management in ancient Greece. *Water Science and Technology: Water Supply*, *10*(4), 618–628. doi:10.2166/ws.2010.105

Blevins, S. M., & Bronze, M. S. (2010). Robert Koch and the 'golden age' of bacteriology. *International Journal of Infectious Diseases*, *14*(9), e744–e751. doi:10.1016/j.ijid.2009.12.003 PMID:20413340

Boylston, A. (2012). The origins of inoculation. *Journal of the Royal Society of Medicine*, *105*(7), 309–313. doi:10.1258/jrsm.2012.12k044 PMID:22843649

Brim, R. L., & Miller, F. G. (2013). The potential benefit of the placebo effect in sham-controlled trials: Implications for risk-benefit assessments and informed consent. *Journal of Medical Ethics*, *39*(11), 703–707. doi:10.1136/medethics-2012-101045 PMID:23239742

Brown, R. C., Savulescu, J., Williams, B., & Wilkinson, D. (2020). Passport to freedom? Immunity passports for COVID-19. *Journal of Medical Ethics*, *46*(10), 652–659. doi:10.1136/medethics-2020-106365 PMID:32817362

Damaso, C. R. (2018). Revisiting Jenner's mysteries, the role of the Beaugency lymph in the evolutionary path of ancient smallpox vaccines. *The Lancet. Infectious Diseases*, *18*(2), e55–e63. doi:10.1016/S1473-3099(17)30445-0 PMID:28827144

Dinc, G., & Ulman, Y. I. (2007). The introduction of variolation 'A La Turca' to the West by Lady Mary Montagu and Turkey's contribution to this. *Vaccine*, *25*(21), 4261–4265. doi:10.1016/j.vaccine.2007.02.076 PMID:17383778

Drew, B. A. (2015). George Washington and smallpox: A revolutionary hero and public health activist. *JAMA Dermatology*, *151*(7), 706–706. doi:10.1001/jamadermatol.2015.1 PMID:25739090

Edsall, G. (1964). Smallpox vaccination vs inoculation. *Journal of the American Medical Association*, *190*(7), 689–690. doi:10.1001/jama.1964.03070200125036

Esparza, J., Nitsche, A., & Damaso, C. R. (2018). Beyond the myths: Novel findings for old paradigms in the history of the smallpox vaccine. *PLoS Pathogens*, *14*(7), e1007082. doi:10.1371/journal.ppat.1007082 PMID:30048524

Fleming, A. (1945, December 10). *Sir Alexander Fleming Banquet speech.* https://www.nobelprize.org/prizes/medicine/1945/fleming/speech/

Flowerdew, J. (1999). Writing for scholarly publication in English: The case of Hong Kong. *Journal of Second Language Writing*, *8*(2), 123–145. doi:10.1016/S1060-3743(99)80125-8

Gaynes, R. (2017). The discovery of penicillin—New insights after more than 75 years of clinical use. *Emerging Infectious Diseases*, *23*(5), 849–853. doi:10.3201/eid2305.161556

Gensini, G. F., Yacoub, M. H., & Conti, A. A. (2004). The concept of quarantine in history: From plague to SARS. *The Journal of Infection*, *49*(4), 257–261. doi:10.1016/j.jinf.2004.03.002 PMID:15474622

Gupta, S., Ashrith, G., Chandra, D., Gupta, A. K., Finkel, K. W., & Guntupalli, J. S. (2008). Acute phenol poisoning: A life-threatening hazard of chronic pain relief. *Clinical Toxicology*, *46*(3), 250–253. doi:10.1080/15563650701438888 PMID:17852157

Hirsch, T., Koerber, A., Jacobsen, F., Dissemond, J., Steinau, H. U., Gatermann, S., Al-Benna, S., Kesting, M., Seipp, H.-M., & Steinstraesser, L. (2010). Evaluation of toxic side effects of clinically used skin antiseptics in vitro. *The Journal of Surgical Research*, *164*(2), 344–350. doi:10.1016/j.jss.2009.04.029 PMID:19726054

Impelluso, G., & Lentzos, F. (2017). The threat of synthetic smallpox: European perspectives. *Health Security*, *15*(6), 582–586. doi:10.1089/hs.2017.0045 PMID:29178813

International Human Genome Sequencing Consortium. (2004). Finishing the euchromatic sequence of the human genome. *Nature*, *431*(7011), 931–945. doi:10.1038/nature03001 PMID:15496913

Jenner, E. (1798). *The Three Original Publications on Vaccination Against Smallpox by Edward Jenner.* https://biotech.law.lsu.edu/cphl/history/articles/jenner.htm

Kahn, K. E., Black, C. L., Ding, H., Williams, W. W., Lu, P. J., Fiebelkorn, A. P., Havers, F., D'Angelo, D. V., Ball, S., Fink, R. V., & Devlin, R. (2018). Influenza and Tdap vaccination coverage among pregnant women—United States, April 2018. *Morbidity and Mortality Weekly Report*, *67*(38), 1055–1059. doi:10.15585/mmwr.mm6738a3 PMID:30260946

Kalbermatten, J. M. (1991). Water and sanitation for all, will it become reality or remain a dream? *Water International*, *16*(3), 121–126. doi:10.1080/02508069108686104

Kemper, A. R., Davis, M. M., & Freed, G. L. (2002). Expected adverse events in a mass smallpox vaccination campaign. *Effective Clinical Practice*, *5*(2). PMID:11990216

Kleisiaris, C. F., Sfakianakis, C., & Papathanasiou, I. V. (2014). Health care practices in ancient Greece: The Hippocratic ideal. *Journal of Medical Ethics and History of Medicine*, *7*, 6. PMID:25512827

Konstantinidou, K., Mantadakis, E., Falagas, M. E., Sardi, T., & Samonis, G. (2009). Venetian rule and control of plague epidemics on the Ionian Islands during 17th and 18th centuries. *Emerging Infectious Diseases*, *15*(1), 39–43. doi:10.3201/eid1501.071545 PMID:19116047

Lee, T. H., & Chen, A. H. (2021). Last-mile logistics of covid vaccination—The role of health care organizations. *The New England Journal of Medicine*, *384*(8), 685–687. doi:10.1056/NEJMp2100574 PMID:33503340

Lino, C. A., Harper, J. C., Carney, J. P., & Timlin, J. A. (2018). Delivering CRISPR: A review of the challenges and approaches. *Drug Delivery*, *25*(1), 1234–1257. doi:10.1080/10717544.2018.1474964 PMID:29801422

Lister, J. (1867). *Modern History Sourcebook: Joseph Lister (1827-1912): Antiseptic Principle Of The Practice Of Surgery, 1867*. https://sourcebooks.fordham.edu/mod/1867lister.asp

Ma, B. (1995). Variolation, pioneer of modern immunology. *Zhonghua Yi Shi Za Zhi, 25*(3), 139-144.

MacIntyre, C. R. (2020). Reevaluating the risk of smallpox reemergence. *Military Medicine*, *185*(7-8), e952–e957. doi:10.1093/milmed/usaa084 PMID:32373931

Mandra, A. M., Superior, M. J., Guagliardo, S. A. J., Hesse, E., Pacha, L. A., Stidham, R. A., Colbeck, D. C., Hrncir, D. E., Hall, N., Petersen, B. W., & Rao, A. K. (2021). Myopericarditis associated with smallpox vaccination Among US Army personnel–Fort Hood, Texas, 2018. *Disaster Medicine and Public Health Preparedness*, 1–7. doi:10.1017/dmp.2020.478 PMID:33719991

Markel, H. (1999). *Quarantine! East European Jewish Immigrants and the New York City Epidemics of 1892*. JHU Press.

McDonald, J. C. (1951). The history of quarantine in Britain during the 19th century. *Bulletin of the History of Medicine*, *25*(1), 22–44. https://www.jstor.org/stable/44443588 PMID:14821636

McLeod, M. A., Baker, M., Wilson, N., Kelly, H., Kiedrzynski, T., & Kool, J. L. (2008). Protective effect of maritime quarantine in South Pacific jurisdictions, 1918–19 influenza pandemic. *Emerging Infectious Diseases*, *14*(3), 468–470. doi:10.3201/eid1403.070927 PMID:18325264

Meyer, H., Ehmann, R., & Smith, G. L. (2020). Smallpox in the post-eradication era. *Viruses*, *12*(2), 138. doi:10.3390/v12020138 PMID:31991671

Montagu, L. M. W. (1717). *Lady Mary Wortley Montagu on Small Pox in Turkey* [Letter]. https://chnm.gmu.edu/cyh/primary-sources/157

Naruszewicz-Lesiuk, D., & Stypułkowska-Misiurewicz, H. (2017). Past and present history of cholera epidemics. Hundred years of operation of National Institute of Hygiene for the prevention and control of cholera. *Przegląd Epidemiologiczny*, *71*(4), 661–670. PMID:29417804

Niu, Y. (2020). Variolation of Traditional Chinese Medicine Diagnosis and Treatment. In J. Hua & L. Feng (Eds.), *Thirty Great Inventions of China*. Springer., doi:10.1007/978-981-15-6525-0_30

Noor, R. (2021). Developmental status of the potential vaccines for the mitigation of the COVID-19 pandemic and a focus on the effectiveness of the Pfizer-BioNTech and Moderna mRNA Vaccines. *Current Clinical Microbiology Reports*, *8*(3), 178–185. Advance online publication. doi:10.100740588-021-00162-y PMID:33686365

Normansell, D. E. (1996). The Erwin Neter Memorial Lecture: Looking to the future of medical laboratory immunology, a personal view. *Clinical and Diagnostic Laboratory Immunology*, *3*(4), 369–370. doi:10.1128/cdli.3.4.369-370.1996 PMID:8807197

Nutton, V. (1983). The seeds of disease: An explanation of contagion and infection from the Greeks to the Renaissance. *Medical History*, *27*(1), 1–34. doi:10.1017/S0025727300042241 PMID:6339840

Nutton, V. (2005). The fatal embrace: Galen and the history of ancient medicine. *Science in Context*, *18*(1), 111–121. doi:10.1017/S0269889705000384 PMID:16075496

Oleckno, W. A. (2008). Remembering Dr. John Snow on the sesquicentennial of his death. *Canadian Medical Association Journal*, *178*(13), 1691–1692. doi:10.1503/cmaj.080772

Pappas, G., Kiriaze, I. J., & Falagas, M. E. (2008). Insights into infectious disease in the era of Hippocrates. *International Journal of Infectious Diseases*, *12*(4), 347–350. doi:10.1016/j.ijid.2007.11.003 PMID:18178502

Paquette, E. T. (2021). In the Wake of a Pandemic: Revisiting School Approaches to Nonmedical Exemptions to Mandatory Vaccination in the US. *The Journal of Pediatrics*, *231*, 17–23. doi:10.1016/j.jpeds.2021.01.022 PMID:33484695

Pasipoularides, A. (2014). Galen, father of systematic medicine. An essay on the evolution of modern medicine and cardiology. *International Journal of Cardiology*, *172*(1), 47–58. doi:10.1016/j.ijcard.2013.12.166 PMID:24461486

Pasteur, L. (1878). *Modern History Sourcebook: Louis Pasteur (1822-1895): Germ Theory and Its Applications to Medicine and Surgery, 1878* (H. Ernst, Trans.). https://sourcebooks.fordham.edu/mod/1878pasteur-germ.asp

Pead, P. J. (2003). Benjamin Jesty: New light in the dawn of vaccination. *Lancet*, *362*(9401), 2104–2109. doi:10.1016/S0140-6736(03)15111-2 PMID:14697816

Pitt, D., & Aubin, J. M. (2012). Joseph Lister: Father of modern surgery. *Canadian Journal of Surgery*, *55*(5), E8–E9. doi:10.1503/cjs.007112 PMID:22992425

Scobie, A. (1986). Slums, sanitation and mortality in the Roman world. *Klio*, *68*(2), 399–433. doi:10.1524/klio.1986.68.68.399

Segre, J. A. (2013). What does it take to satisfy Koch's postulates two centuries later? Microbial genomics and Propionibacteria acnes. *The Journal of Investigative Dermatology*, *133*(9), 2141–2142. doi:10.1038/jid.2013.260 PMID:23842116

Sheng, J. (2008). On the Earliest Chinese Record of 1522 on Inoculation Against Smallpox and the Legends on Its Inventor. *Studies in the History of Natural Sciences*, *1*, 123–130.

Simpson, K., Heymann, D., Brown, C. S., Edmunds, W. J., Elsgaard, J., Fine, P., Hochrein, H., Hoff, N. A., Green, A., Ihekweazu, C., Jones, T. C., Lule, S., Maclennan, J., McCollum, A., Mühlemann, B., Nightingale, E., Ogoina, D., Ogunleye, A., Petersen, B., ... Wapling, A. (2020). Human monkeypox–After 40 years, an unintended consequence of smallpox eradication. *Vaccine*, *38*(33), 5077–5081. doi:10.1016/j.vaccine.2020.04.062 PMID:32417140

Šimunić Buršić, M. (2018). Knowledge transfer in the early medieval art of vaulting in Dalmatia. *6th International Congress on Construction History (6ICCH 2018),* 1219-1227.

Snow, J. (1855). *On the Mode of Communication of Cholera.* http://www.ph.ucla.edu/epi/snow/snowbook2.html

Spitale, G. (2020). COVID-19 and the ethics of quarantine: A lesson from the Eyam plague. *Medicine, Health Care, and Philosophy*, *23*(4), 603–609. doi:10.100711019-020-09971-2 PMID:32761351

Tankersley, K. B., Dunning, N. P., Carr, C., Lentz, D. L., & Scarborough, V. L. (2020). Zeolite water purification at Tikal, an ancient Maya city in Guatemala. *Scientific Reports*, *10*(1), 1–7. doi:10.103841598-020-75023-7 PMID:33093562

Thomas, S. B., & Quinn, S. C. (1991). The Tuskegee Syphilis Study, 1932 to 1972: Implications for HIV education and AIDS risk education programs in the black community. *American Journal of Public Health*, *81*(11), 1498–1505. doi:10.2105/AJPH.81.11.1498 PMID:1951814

Tognotti, E. (2013). Lessons from the history of quarantine, from plague to influenza A. *Emerging Infectious Diseases*, *19*(2), 254–259. doi:10.3201/eid1902.120312 PMID:23343512

Trevisanato, S. I. (2007). The 'Hittite plague', an epidemic of tularemia and the first record of biological warfare. *Medical Hypotheses*, *69*(6), 1371–1374. doi:10.1016/j.mehy.2007.03.012 PMID:17499936

Tschanz, D. W. (2003). Arab roots of European medicine. *Heart Views*, *4*(2), 9.

Tulchinsky, T. H. (2018). John Snow, Cholera, the Broad Street Pump; Waterborne Diseases Then and Now. *Case Studies in Public Health*, 77–99. doi:10.1016/B978-0-12-804571-8.00017-2

Vanderslott, S., & Marks, T. (2021). Travel restrictions as a disease control measure: Lessons from yellow fever. *Global Public Health: An International Journal for Research, Policy and Practice*, *16*(3), 340–353. doi:10.1080/17441692.2020.1805786 PMID:32772788

Vetter, V., Denizer, G., Friedland, L. R., Krishnan, J., & Shapiro, M. (2018). Understanding modern-day vaccines: What you need to know. *Annals of Medicine*, *50*(2), 110–120. doi:10.1080/07853890.2017.1407035 PMID:29172780

Walkowiak, M. P., Walkowiak, J. B., & Walkowiak, D. (2021). COVID-19 passport as a factor determining the success of national vaccination campaigns: Does it work? The case of Lithuania vs. Poland. *Vaccines*, *9*(12), 1498. doi:10.3390/vaccines9121498 PMID:34960245

Whittles, L. K., & Didelot, X. (2016). Epidemiological analysis of the Eyam plague outbreak of 1665-1666. *Proceedings. Biological Sciences, 283*(1830). doi:10.1098/rspb.2016.0618

Yapijakis, C. (2009). Hippocrates of Kos, the father of clinical medicine, and Asclepiades of Bithynia, the father of molecular medicine. *In Vivo (Athens, Greece), 23*(4), 507–514. PMID:19567383

Yu, X. (2020). Response to epidemic disease in ancient China and its characteristics. *Chinese Medicine and Culture*, *3*(2), 55–59. doi:10.4103/CMAC.CMAC_22_20

Yürüyen, M., Ayan, G., Demirdağ, F., Kara, Z., Avcı, S., Yavuzer, H., ... Erdinçler, D. S. (2018). Why is vaccination frequency low in elderly patients? *Journal of Clinical and Analytical Medicine*, *9*(02), 138–142. doi:10.4328/JCAM.5611

Chapter 5
Quantifying the Lethality of Infectious Disease

ABSTRACT

Fatality risk, in general, is a fraught concept, with many misconceptions about chances of harm rising in contrast to actual harm. Additionally, even in situations where a disease is clearly highly fatal, there are different ways to think about fatality. Is the most dangerous disease the one that is the least likely for a patient to survive, or is the most dangerous disease one that kills the most people? How do phenomena like environmental sanitation and individual risk factors play into this, since differing "preparedness landscapes" may lead to wildly different disease outcomes in a population? The goal of this chapter is to unpack the toll of disease in as statistically minded a manner as possible.

INTRODUCTION

Two basic ways of understanding lethality are total deaths, and chance of death within a given illness. Transmission rate is an important part of the context.

Context is critical to understanding infectious disease. Statistics can be manipulated in a variety of ways, and they can even be manipulated accidentally. Consider a basic example of distribution, and how it interacts with representativeness. Between Bill and Bob, they share one hundred marbles. On average, Bill and Bob each have fifty marbles. And yet, one level deeper in terms of analysis, Bill may have all one hundred marbles, while Bob has

DOI: 10.4018/978-1-7998-8689-1.ch005

zero. This may seem superficially silly. In the hypothetical, anyone who meets Bill and Bob, and sees their marble collections, will notice clearly that it is Bill who actually has marbles. However, the average statistic about marbles comparing the two people in the example is perfectly legitimate math, math that can be deceptive either by accident or deliberately.

Dynamic lethality--the idea that in certain contexts an infectious disease can be much more dangerous than others--is an important concept that highlights the need to look at statistics carefully. One of the way to understand the dynamic lethality of infectious disease, and how caseload and fatalities can change drastically depending on the environmental context, is to look at the twentieth century annual morbidity of specific vaccine-preventable infectious diseases in the United States, and compare those numbers with recent reported cases in the United States (Notifiable Diseases and Mortality Tables, 2016; Orenstein & Ahmed, 2017; Roush et al., 2007). The following numbers compare twentieth century morbidity with reported cases from 2016. Smallpox: 29,005 twentieth century annual morbidity, and 0 reported cases from 2016. Measles: 530,217 twentieth century annual morbidity, and 69 reported cases from 2016. Pertussis: 200,752 twentieth century annual morbidity, and 15,737 reported cases from 2016. It is evident that within the remit of these numbers, disease burden has drastically reduced.

DISEASES BY TOTAL PRESENT LETHALITY

Creating categories of disease lethality is itself a problematic abstraction, for at least two different reasons. First, disease does not exist in isolation. It is common for someone who dies to have multiple causes of death, and this is a complication of the world--the fact that really all facets within it are multicausal (Wall et al., 2005). The second reason discrete statistics are problematic is in how they separate the effect of disease from its human impact. Disease is only important because of the patients it impacts, and yet, paradoxically, one simple shorthand for summarizing that impact, count, reduces the experience of infectious disease to a tally that contains nothing of the experience motivating the tally to be collected in the first place. Physicians and other individuals on the front lines of treating infectious disease run the risk of missing the personal context by focusing too narrowly on a specific disease. All that said, there is value in focusing on statistics because they provide a sense of what diseases are present. Here is a list of the ten largest infectious disease causes of death worldwide in 2019:

1. Lower respiratory infections 2,593,098
2. Diarrheal diseases 1,519,229
3. Tuberculosis 1,208,044
4. HIV/AIDS 674,662
5. Malaria 410,762
6. Hepatitis C 351,313 (cirrhosis) + 22,147 (acute)
7. Hepatitis B 311,622 (cirrhosis) + 36,036 (acute)
8. Meningitis 233,303
9. Measles 165,756
10. Whooping Cough 111,317 (World Health Organization, 2020a)

A context to these numbers is not only the fact that major causes of death have shifted over time--note that smallpox and plague are missing--but also that data collection has limitations. There is limited information on, for example, understanding the amount of lower respiratory tract infection attributable to influenza, and this makes it difficult to understand the actual benefits of influenza vaccines (Malosh et al., 2018). Staying on influenza as the example, it is also difficult to peer within the category to view the subtypes--each new influenza epidemic is generally linked to a new variant that comes from viral evolution, creating limitations in seeing the disease as consistently one category (Earn et al., 2002). The 1918 flu pandemic had a death rate around 2 or 3%, while seasonal flu epidemics often have a mortality rate around 0.1% (Billings, 1997; Chiolero, 2020).

It should be valuable at this point to give an overview of the nature of each of the ten leading causes of infectious disease death in 2019, to give a better profile of what the threat looks like.

Lower respiratory infections are associated with a number of different pathogens, with certain pathogens being more common depending on the etiology (Carroll & Adams, 2016). Lower respiratory infections commonly manifest as pneumonia. In pneumonia, there is radiological evidence of infiltrate in the lungs (dense material that should not be there), as well as a symptom like fever, hypothermia, cough, rapid or difficult breathing (tachypnea or dyspnea, respectively), spitting up of blood (hemoptysis), or hypoxemia (low tissue saturation of oxygen). Typically, the same species cause pneumonia in those who are immunocompromised and particularly susceptible, as well as those who have no particular risk factors. This overlap seems linked to what pathogens are simply common in communities. Around 85% of community-acquired pneumonia comes from *Streptococcus pneumoniae, Haemophilus influenzae*, and *Moraxella catarrhalis*. Individuals with more specific risks may be more susceptible to a wide variety of other pathogens. *Streptococcus pneumoniae* and *Haemophilus influenzae* are bacterial pathogens that also cause meningitis (Prager et al., 2017). *Moraxella catarrhalis*, meanwhile, is another bacterium, which is also known to cause otitis media (ear infection), as well as exacerbations of chronic obstructive pulmonary disease (Murphy & Parameswaran, 2009).

Diarrheal diseases with a pathology associated with the respiratory tract and not breath, have another, even more pernicious link--to poverty (Guerrant et al., 2002). A common treatment to this class of disease is simple rehydration. However, sufficient rehydration can be beyond reach for many with this class of condition. Especially vulnerable are the very young.

Tuberculosis, caused by *Mycobacterium tuberculosis*, travels by air, and can be the cause of a lower respiratory disease, despite the fact that it is placed into a separate category by the World Health Organization (Carroll & Adams, 2016; Pai et al., 2016). While tuberculosis and its pathogen is primarily linked to the lungs, the pathogen can travel to nearly anywhere in the body (Pai et al., 2016). Tuberculosis is characterized by a contained state, which involves *M. tuberculosis* trapped in granulomas, which develops into a contiguous state where *M. tuberculosis* is limited by no such barrier, and is characterized by symptoms like cough, fever, night sweats, and weight loss. Vaccination is available, as well as treatment that can take the form of multiple rounds of antimicrobials, but ongoing mutation in *M. tuberculosis* has caused the emergence of multidrug resistance, which is associated with notably severe symptoms. Because of the tendency of *M. tuberculosis* to enter a quintencent granuloma-contained state, the mere presence of the pathogen does not necessitate symptoms. However, tuberculosis can be a lifetime problem for individuals infected with the pathogen, as it can potentially overcome granuloma containment at any time. Despite this, many individuals even with active infections do not show symptoms, which can contribute to the spread of the disease. Because tuberculosis can have drastically different levels of symptoms depending on the person and the phase of the disease, tuberculosis is especially dangerous in combination with HIV. Around 12% of new tuberculosis cases occur in HIV-positive individuals, as well as 25% of deaths. The linkages between the pathogens underlying the most fatal infectious diseases in the world are quite sophisticated, and complex, as it should be recalled that tuberculosis can sometimes be characterized as a lower respiratory infection, even if the World Health Organization (WHO) statistics classify it separately. Meanwhile, HIV/AIDS is the next most lethal disease on the World Health Organization's list.

HIV/AIDS, or, in extended form, human immunodeficiency virus/acquired immunodeficiency syndrome, is a positive-sense RNA retrovirus, containing two single-stranded genetic provirus copies, that transmits by various forms of intimate or approximately intimate contact, which can involve normal intercourse, or a blood transfusion or intravenous injection contaminated with the pathogen (Germany Advisory Committee Blood, 2016; Moore & Hu, 2009). Specifically, HIV can enter the body through intact mucous membranes, injured skin, skin experiencing eczema, or injection. Positive-sense RNA (unlike negative-sense RNA) means that the viral genetic material is written in such a way that it could be directly translated by a cellular ribosome to create viral proteins, but, being a retrovirus, HIV operates through the more nuanced process of reverse transcription, which involves a viral DNA intermediate. Organ transplants can be a vector for acquiring HIV, which, while a rare outcome, is especially impactful for the patient (Mukhopadhyay et al., 2012). Breast milk is another potential vector (Wahl et al., 2015). HIV has an extended progression (Germany Advisory Committee Blood, 2016). In an initial phase, three to six weeks after infection, there is usually a period (of two to six weeks) involving relatively nonspecific influenza-like symptoms, including fever, fatigue, and lymph node enlargement. The symptoms are nonspecific because they are linked to the body's antibody or humoral response to the HIV infection. However, after this round of symptoms diminish, the virus is expected to remain in the body in a largely asymptomatic phase for many years. Eventually, since its reproductive behavior involves attachment to CD4 molecules that are present on the surface of immune cells like T helpers, macrophages, and dendritic cells, as well as astrocytes, severe symptoms emerge in untreated cases. The asymptomatic phase can last from two years to twenty-five or more, but if it ends, and the condition converts to AIDS, the destruction of immune cells allows for other pathogens to become more deadly to the health of the patient. Currently, drug cocktails exist that can essentially halt the progression of HIV (Kemnic & Gulick, 2020) and essentially remove transmission risk even with unprotected sex (Eriksen et al., 2020), but these cocktails require adequate health infrastructure and funding to be available, and so the burden of HIV falls disproportionately on countries with limited resources.

Malaria comes from parasitic protozoans of the genus *Plasmodium* (Alven & Aderibigbe, 2019). These protozoans are tiny, but are microscopic animals, not bacteria or viruses. The impact of malaria can be controlled by antimicrobials, and the lifecycle of the parasites does not require the death of the host. *Plasmodium* specimens have a complicated lifecycle, involving a variety of forms, that takes them to different parts of human and mosquito hosts, and the death of either would remove the space the protozoans use to spread and grow. It is telling that while, contemporarily, there are hundreds of thousands of annual deaths from malaria, there have been around 230 million cases annually since 2016 (Dyer, 2020). The burden of malaria stems from the depths to which it is endemic in terrain where mosquitos carrying the malaria parasite inhabit, largely but not exclusively in sub-Saharan Africa.

Hepatitis C, caused by a positive-sense, single-stranded, and enveloped RNA virus, is extremely prevalent, and infects almost 3% of the world's population (Kim & Chang, 2013; Li & Lo, 2015; Moosavy et al., 2017). Unlike hepatitis B, most who are infected cannot clear the underlying virus. Individuals who have HIV are even more likely to have a chronic hepatitis C condition. Transmision is generally through blood, such as via injections or unsterile medical devices. High risk populations include IV drug users, dialysis patients, and hemophiliacs. The nature of hepatitis C transmission underscores how vulnerable populations can often be at risk to acquire even more vulnerability. Symptoms can include jaundice, fatigue, abdominal pain, and dyspepsia (Deutsch et al, 2013).

Hepatitis B, as is typical of the diseases on this list, is caused by a pathogen with a relatively low mortality rate, and makes up its numbers by being so widespread (Liang, 2019). There are more than 300 million hepatitis B infections currently worldwide. Hepatitis B is caused by a specific DNA virus of the Hepadnaviridae family, and can cause a wide variety of liver-related conditions or symptoms, including acute and chronic hepatitis (hepatitis means inflammation), cirrhosis, and hepatocellular carcinoma. However, between 90% and 95% of people who are infected with the hepatitis B virus recover, and of the remainder, who experience chronic infections, hepatitis B can still be asymptomatic, and many cases are mild. Transmission can occur through blood and open cuts, and perinatal transmission, from mother to newborn, makes up the majority of cases worldwide (Nelson et al., 2016).

In the so-called developed world, two-thirds of meningitis cases may be caused by *Streptococcus pneumoniae* (Prager et al., 2017). Meningitis can come from bacteria (including *M. tuberculosis*), viruses, or fungi, and typical symptoms include fever, drowsiness/confusion, severe headache, stiff neck, sensitivity to light, nausea, and vomiting ("Meningitis", 2001). In 2015, there were 8.7 million reported cases worldwide, as well as 379,000 deaths that year, for a mortality rate of over 4% (Hersi et al, 2021). Typically, pathogens of meningitis a space where they create meningitis through one of two pathways--in bacteria, through mucosal invasion after colonizing the nasopharynx, and otherwise, through entry into the cerebrospinal fluid by way of adjacent body structures or forieign objects. A wide variety of the causative agents of meningitis can be blocked by vaccination, including *S. pneumoniae*, *H. influenzae* type B, *N. meningitidis*, the measles agent, and varicella. Some of the agents have particularly high case fatality (CFR) rates--*S. Pnemoniae*'s in the United States is 17.9% (Thigpen et al., 2011). This underlines the importance of vaccination. While there are a variety of treatments available depending on the precise pathogen that is causative, incomplete vaccinations along with immunosuppression, living in close contact housing like that of a military barracks or college dorm, age of less than 5 or greater than 65 years, and alcohol use disorder all increase risk (Hersi et al, 2021).

A negative-sense, single-stranded RNA virus causes measles (Plumet et al. 2005). This virus, like many causative agents of meningitis, can be headed off by use of an existing vaccine (Misin et al., 2020). Despite the scientific availability of vaccination, difficulties in dispersal, as well as a very high case fatality rate, have made measles persistent as a leading cause of death. In 2018, there were about 350,000 measles cases and an estimated 142,300 deaths, leading to a CFR of just over 40%. Measles virus is of the family Paramyxoviridae, and the genus *Morbillvirus*. The measles virus is transmitted through respiratory droplets, and the disease itself tends towards epidemic patterns based on situational factors that modify its ease of spread. For example, it spreads better in winter due to the congregation of individuals into enclosed spaces like schools. Longer cycles can be due to patterns of human movement creating new opportunities for the virus to infect concentrations of hosts. The virus itself has an incubation period of around 10 to 14 days, and then typical symptoms include fever that may be over 40 °C, as well as cough, coryza, and conjunctivitis. Measles is an acute infection, and symptoms generally persist for 5 or 6 days (Desai et al., 2012). However, measles is associated with a wide variety of complications, including pneumonia, which is associated with most measles-linked deaths (Misin et al., 2020). The fact that lower respiratory infections are the top of the 2019 WHO list reinforces how linked the items are.

Whooping cough is also known as pertussis (Kilgore et al., 2016). This is a respiratory infection caused by the bacterium *Bordetella pertussis*. With 16 million cases reported in 2008, its modern case fatality rate is approximately 1.2%. The first vaccines were made available in the 1940s, but, like with measles, difficulties in making vaccination sufficiently widespread have contributed to the persistence of this disease. Additionally, vaccination from whooping cough does not grant lifelong immunity. Rather, with vaccination, immunity does not seem likely to persist beyond 14 years, while natural infection grants an estimated immunity duration of between 3.5 and 30 years. Coughing and sneezing can spread this disease, which carries a risk of infection within a hospital context.

Beyond the list of leading causes of infectious-disease-related death in 2019, there may be *reductions* in certain categories of death that come from certain patterns associated with infectious disease--not necessarily anywhere close to enough to offset the total negative impact, but enough to make a meaningful actuarial difference. During the time of the early outbreak of coronavirus COVID-19, for example, ischaemic heart disease death reported in England and Wales was down 26%, while cerebrovascular disease mortality was down 18% and chronic lower respiratory disease mortality was down 10% (Appleby, 2020). This may be due to those who would have died to other conditions succumbing to COVID-19.

DISEASES BY EPIDEMIC LETHALITY

Another way of looking at the most deadly infectious diseases is by looking at the worst historical epidemics. It is difficult to get a measure of this because of obvious limitations in record-keeping over the span of all of human history, but *The Washington Post* made an effort that is worth listing the top of because of how it sheds another light on this complicated topic.

1. Black Death 1347-1352 75 to 200 million
2. 1918 influenza 1918-1920 50 million
3. HIV/AIDS 1981-current 35 million
4. Plague of Justinian 541-542 A.D. 30 to 50 million
5. New World smallpox 1520-unknown 25 to 55 million
6. Third Plague 1885 12 million
7. Antonine Plague 165-180 A.D. 5 million
8. Coronavirus pandemic 2020-current About 5 million (*Washington Post* estimate as of October 3, 2021)
9. Italian Plague 1629-1631 1 million
10. Russian influenza 1889-1890 1 million
11. Asian influenza 1957-1958 1 million

12. Hong Kong influenza 1968-1970 1 million (Rosenwald, 2021)

The above list is comprehensive of *The Washington Post*'s entries for pandemics that took one million or more lives. It is sorted by the low-bound estimate of fatalities, and then by earliest incident. While the biggest caveat of the World Health Organization's ten most lethal infectious diseases of 2019 is that it does not look back at the historical record, two big caveats with the *Washington Post* list are (1) the questionable comprehensiveness of the list, and (2) the fact that the list counts epidemic incidents, and thus does not include cumulative endemic infectious disease death tolls, such as from malaria, that may be far higher. However, the hope that goes along with providing the list is that an additional lens of the topic of lethality is useful. A secondary purpose is to get a sense of what epidemics have entered into the historical record in the United States.

Caveats aside, what can be said about the *Washington Post* list? First of all, it is substantively different from the 2019 list of the ten most lethal infectious diseases. The first epidemic on this list is the Black Death, caused by plague, which has a wide estimate because of the difficulties in measuring something so far back in history that was so wide scale, and caused so much devastation. The fourth, sixth, seventh, and ninth epidemics are also plague. Plague, however, does not make it onto the 2019 list at all, likely showcasing the power of antibiotics. The second item, however, the flu of 1918, with its influenza pathogen, is matched by the top item on the 2019 list--lower respiratory infections. Lower respiratory infections include the flu. The tenth, eleventh, and twelfth items on *The Washington Post*'s list are also flu. Clearly influenza has been ubiquitous for a long time, at very high background rates that occasionally surpass even their high norms.

Third on *The Washington Post*'s list is HIV/AIDS (human immunodeficiency virus/acquired immunodeficiency syndrome). This is a modern disease that became known worldwide starting in the 1980s, and, unlike the first two diseases on *The Washington Post*'s list, is predominantly transmitted by bodily fluids, as opposed to transmitted by air. The high number of lethal cases of HIV/AIDS, combined with its spread in the modern world, and its intimate mode of transmission, combines to point out how singularly significant HIV/AIDS is--it seems to be part of a class of disease that does not have many parallels, which may account for the strong social reaction to the HIV/AIDS pandemic. The fact that the 2019 list has a number of fatalities accorded to HIV/AIDS that is 77% of the expected annual average that can be derived from *The Washington Post*'s list (35,000,000 / (2021 - 1981) = 875,000 versus 674,662) asserts that the HIV/AIDS pandemic is not over yet.

Smallpox is the next most lethal unique disease on *The Washington Post*'s list. Smallpox is one of the components of the disease combination that ravaged the New World after Columbus. Smallpox is notable on this list because it shows up as an epidemic only in the context of the Columbian exchange, and not in the context of the lives it took in the Eastern Hemisphere. On that side of the world, it was long known as a killer of children, but was endemic until innovations in inoculation and vaccination were capable enough of removing it that it is excluded from the 2019 list.

Eighth on *The Washington Post*'s list, after two instances of plague, is the coronavirus disease 2019 or COVID-19 pandemic. This number is clearly an undercount of the full cost--as of 7:01 PM CEST, 8 April 2022, the World Health Organization reports receiving records of 6,170,283 deaths (World Health Organization, 2021). That World Health Organization number itself is likely still an undercount, first, because you are reading these words well after they were written, and second, because of natural problems with case count transfer. The WHO itself believes in the plausibility of the second argument, and has estimated that the actual COVID-19 fatality count may be two or three times higher than reported (Revill & Farge, 2021). Thusly, the COVID-19 pandemic should arguably be higher on *The Washington Post*'s list, above the Antonine Plague. However, it should not be said that COVID-19 necessarily had a greater world impact than the Antonine Plague, because the population around eighteen centuries ago was much lower.

DISEASE BY INDIVIDUAL SURVIVAL

Aside from looking at annual mortality, or mortality associated with an epidemic, another way of assessing the lethality question is from an individual perspective. That is, what infectious disease, if acquired, is most likely to be fatal? This question is difficult because it introduces diseases that may have very low incidence rates, and thus not be well known, or even, hypothetically, diseases that do not exist yet. As an example, the prion condition known as Creutzfeldt–Jakob disease is considered uniformly fatal at the time of this writing (Groverman et al., 2021). Despite the bleak outcomes associated with this disease, it is not particularly common, with 575 patients linked with disease cases between the years 1993 and 1995 in France, Germany, Italy, The Netherlands, Slovakia, and the United Kingdom (Will et al., 1998). Another factor that should be considered in the context of Creutzfeldt-Jakob disease's lethality is that it does not spread through typical methods of contagion. Most cases emerge in an individual spontaneously, and 15% emerge in individuals with a family history of the disease (Mayo Clinic, 2021). However, in extremely rare cases, transmission can occur, including through exposure to infected tissue via a skin or cornea transplant, via brain surgery, or by consuming contaminated beef. A particularly famous incident occurred in the 1990s in the United Kingdom pertaining to contaminated beef, but this form of transmission, while possible, is not characteristic of the mainstream version of the disorder. Does Creutzfelt-Jakob disease qualify as infectious? Certainly, the answer is yes, but just as the disease rarely spreads contagiously even to those affected, it is not particularly characteristic of most infectious diseases, itself. As should be clear from the statistics, far more people die of respiratory infections than die of this prion condition, but regardless of this fact, Creutzfeldt-Jakob disease is more dangerous to have.

DISEASES BY TRANSMISSION RATE

Another valuable way to think of infectious disease lethality is through transmission rate. The reproduction number of a contagious disease, or R_0, refers to the number of new infections that can be expected to be generated from one infection (Najafimehr et al., 2020). While the infectivity of a disease is not the same as its lethality across a population, infectivity rate times lethality rate in an individual is a reasonable proxy for aggregate mortality. Further, given the ability of infectious diseases to mutate, one defense of using R_0 as a proxy here is that it is fairly uncontroversially a proxy for potential lethality. A disease with a high R_0, which changes to become more lethal on an individual case basis, should be expected to have a multiplier effect on its lethality. Given that a key way new infectious diseases arise is through mutation, thinking of mortality risk in this foreshadowable way might be heterodox, but is useful in understanding the scope of risk.

The future of the relationship between humans and infectious diseases will have something to do with the history, but the correlation may not be direct. Importantly, diseases with lower R_0 values but high individual mortality are far less devastating on a world scale than the other way around. A disease with low R_0 and high individual mortality may be more likely, in individual outbreaks, to burn itself out, with the high individual mortality even contributing to the low R_0 by giving infected individuals less time and health to infect other people. In the most dangerous diseases on a world scale, there is a balance between the lethality and the opportunities the disease affords those with the condition to spread the condition. Consider how in HIV/AIDS, even untreated, there is typically a gap of about ten to fifteen years between HIV transmission and the AIDS diagnosis that accompanies the more deadly stage of the condition (Word Health Organization, 2020b).

RELEVANCE BY SECONDARY EFFECT AND LETHAL DISEASES INDIRECTLY IMPACTING HUMANS

One last topic is the lethal impact of diseases that only indirectly affect humans. There are about 1.3 billion cattle in the world, as well as one billion pigs, and 50 billion poultry grown annually for food (Toomly & Shirley, 2009). Conditions that can harm these animals can have impacts on humans, in addition to harm and suffering experienced by the animals themselves. Epidemic diseases that target domestic animals can cause famine and ravage the livelihoods of farmers (Toomly & Shirley, 2009). For example, rinderpest was a historically deadly viral disease of livestock that caused widespread famine and poverty, but was eradicated after a worldwide campaign in 2011, being only the second disease to be eradicated, after smallpox (Roeder et al., 2013). The indirect impact of infectious disease via famine is immense. For the Irish Potato Famine, caused by the oomycete (fungus-like) *Phytophthora infestans* (Yoshida et al., 2013), traditional historiography posits around 1 million deaths, and recent revisions to that number, while lower, are still in the hundreds of thousands (Nusteling, 2009). More recently, wheat stem rust fungus has been noted as a particular danger to global food supplies (Singh et al., 2015). No single statistic can provide a full picture of the impact of an infectious disease.

REFERENCES

Alven, S., & Aderibigbe, B. (2019). Combination therapy strategies for the treatment of malaria. *Molecules (Basel, Switzerland)*, *24*(19), 3601. doi:10.3390/molecules24193601 PMID:31591293

Appleby, J. (2020). What is happening to non-covid deaths? *BMJ (Clinical Research Ed.)*, *369*, m1607. doi:10.1136/bmj.m1607 PMID:32332059

Billings, M. (1997). *The influenza pandemic of 1918*. Human virology at Stanford. https://virus.stanford.edu/uda/

Carroll, K. C., & Adams, L. L. (2016). Lower respiratory tract infections. *Microbiology Spectrum*, *4*(4), 4.4.21. Advance online publication. doi:10.1128/microbiolspec.DMIH2-0029-2016 PMID:27726814

Chiolero, A. (2020). What is happening to non-covid death?: Rapid response. *BMJ (Clinical Research Ed.)*, *369*, m1607. doi:10.1136/bmj.m1607 PMID:32332059

Desai, S., Shane, A., & Lewis, R. (2012). Measles. *CMAJ: Canadian Medical Association Journal = Journal de l'Association Medicale Canadienne*, *184*(16), 1811. doi:10.1503/cmaj.111574

Deutsch, M., Papadopoulos, N., Hadziyannis, E. S., & Koskinas, J. (2013). Clinical characteristics, spontaneous clearance and treatment outcome of acute hepatitis C: A single tertiary center experience. *Saudi Journal of Gastroenterology: Official Journal of the Saudi Gastroenterology Association*, *19*(2), 81–85. doi:10.4103/1319-3767.108479 PMID:23481134

Diseases, N., & Tables, M. (2016).. . *MMWR. Morbidity and Mortality Weekly Report*, *65*(3).

Dyer, O. (2020). African malaria deaths set to dwarf covid-19 fatalities as pandemic hits control efforts, WHO warns. *BMJ (Clinical Research Ed.)*, *371*, m4711. doi:10.1136/bmj.m4711 PMID:33268334

Earn, D. J., Dushoff, J., & Levin, S. A. (2002). Ecology and evolution of the flu. *Trends in Ecology & Evolution*, *17*(7), 334–340. doi:10.1016/S0169-5347(02)02502-8

Eriksen, J., Carlander, C., Albert, J., Flamholc, L., Gisslén, M., Navér, L., Svedhem, V., Yilmaz, A., & Sönnerborg, A. (2020). Antiretroviral treatment for HIV infection: Swedish recommendations 2019. *Infectious Diseases*, *52*(5), 295–329. doi:10.1080/23744235.2019.1707867 PMID:31928282

German Advisory Committee Blood (Arbeitskreis Blut). (2016). Human Immunodeficiency Virus (HIV). *Transfusion Medicine and Hemotherapy; Offizielles Organ der Deutschen Gesellschaft fur Transfusionsmedizin und Immunhamatologie*, *43*(3), 203–222. doi:10.1159/000445852 PMID:27403093

Groveman, B. R., Ferreira, N. C., Foliaki, S. T., Walters, R. O., Winkler, C. W., Race, B., Hughson, A. G., Zanusso, G., & Haigh, C. L. (2021). Human cerebral organoids as a therapeutic drug screening model for Creutzfeldt–Jakob disease. *Scientific Reports*, *11*(1), 1–9. doi:10.103841598-021-84689-6 PMID:33727594

Guerrant, R. L., Kosek, M., Moore, S., Lorntz, B., Brantley, R., & Lima, A. A. (2002). Magnitude and impact of diarrheal diseases. *Archives of Medical Research*, *33*(4), 351–355. doi:10.1016/S0188-4409(02)00379-X PMID:12234524

Hersi, K., Gonzalez, F. J., & Kondamudi, N. P. (2021). *Meningitis, StatPearls. (2021 Jan-)*. StatPearls Publishing. https://www.ncbi.nlm.nih.gov/books/NBK459360/

Hersi, K., Gonzalez, F. J., & Kondamudi, N. P. (2021). *Meningitis, StatPearls. (2021 Jan-)*. StatPearls Publishing. https://www.ncbi.nlm.nih.gov/books/NBK459360/

Kemnic, T. R., & Gulick, P. G. (2020). *HIV antiretroviral therapy, StatPearls. (2021 Jan-)*. StatPearls Publishing. https://www.ncbi.nlm.nih.gov/books/NBK513308/

Kilgore, P. E., Salim, A. M., Zervos, M. J., & Schmitt, H. J. (2016). Pertussis: Microbiology, disease, treatment, and prevention. *Clinical Microbiology Reviews*, *29*(3), 449–486. doi:10.1128/CMR.00083-15 PMID:27029594

Kim, C. W., & Chang, K. M. (2013). Hepatitis C virus: Virology and life cycle. *Clinical and Molecular Hepatology*, *19*(1), 17–25. doi:10.3350/cmh.2013.19.1.17 PMID:23593605

Li, H. C., & Lo, S. Y. (2015). Hepatitis C virus: Virology, diagnosis and treatment. *World Journal of Hepatology*, *7*(10), 1377–1389. doi:10.4254/wjh.v7.i10.1377 PMID:26052383

Liang, T. J. (2009). Hepatitis B: The virus and disease. *Hepatology (Baltimore, Md.)*, *49*(5, Suppl), S13–S21. doi:10.1002/hep.22881 PMID:19399811

Malosh, R. E., Martin, E. T., Ortiz, J. R., & Monto, A. S. (2018). The risk of lower respiratory tract infection following influenza virus infection: A systematic and narrative review. *Vaccine*, *36*(1), 141–147. doi:10.1016/j.vaccine.2017.11.018 PMID:29157959

Mayo Clinic. (2021). *Creutzfeldt-Jakob Disease*. https://www.mayoclinic.org/diseases-conditions/creutzfeldt-jakob-disease/symptoms-causes/syc-20371226

Meningitis. (2001). *Paediatrics & Child Health, 6*(3), 126–127. doi:10.1093/pch/6.3.126

Misin, A., Antonello, R. M., Di Bella, S., Campisciano, G., Zanotta, N., Giacobbe, D. R., Comar, M., & Luzzati, R. (2020). Measles: An overview of a re-emerging disease in children and immunocompromised patients. *Microorganisms, 8*(2), 276. doi:10.3390/microorganisms8020276 PMID:32085446

Moore, M. D., & Hu, W. S. (2009). HIV-1 RNA dimerization: It takes two to tango. *AIDS Reviews, 11*(2), 91–102. PMID:19529749

Moosavy, S. H., Davoodian, P., Nazarnezhad, M. A., Nejatizaheh, A., Eftekhar, E., & Mahboobi, H. (2017). Epidemiology, transmission, diagnosis, and outcome of Hepatitis C virus infection. *Electronic Physician, 9*(10), 5646–5656. doi:10.19082/5646 PMID:29238510

Mukhopadhyay, P., Kumar, V., Rathi, M., Kohli, H. S., Jha, V., & Sakhuja, V. (2012). Transmission of human immunodeficiency virus infection by renal transplantation. *Indian Journal of Nephrology, 22*(2), 133–135. doi:10.4103/0971-4065.97135 PMID:22787317

Murphy, T. F., & Parameswaran, G. I. (2009). Moraxella catarrhalis, a human respiratory tract pathogen. *Nephrology, Dialysis, Transplantation, 49*(1), 124–131. doi:10.1086/599375 PMID:19480579

Najafimehr, H., Mohamed Ali, K., Safari, S., Yousefifard, M., & Hosseini, M. (2020). Estimation of basic reproduction number for COVID-19 and the reasons for its differences. *International Journal of Clinical Practice, 74*(8), e13518. doi:10.1111/ijcp.13518 PMID:32301199

Nelson, N. P., Easterbrook, P. J., & McMahon, B. J. (2016). Epidemiology of hepatitis B Virus infection and impact of vaccination on disease. *Clinics in Liver Disease, 20*(4), 607–628. doi:10.1016/j.cld.2016.06.006 PMID:27742003

Nusteling, H. P. (2009). How many Irish potato famine deaths?: Toward coherence of the evidence. *Historical Methods: A Journal of Quantitative and Interdisciplinary History, 42*(2), 57-80. doi:10.3200/HMTS.42.2.57-80

Orenstein, W. A., & Ahmed, R. (2017). Simply put: Vaccination saves lives. *Proceedings of the National Academy of Sciences of the United States of America*, *114*(16), 4031–4033. doi:10.1073/pnas.1704507114 PMID:28396427

Pai, M., Behr, M., Dowdy, D., & Raviglione, M. (2016). Tuberculosis. *Nature Reviews. Disease Primers*, *2*(1), 16076. doi:10.1038/nrdp.2016.76 PMID:27784885

Plumet, S., Duprex, W. P., & Gerlier, D. (2005). Dynamics of viral RNA synthesis during measles virus infection. *Journal of Virology*, *79*(11), 6900–6908. doi:10.1128/JVI.79.11.6900-6908.2005 PMID:15890929

Prager, O., Friedman, A., & Nebenzahl, Y. M. (2017). Role of neural barriers in the pathogenesis and outcome of *Streptococcus pneumoniae* meningitis. *Experimental and Therapeutic Medicine*, *13*(3), 799–809. doi:10.3892/etm.2017.4082 PMID:28450902

Revill, J., & Farge, E. (2021, May 21). *Real COVID-19 death toll could be 'two to three' times above official stats: WHO*. https://www.reuters.com/world/covid-19-death-tolls-are-likely-significant-undercount-who-says-2021-05-21/

Roeder, P., Mariner, J., & Kock, R. (2013). Rinderpest: The veterinary perspective on eradication. *Philosophical Transactions of the Royal Society of London. Series B, Biological Sciences*, *368*(1623), 20120139. doi:10.1098/rstb.2012.0139 PMID:23798687

Rosenwald, M. (2021, February 22). *History's deadliest pandemics, from ancient Rome to modern America*. https://www.washingtonpost.com/graphics/2020/local/retropolis/coronavirus-deadliest-pandemics/

Roush, S. W., & Murphy, T. V.Vaccine-Preventable Disease Table Working Group. (2007). Historical comparisons of morbidity and mortality for vaccine-preventable diseases in the United States. *Journal of the American Medical Association*, *298*(18), 2155–2163. doi:10.1001/jama.298.18.2155 PMID:18000199

Singh, R. P., Hodson, D. P., Jin, Y., Lagudah, E. S., Ayliffe, M. A., Bhavani, S., Rouse, M. N., Pretorius, Z. A., Szabo, L. J., Huerta-Espino, J., Basnet, B. R., Lan, C., & Hovmøller, M. S. (2015). Emergence and spread of new races of wheat stem rust fungus: Continued threat to food security and prospects of genetic control. *Phytopathology*, *105*(7), 872–884. doi:10.1094/PHYTO-01-15-0030-FI PMID:26120730

Thigpen, M. C., Whitney, C. G., Messonnier, N. E., Zell, E. R., Lynfield, R., Hadler, J. L., Harrison, L. H., Farley, M. M., Reingold, A., Bennett, N. M., Craig, A. S., Schaffner, W., Thomas, A., Lewis, M. M., Scallan, E., & Schuchat, A. (2011). Bacterial meningitis in the United States, 1998–2007. *The New England Journal of Medicine*, *364*(21), 2016–2025. doi:10.1056/NEJMoa1005384 PMID:21612470

Tomley, F. M., & Shirley, M. W. (2009). Livestock infectious diseases and zoonoses. *Philosophical Transactions of the Royal Society of London. Series B, Biological Sciences*, *364*(1530), 2637–2642. doi:10.1098/rstb.2009.0133 PMID:19687034

Wahl, A., Baker, C., Spagnuolo, R. A., Stamper, L. W., Fouda, G. G., Permar, S. R., Hinde, K., Kuhn, L., Bode, L., Aldrovandi, G. M., & Garcia, J. V. (2015). Breast Milk of HIV-Positive Mothers Has Potent and Species-Specific In Vivo HIV-Inhibitory Activity. *Journal of Virology*, *89*(21), 10868–10878. doi:10.1128/JVI.01702-15 PMID:26292320

Wall, M. M., Huang, J., Oswald, J., & McCullen, D. (2005). Factors associated with reporting multiple causes of death. *BMC Medical Research Methodology*, *5*(1), 1–13. doi:10.1186/1471-2288-5-4 PMID:15655070

Will, R. G., & Annick Alperovitch, S. (1998). Descriptive epidemiology of Creutzfeldt-Jakob disease in six European countries, 1993–1995. *Annals of Neurology*, *43*(6), 763–767. doi:10.1002/ana.410430611 PMID:9629846

World Health Organization. (2020a). *Global Health Estimates 2020: Deaths by Cause, Age, Sex, by Country and by Region, 2000-2019*. https://www.who.int/data/gho/data/themes/mortality-and-global-health-estimates/ghe-leading-causes-of-death

World Health Organization. (2020b, November 30). *HIV/AIDS*. https://www.who.int/news-room/q-a-detail/hiv-aids

World Health Organization. (2022, April 8). *WHO Coronavirus (COVID-19) Dashboard*. https://covid19.who.int/

Yoshida, K., Schuenemann, V. J., Cano, L. M., Pais, M., Mishra, B., Sharma, R., Lanz, C., Martin, F. N., Kamoun, S., Krause, J., Thines, M., Weigel, D., & Burbano, H. A. (2013). The rise and fall of the Phytophthora infestans lineage that triggered the Irish potato famine. *eLife*, *2*, e00731. doi:10.7554/eLife.00731 PMID:23741619

Chapter 6
Nonlethality in Infectious Disease

ABSTRACT

This chapter describes and analyzes impacts of infectious disease that do not rise to the level of death. Earth exists in a landscape filled with infectious disease, and anyone who has ever had the common cold, or the flu, has experienced a fragment of the larger narrative presented in so many ways earlier in the book, but it is easy enough for so many who get sick to escape relatively unscathed, or at least alive, that the context of nonlethal experiences may seem very much removed from the context of those who lose their lives. Four themes are emphasized: environment, illness, pathogen, and the immune.

INTRODUCTION

There is a totalizing impulse in human society to count harm done in terms of final harm. It is extremely common to see terrible events expressed in terms of the number of lives taken. However, the impact of harmful events goes beyond a single statistic. Just as a natural disaster, or an act of terrorism, can result in trauma and displacement, so too can infectious disease, in terms of displacement from home to hospital, loss of a sense of safety, or similar. Polio, a particularly feared disease in the United States in the first part of the twentieth century, was feared largely not because of its death rate, but because of its tendency to leave a substantial number of those who caught the disease with paralysis significant enough to leave the patient with need

DOI: 10.4018/978-1-7998-8689-1.ch006

for a wheelchair, or an encasing iron lung. Obviously lethality is a dire result of infectious disease, but it is not the only result.

EXPERIENCES OF INFECTIOUS DISEASE

The progression of infectious disease in an individual can be split into four basic experiences. First, the risk environment. By what vector is a given person likely to acquire the disease? What factors in their life either contribute to, or put a drag on their health? Second, the illness from the perspective of the person who acquired the pathogen. How do they feel? What parts of their day-to-day experience are impacted? What short-term and long-term consequences are present? Third, the disease from the perspective of the pathogen. What is its physical nature? How does it reproduce? What are its strategies for attempting to evade the immune system? Fourth, the disease from the perspective of the immune system. What defenses are triggered by the pathogen entering the body? What events proceed? How is the pathogen eventually overcome, if it is indeed overcome?

By focusing on these four experiences--environmental, illness, pathogen, and immune--a complementary picture of the experience of acquiring and having an infectious disease can be built up. One important part of this quartet is what it does not include--statistics about lethality, which is an extremely common way of understanding infectious disease from an outside perspective. The problem with such an approach is that, even in the worst fatal outcomes, a tally mark does not do much to explain what the process of the disease was actually like. There are a number of other statistics that are relevant, such as case numbers, and disease geography, but these factors also are more of a summary than is relevant to the main thrust of this chapter, which is on the experience and not the context of the experience from a demographic perspective.

Goal of the chapter settled, and caveats given, the body of the chapter begins with the *environmental* context of disease.

ENVIRONMENT

How does the environment interact with the experience of infectious disease? The opposite question, about how it could not, is probably harder--pathogens and individuals susceptible to infection necessarily exist in an environmental context. A virus, bacterium, or other pathogen does not find a human in a sort of perfectly neutral space with no distinguishing characteristics. Three subcategories here are (1), the actual climate where a person lives, (2), where a person works or travels, and (3), unique factors related to a person's body or genetic predisposition.

There is always a relevant climate, with various endemic species and strains, as well as a whole ecosystem of behaviors and patterns. Every disease must be caught from a vector, and that vector, which, it must be noted, is a physical word implying a physical source, might be something like a friend, a neighbor, or a jaunt in the woods that involved an insect bite. Those sources, too, need to have their own sources.

The idea of an insect bite opens the door to a new level of analysis on the word "ecosystem." Fundamentally, acquiring an infectious disease is all about acquiring the disease from a context, and any pathogen that enters the body either comes from the environment "at large" or makes the transition from another host.

Animals and nonhuman organisms are worth a mention as hosts in their own right. Which this book is focused on the context of disease from a human perspective, and it is arguable that, insofar as illness involves a particular experience of a disease, animals do not get sick in the same way people do, it is nevertheless important to point out that pathogens can infect virtually anything in theory. In practice, specific pathogens are targeted to specific hosts and climes, but the overall topic is very broad. So too is the indirect effect of infectious disease on human civilization, as seen through diseases of crops, as well as diseases in animals raised by humans.

The Irish Potato Famine, which fundamentally shaped the experience of millions of people who today have Irish ancestry, is one example of infectious disease causing such an impact. While the Potato Famine was experienced as a famine from the perspective of the giant wave of emigrants pushed off the island by hunger, to the potatoes, the Irish Great Famine of the 1840s was caused by the mold *Phytophthora infestans* (Yoshida et al., 2013). The famine developed in part because of lack of concern by the British, who controlled Ireland at the time, but the crucible through which human and political behavior occurred was created by mold (Edwards & Luckie, 2014). Traditional historiography posits around 1 million deaths, and around 1.5 million migrants, while recent evidence suggests the number of fatalities may have been lower, and the number of migrants higher (Nusteling, 2009).

Infectious disease has struck humans indirectly in other parts of the world, too, and in other shapes. It seems Mexico was the source of the potato-blight-causing *Phytophthora infestans*, as well as other *Phytophthora* species (Grünwald & Flier, 2005). There is also Potato Virus Y of the family *Potyviridae*, as another example, which is commonly transferred between plants by aphids, or by planting contaminated tubers (Quenouille et al., 2013). A wheat pathogen is the fungus *Zymoseptoria tritici* (Feurtey et al., 2019). The existence of nature has a complicated relationship with human crops--landscape structures supporting large wild pathogen populations naturally foster the creation of crop pathogens, but at the same time, reduce the ability for these crop pathogens to specifically target the crops, which would seem more likely in more broad monoculture agricultures (Papaïx et al., 2015).

Another major role of nonhuman organisms, particularly animals, in preserving infectious disease with effects that may make their way back to humans, is in the idea of a reservoir. In a reservoir, infectious disease circulates adjacent to a population that is not currently being infected. Consider, for example, rats passing plague amongst themselves for many years without spreading the disease to humans (Reluga et al., 2007). Migratory animals are a relevant vector, as animals trying to escape disease may also spread it, and the disease pathogen may mutate (Altizer et al., 2011).

Moving away from animals, air pollutants can contribute to immune responses (Glencross, 2020). In terms of occupations, healthcare workers, workers who engage with animals, workers who are in laboratories, and workers who work with waste or public service, are more likely than others to be infected with pathogens (Haagsma et al., 2012; Su et al., 2019). This sort of relationship can be even more specific--leptospirosis often involves being near small animals or meat products at work, and people who acquire hepatitis A often have contact with raw sewage, while hepatitis B or C risk increases with jobs that involve exposure to human blood, and (Aw & Blair, 2010). Thirty-year infection risk for hepatitis C among police, fire, and corrections workers is less than 0.1%, but 1.9% for paramedics and emergency response personnel in communities of high risk (Rischitelli et al., 2005). HIV exposure as a medical worker is linked to the frequency of patients with HIV in the area of work (Buro et al., 2001). Work seems to have an influence on the propensity of people to get vaccinated--within the healthcare space in the United States, seasonal influenza vaccination is greatest among individuals in the fields of health diagnosing and treating, at 52.3%, and lowest in healthcare support, at 32.0% (Caban-Martinez et al., 2010). Outside of healthcare, vaccination rates for influenza are greatest in the white collar category, at 24.7%, and reach a minimum for farm workers, at 11.7%.

In terms of the environment as unique aspects of a human body, obesity is linked to increased hospital admission and critical care need, including for the coronavirus COVID-19 (Lighter et al., 2020). Genetics can also play a major role in disease susceptibility (Cooke & Hill, 2001). Infectious disease can be seen as a system of input, throughput, and output, with the full range of environmental factors creating various direct or subtle vulnerabilities and resistances.

ILLNESS

The next major way to experience infectious disease is through the lens of illness. Earlier in this book, a good deal of attention was placed on the ways in which the "illness experience" is a phenomenon in its own right, and that the personal and social circumstances of an individual can have an overwhelming impact on the course of a disease. A person who is supported, has health insurance, and can take time off to rest, as appropriate, is someone who, all other things being equal, is likely to have a meaningfully different experience for practically any illness than someone who is uninsured, has nutritional deficiencies in their diet, and is chronically stressed. Stress is a physical phenomenon that can be explained as the body running 'hot' for long periods of time, with fairly straightforward limitations on its ability to react to further difficult conditions. Meanwhile, access to care is an even more obvious game-changer. Vaccinations can make the difference between a pathogen not being able to cause a noticeable illness, and a situation that leads to death. So too can access to antibiotics. Plague is a powerful example of that last case--the world of today is not at as much risk of plague as in the days of the Black Death. However, there must always be some illness experience when disease is present.

In an institution for children and adolescents in São Paulo, Brazil, providing housing for some with perinatally acquired HIV, those with the infection adapt to taking medication but may have difficulty understanding the implications about the condition, in part because of limitations of efforts by staff (Abadía-Barrero & LaRusso, 2006).

In effort to address some of the issues tied to that example, Narrative Medicine exists, which strives to connect patients' personal stories to their medical histories, but this field is still in development (Fioretti et al., 2016). Similarly, there is a biographical approach to understanding the individual response to risk in illness (Zinn, 2005). The point is that uncertainty tied to a health condition may well contribute significantly to mental health and overall quality of life (Brashers et al., 2003). This feature is very common in disease, as uncertainty may be considered typical in any long-term illness condition, which, in the infectious disease space, may include HIV or other viruses (Mishel, 1990). Work by Mishel (1988) highlights three themes of response to health difficulty--the source of uncertainty, the process of uncertainty, and how to cope with uncertainty (Mishel, 1988).

The risk is measurable. Illness as an experience is connected to the concept of quality of life, with indication that chronic illness is particularly influential in this domain–for patients completing an intensive care unit (ICU) stay, preexisting comorbidities and not severity of acute condition is linked with longer-term healthful quality of life indicators (Griffith et al., 2018). Adult survivors of ICUs generally do show quality of life improvements, but overall metrics in this space remain lower than that of the general population (Dowdy et al., 2005).

In a metaanaysis investigating psychosocial responses of the general population towards epidemic, themes of anxiety, anger, stress, and guilt showed up, in addition to some degree of empowerment to respond with increased compassion towards others (Chew et al., 2020). Severe chronic stressors (lasting one month or more in duration) are associated with substantial increase in risk of disease (Cohen et al., 1998). The source of these stressors is largely underemployment, unemployment, or interpersonal difficulties with family or friends.

PATHOGEN

This chapter has so far discussed the way normal courses of infectious disease exist and come from an environmental context, and then, how a course of illness can impact a patient. One important element deserving of discussion is the course of infectious disease from the perspective of a pathogen, itself. Diseases are disruptions of functioning that are essentially side-effects of an actual physical pathogen.

One straightforward way of understanding the immune system is in the order in which pathogens come across immune defenses. The first defense, and the only defense needed in a vast number of cases, is the skin itself. The skin as an immune defense is indeed so obviously a preliminary protection that its relevance may be best understood by the actions often taken when a breach is made, such as a cut during a fall. In such a case, a standard course of action is to clean and bandage the wound, and even to receive attention for stitches, if so required. Why are these steps necessary? The cleaning is done to prevent potential pathogens that exist in the air, the soil, or any other location that may come in contact with the wound, including scraped bits of outer flesh itself, from infecting the body, and then one of the primary purposes of bandaging and stitching is to prevent further chance of infection. Indeed, even the more obvious reason for bandaging and stitching--it is important to keep the inside of the body inside the body--is tied fundamentally rather than peripherally to infection, because the key purpose of an external barrier is sorting the outside from the inside.

As an example of the journey a pathogen can take, it may be valuable to consider rhinovirus, which can cause what is known as the common cold. Rhinovirus can transfer via cough, which the virus itself stimulates, possibly through excess mucus production or disruption of epithelial lining (Atkinson et al., 2016). Rhinovirus targets the upper and lower airways, and may often lead to subclinical results, but can end in life-threatening infections in some cases (Kennedy et al., 2012; To et al., 2017). The point of the virus, from a propagation standpoint, is to have its lineage survive and spread, not necessarily cause great damage to its host. Rhinoviruses do, however, need to enter cells to promulgate the standard virus life cycle, and use low density lipoprotein receptors on the outside of cells to facilitate their entry (Bayer et al., 2001). Viruses inside cells can modify their processes extensively including pushing host cell metabolism towards an anabolic state (Gualdoni et al., 2018). Respiratory viruses are common (Hao et al., 2012; Griggs et al., 2017), likely because they exploit a vulnerable access point to the human body.

IMMUNE

Once a pathogen is inside the human body, there are two basic levels of immune response--the innate, and adaptive. Based on strict definitions, it is straightforward to line the skin to the innate immune system. The essential difference is--in the innate immune system, the body combats a pathogen with responses that are ready to go from the moment of first contact, while the adaptive immune system involves a training period where the body readies itself to produce antibodies. As mentioned, skin is a critical preliminary barrier (Tsepkolenko et al., 2019). However, there are many other components. The innate immune system includes phagocytic cells like neutrophils, monocytes, and macrophages, as well as cells which release inflammatory mediators--basophils, mast cells, and eosinophils, along with natural killer cells (Delves & Roitt, 2000) Molecules like complement, acute-phase proteins, and complement also contribute to hinder or destroy invaders. Neutrophils are particularly interesting--they can directly destroy pathogens, but also help trigger other parts of the innate immune response, as well as possibly the adaptive immune system (Kubes, 2018). Meanwhile, the adaptive side is mediated by T lymphocytes and B lymphocytes, and can store memory of previous infections (Parkin & Cohen, 2001). Regulatory B cells engage in their control of immune responses in key part through release of the immune cell secretion IL-10 (Mauri & Menon, 2017). Many other ILs, or interleukins, part of a class of proteins called cytokines that mediate intercellular communication, are critical in immune functioning as well.

On a scale much broader than proteins, human immune systems function to various degrees based on inherited influences, as well as non-heritable influences, with the second category tied largely to the impact of symbiotic and pathogenic microbes--consider HIV, or the concept of opportunistic infections (Brodin & Davis, 2017). Meanwhile, age can impact or damage cellular processes of the immune system, particularly the adaptive immune system (Nikolich-Žugich, 2018).

Through interactions with the immune system, and beyond, infectious disease harms humans through mechanisms that cannot easily be reduced to statistics.

REFERENCES

Abadía-Barrero, C. E., & LaRusso, M. D. (2006). The disclosure model versus a developmental illness experience model for children and adolescents living with HIV/AIDS in Sao Paulo, Brazil. *AIDS Patient Care and STDs*, *20*(1), 36–43. doi:10.1089/apc.2006.20.36 PMID:16426154

Altizer, S., Bartel, R., & Han, B. A. (2011). Animal migration and infectious disease risk. *Science, 331*(6015), 296–302. doi:10.1126cience.1194694 PMID:21252339

Atkinson, S. K., Sadofsky, L. R., & Morice, A. H. (2016). How does rhinovirus cause the common cold cough? *BMJ Open Respiratory Research, 3*(1). doi:10.1136/bmjresp-2015-000118

Aw, T. C., & Blair, I. (2010). Occupational infections. *Infectious Diseases*, 715–726. doi:10.1016/B978-0-323-04579-7.00067-8

Bayer, N., Schober, D., Hüttinger, M., Blaas, D., & Fuchs, R. (2001). Inhibition of clathrin-dependent endocytosis has multiple effects on human rhinovirus serotype 2 cell entry. *The Journal of Biological Chemistry, 276*(6), 3952–3962. doi:10.1074/jbc.M004722200 PMID:11073943

Brashers, D. E., Neidig, J. L., Russell, J. A., Cardillo, L. W., Haas, S. M., Dobbs, L. K., Garland, M., McCartney, B., & Nemeth, S. (2003). The medical, personal, and social causes of uncertainty in HIV illness. *Issues in Mental Health Nursing*, *24*(5), 497–522. doi:10.1080/01612840305292 PMID:12775548

Brodin, P., & Davis, M. M. (2017). Human immune system variation. *Nature Reviews. Immunology*, *17*(1), 21–29. doi:10.1038/nri.2016.125 PMID:27916977

Caban-Martinez, A. J., Lee, D. J., Davila, E. P., LeBlanc, W. G., Arheart, K. L., McCollister, K. E., Christ, S. L., Clarke, T., & Fleming, L. E. (2010). Sustained low influenza vaccination rates in US healthcare workers. *Preventive Medicine*, *50*(4), 210–212. doi:10.1016/j.ypmed.2010.01.001 PMID:20079761

Chew, Q. H., Wei, K. C., Vasoo, S., Chua, H. C., & Sim, K. (2020). Narrative synthesis of psychological and coping responses towards emerging infectious disease outbreaks in the general population: Practical considerations for the COVID-19 pandemic. *Tropical Journal of Pharmaceutical Research*, *61*(7), 350–356. Advance online publication. doi:10.11622medj.2020046 PMID:32241071

Cohen, S., Frank, E., Doyle, W. J., Skoner, D. P., Rabin, B. S., & Gwaltney, J. M. Jr. (1998). Types of stressors that increase susceptibility to the common cold in healthy adults. *Health Psychology*, *17*(3), 214–223. doi:10.1037/0278-6133.17.3.214 PMID:9619470

Cooke, G. S., & Hill, A. V. (2001). Genetics of susceptibility to human infectious disease. *Nature Reviews. Genetics*, *2*(12), 967–977. doi:10.1038/35103577 PMID:11733749

Delves, P. J., & Roitt, I. M. (2000). The immune system. *The New England Journal of Medicine*, *343*(1), 37–49. doi:10.1056/NEJM200007063430107 PMID:10882768

Dowdy, D. W., Eid, M. P., Sedrakyan, A., Mendez-Tellez, P. A., Pronovost, P. J., Herridge, M. S., & Needham, D. M. (2005). Quality of life in adult survivors of critical illness: A systematic review of the literature. *Intensive Care Medicine*, *31*(5), 611–620. doi:10.100700134-005-2592-6 PMID:15803303

Edwards, J. A., & Luckie, A. (2014). British Prime Minister Tony Blair's Irish Potato Famine Apology. *Journal of Conflictology*, *5*(1), 43–51. doi:10.7238/joc.v5i1.1863

Feurtey, A., Stevens, D. M., Stephan, W., & Stukenbrock, E. H. (2019). Interspecific gene exchange introduces high genetic variability in crop pathogen. *Genome Biology and Evolution*, *11*(11), 3095–3105. doi:10.1093/gbe/evz224 PMID:31603209

Fioretti, C., Mazzocco, K., Riva, S., Oliveri, S., Masiero, M., & Pravettoni, G. (2016). Research studies on patients' illness experience using the narrative medicine approach: A systematic review. *BMJ Open*, *6*(7), e011220. doi:10.1136/bmjopen-2016-011220 PMID:27417197

Glencross, D. A., Ho, T. R., Camina, N., Hawrylowicz, C. M., & Pfeffer, P. E. (2020). Air pollution and its effects on the immune system. *Free Radical Biology & Medicine*, *151*, 56–68. doi:10.1016/j.freeradbiomed.2020.01.179 PMID:32007522

Griffith, D. M., Salisbury, L. G., Lee, R. J., Lone, N., Merriweather, J. L., & Walsh, T. S. (2018). Determinants of health-related quality of life after ICU: Importance of patient demographics, previous comorbidity, and severity of illness. *Critical Care Medicine*, *46*(4), 594–601. doi:10.1097/CCM.0000000000002952 PMID:29293149

Griggs, T. F., Bochkov, Y. A., Basnet, S., Pasic, T. R., Brockman-Schneider, R. A., Palmenberg, A. C., & Gern, J. E. (2017). Rhinovirus C targets ciliated airway epithelial cells. *Respiratory Research*, *18*(1), 1–11. doi:10.118612931-017-0567-0 PMID:28472984

Grünwald, N. J., & Flier, W. G. (2005). The biology of Phytophthora infestans at its center of origin. *Annual Review of Phytopathology*, *43*(1), 171–190. doi:10.1146/annurev.phyto.43.040204.135906 PMID:16078881

Gualdoni, G. A., Mayer, K. A., Kapsch, A. M., Kreuzberg, K., Puck, A., Kienzl, P., Oberndorfer, F., Frühwirth, K., Winkler, S., Blaas, D., Zlabinger, G. J., & Stöckl, J. (2018). Rhinovirus induces an anabolic reprogramming in host cell metabolism essential for viral replication. *Proceedings of the National Academy of Sciences of the United States of America*, *115*(30), E7158–E7165. doi:10.1073/pnas.1800525115 PMID:29987044

Haagsma, J. A., Tariq, L., Heederik, D. J., & Havelaar, A. H. (2012). Infectious disease risks associated with occupational exposure: A systematic review of the literature. *Occupational and Environmental Medicine*, *69*(2), 140–146. doi:10.1136/oemed-2011-100068 PMID:22006935

Hao, W., Bernard, K., Patel, N., Ulbrandt, N., Feng, H., Svabek, C., Wilson, S., Stracener, C., Wang, K., Suzich, J. A., Blair, W., & Zhu, Q. (2012, December 15). Infection and propagation of human rhinovirus C in human airway epithelial cells. *Journal of Virology*, *86*(24), 13524–13532. doi:10.1128/JVI.02094-12 PMID:23035218

HaoW.BernardK.PatelN.UlbrandtN.FengH.SvabekC.ZhuQ. (2012).

Kennedy, J. L., Turner, R. B., Braciale, T., Heymann, P. W., & Borish, L. (2012). Pathogenesis of rhinovirus infection. *Current Opinion in Virology*, *2*(3), 287–293. doi:10.1016/j.coviro.2012.03.008 PMID:22542099

Kubes, P. (2018). The enigmatic neutrophil: What we do not know. *Cell and Tissue Research*, *371*(3), 399–406. doi:10.100700441-018-2790-5 PMID:29404726

Lighter, J., Phillips, M., Hochman, S., Sterling, S., Johnson, D., Francois, F., & Stachel, A. (2020). Obesity in patients younger than 60 years is a risk factor for Covid-19 hospital admission. *Clinical Infectious Diseases*, *71*(15), 896–897. doi:10.1093/cid/ciaa415 PMID:32271368

Mauri, C., & Menon, M. (2017). Human regulatory B cells in health and disease: Therapeutic potential. *The Journal of Clinical Investigation*, *127*(3), 772–779. doi:10.1172/JCI85113 PMID:28248202

Mishel, M. H. (1988). Uncertainty in illness. *Image—the Journal of Nursing Scholarship*, *20*(4), 225–232. doi:10.1111/j.1547-5069.1988.tb00082.x PMID:3203947

Mishel, M. H. (1990). Reconceptualization of the uncertainty in illness theory. *Image—the Journal of Nursing Scholarship*, *22*(4), 256–262. doi:10.1111/j.1547-5069.1990.tb00225.x PMID:2292449

Nikolich-Žugich, J. (2018). The twilight of immunity: Emerging concepts in aging of the immune system. *Nature Immunology*, *19*(1), 10–19. doi:10.103841590-017-0006-x PMID:29242543

Nusteling, H. P. (2009). How many Irish potato famine deaths?: Toward coherence of the evidence. *Historical Methods: A Journal of Quantitative and Interdisciplinary History, 42*(2), 57-80. doi:10.3200/HMTS.42.2.57-80

Papaïx, J., Burdon, J. J., Zhan, J., & Thrall, P. H. (2015). Crop pathogen emergence and evolution in agro-ecological landscapes. *Evolutionary Applications*, *8*(4), 385–402. doi:10.1111/eva.12251 PMID:25926883

Parkin, J., & Cohen, B. (2001). An overview of the immune system. *Lancet*, *357*(9270), 1777–1789. doi:10.1016/S0140-6736(00)04904-7 PMID:11403834

Puro, V., De Carli, G., Petrosillo, N., & Ippolito, G. (2001). Risk of exposure to bloodborne infection for Italian healthcare workers, by job category and work area. *Infection Control and Hospital Epidemiology*, *22*(4), 206–210. doi:10.1086/501890 PMID:11379710

Quenouille, J., Vassilakos, N., & Moury, B. (2013). Potato virus Y: A major crop pathogen that has provided major insights into the evolution of viral pathogenicity. *Molecular Plant Pathology*, *14*(5), 439–452. doi:10.1111/mpp.12024 PMID:23480826

Reluga, T., Meza, R., Walton, D. B., & Galvani, A. P. (2007). Reservoir interactions and disease emergence. *Theoretical Population Biology*, *72*(3), 400–408. doi:10.1016/j.tpb.2007.07.001 PMID:17719617

Rischitelli, G., Lasarev, M., & McCauley, L. (2005). Career risk of hepatitis C virus infection among US emergency medical and public safety workers. *Journal of Occupational and Environmental Medicine*, *47*(11), 1174–1181. doi:10.1097/01.jom.0000174295.66308.92 PMID:16282879

Su, C. P., de Perio, M. A., Cummings, K. J., McCague, A. B., Luckhaupt, S. E., & Sweeney, M. H. (2019). Case Investigations of Infectious Diseases Occurring in Workplaces, United States, 2006-2015. *Emerging Infectious Diseases*, *25*(3), 397–405. doi:10.3201/eid2503.180708 PMID:30789129

To, K. K., Yip, C. C., & Yuen, K. Y. (2017). Rhinovirus–from bench to bedside. *Journal of the Formosan Medical Association*, *116*(7), 496–504. doi:10.1016/j.jfma.2017.04.009 PMID:28495415

Tsepkolenko, A., Tsepkolenko, V., Dash, S., Mishra, A., Bader, A., Melerzanov, A., & Giri, S. (2019). The regenerative potential of skin and the immune system. *Clinical, Cosmetic and Investigational Dermatology*, *12*, 519–532. doi:10.2147/CCID.S196364 PMID:31410045

Yoshida, K., Schuenemann, V. J., Cano, L. M., Pais, M., Mishra, B., Sharma, R., Lanz, C., Martin, F. N., Kamoun, S., Krause, J., Thines, M., Weigel, D., & Burbano, H. A. (2013). The rise and fall of the Phytophthora infestans lineage that triggered the Irish potato famine. *eLife*, *2*, e00731. doi:10.7554/eLife.00731 PMID:23741619

Zinn, J. O. (2005). The biographical approach: A better way to understand behaviour in health and illness. *Health Risk & Society*, *7*(1), 1–9. doi:10.1080/13698570500042348

Chapter 7
COVID-19 and Historical Parallels

ABSTRACT

This chapter covers COVID-19 as it is understood at the time of writing, and compares and contrasts COVID-19 to prior epidemics with respiratory vectors. While the coronavirus underlying COVID-19 is not the same type of virus involved in the influenza pandemic starting around 1918, processes surrounding epidemics, including principles surrounding spread and human response tendencies, have important similarities. Epidemics and pandemics, regardless of the pathogen behind them, spread through populations in similar ways, and pandemics that impact humans meet the variety of responses in the human toolkit. This text was prepared in 2022, and the coronavirus pandemic has not yet clearly transitioned to a well-defined endemic state. However, as science is not structured to offer final conclusions, this chapter may serve as a foundation from a certain period of medical and social history.

INTRODUCTION

There are certain characteristics that are essential to the experience and transmission of the 2019-originated coronavirus disease COVID-19. It is highly transmissible, airborne, and by 2020, was understood to be present as a global pandemic (Muralidar et al., 2020). Pandemics with respiratory vectors did not begin with COVID-19. One clear point of contrast is the influenza pandemic beginning in 1918, which caused similar shutdowns

DOI: 10.4018/978-1-7998-8689-1.ch007

and mass death almost exactly a hundred years before. Respiratory viruses travel by contact, droplets, or smaller aerosol methods, and knowledge of the precise mechanisms of human-to-human transmission is still developing (Kutter et al., 2018).

COMPARISON STATISTICS

At this point it may be useful to compare basic statistics surrounding well-known outbreaks of coronavirus and influenza. R_0, a value which estimates the number of new infections an existing infection is likely to cause, is thought to have been about 2.5 for the early stages of the COVID-19 outbreak (Petersen et al., 2020). COVID-19 is caused by SARS-CoV-2, which stands for severe acute respiratory syndrome coronavirus 2. The SARS-CoV outbreak of 2003, known generally as SARS, had an R_0 of 2.4 before mitigation steps. Meanwhile, the 1918 pandemic had an R_0 of 2.0, and the influenza pandemic of 2009 had an R_0 of 1.7. By these numbers, it is not obvious why SARS of 2003 did not leave the same impact as COVID-19. The answer appears to be linked to a counterintuitive implication of severity. The 2003 SARS outbreak, unlike the 1918 and 2009 pandemics of influenza, and COVID-19, resulted in a low proportion of patients with mild illness. Most, over 70%, of SARS 2003 patients required hospitalization, while proportionally few patients required hospitalization in any of the known stages of the other three outbreaks. About 40% of SARS 2003 patients also required intensive care. How is it possible that the SARS 2003 outbreak, being on an individual case basis the most severe infection, did not reach the same critical mass as COVID-19? From the data already presented, the clearest answer is that COVID-19 is far more susceptible to undetected transmission.

When looking at diseases as epidemics, rather than individual cases, traits that are a relief to the individual may not be at all a relief to the population as a whole. Asymptomatic or nearly-asymptomatic carriers have a much-clearer natural ability to spread infection than do those who are both hampered by symptoms and visible as having symptoms. Those who have apparent symptoms may be both more likely to get treated, as well as avoided by those who do not wish to catch what is an apparently contagious illness. This situation makes a clear distinction between a model of health that is built around interactions between a patient and their providers, and a model of health that is built around a patient's interaction with the environment, including other people.

Ultimately, the SARS 2003 outbreak resulted in 8,098 cases reported globally, and 774 deaths, creating a case fatality rate of 9.7% (Petersen et al., 2020). In contrast, as of 7:01 PM CEST, April 8, 2022, the World Health Organization (2022b) reported 6,170,283 deaths from COVID-19, and 494,587,638 confirmed cases. This is a case fatality rate of about 1.2%. COVID-19, by these statistics, is both significantly less deadly on an individual basis, and drastically more deadly on a worldwide basis–a lower fatality rate impacting a much larger population.

The 2009 influenza outbreak, while having significant disparity in estimates of case fatality rate, resulted in an early estimate of 0.5% mortality (Nishiura, 2010). While the World Health Organization only reported 18,631 laboratory-confirmed deaths from this outbreak, because of difficulties in data capture, the number of deaths may have been ten times higher (Simonsen et al., 2013). The 1918-1919 influenza pandemic, meanwhile, encompassed approximately 500 million cases, a case fatality rate of greater than 2.5%, and total deaths estimated around 50 million, with an arguable upper bound around 100 million (Taubenberger & Morens, 2006).

While difficulties in tracking disease often make exact quantifications of scale and harm difficult, what should be more clear is that, if epidemics get out of control, given the modern global ecosystem, their underlying diseases can effectively spread worldwide. At that point, until effective treatments are found, whole populations are in danger in proportion to the pandemic's innate lethality. As an example of what this might mean, consider that deaths in both influenza pandemics mentioned above were present broadly in non-elderly populations (Petersen et al., 2020). Meanwhile, in early COVID-19 (D'ascanio et al., 2021), as well as 2003 SARS, mortality was heavily concentrated in those above 65 years of age (Petersen et al., 2020). Of these four epidemics, the two coronavirus outbreaks displayed disproportionate danger to the elderly, but all of the four had or have been deadly.

INFLUENZA

What is flu, or influenza? Influenza is an acute disease of the respiratory tract that can be caused by influenza viruses of three main types–A, B, and C–with type C causing more mild symptoms (Moghadami, 2017). In the United States, a relatively wealthy country that makes up about 5% of the world's population, influenza causes around 200,000 hospitalizations and 36,000 deaths in a standard winter influenza season (Taubenberger &

Morens, 2008; Thompson et al., 2003). These "flu seasons" should not be confused with pandemic outbreaks of influenza. Motivated by specific viral strains, the pandemics occur around every 8 to 41 years, can infect half the world's population, and can lead to mortality far in excess of what is typically expected for seasonal flu illnesses. Major influenza pandemics occurred in 1889, 1957, and 1968, in addition to 1918 and 2009.

In terms of form, influenza is a negative-sense single-stranded RNA virus covered in an envelope, and, in types A and B, studded with particular patterns of the glycoproteins hemagglutinin (H) and neuraminidase (N) (Dawson et al., 2018; Moghadami, 2017; Wang & Veit, 2016). How and when these glycoproteins occur is particularly relevant to different forms of influenza type A--the strain that caused the 2009 pandemic was of the form H1N1, for example (Al-Muharrmi, 2010). Influenza type A can occasionally remodel its surface glycoproteins in quite striking ways, and this antigenic shift can evade existing adaptive immune responses in the human population (Moghadami, 2017). In general, because the influenza virus genome is patterned in a segmented fashion, it is subject to high rates of reassortment, including through influence of influenza more commonly spreading in nonhuman populations. The idea that reassortment between different influenza strains can make typically nonhuman influenza strains suddenly deadly to humans is a key idea behind concern on "bird flu," or "avian flu" (Castrucci et al., 1993).

Influenza virus may propagate primarily through large droplets greater in size than five micrometers, though understanding transmission better is an important area of research, and smaller aerosol particles that may stay suspended in air for extended periods of time may also be important (Moghadami, 2017). In any event, because of the importance of the respiratory transmission vector, relatively close contact with the same air is required. Virus shedding begins one or two days before an often-sharp symptom onset, and, in uncomplicated cases, generally lasts for six or seven days. One or two days is also a standard incubation period of influenza before onset of symptoms. These symptoms are body-wide, or systemic, and commonly include fever, chills, headache, myalgia, malaise, and anorexia. Respiratory components include dry cough, runny nose, and sore throat. The most critical potential symptom of influenza for the individual patient, however, is pneumonia, where influenza aggressively reaches the lungs and causes complications with breathing.

Annual influenza vaccination is recommended for adults both because of the underlying pathogenic mutation rate, and because antiviral therapies have proven moderately effective at controlling symptom duration, and historically ineffective at controlling shedding and complications (Robson et al., 2019). Ventilator stockpiling, to assist in a spike of severe cases requiring mechanical intervention, was identified as an action item well in advance of the COVD-19 outbreak, for a hypothetical future influenza pandemic (Huang et al., 2017).

CORONAVIRUS

What of COVID-19, or SARS-CoV-2? COVID-19 is the third major coronavirus introduction to the human population from a zoonotic disease, after earlier outbreaks of SARS-CoV and MERS-CoV (Middle East respiratory syndrome coronavirus) (V'kovski et al., 2021). Coronaviruses are positive-sense single-stranded RNA viruses. Coronaviruses are enveloped, come in a variety of forms, and can infect a variety of species aside from humans, including other mammals and birds. Livestock can be targeted by coronaviruses. Because the family of coronaviruses is so diverse, various human coronaviruses, such as HCoV-229E, HCoV-OC43, HCoV-NL63, and HCoV-HKU1 circulate seasonally causing generally-mild respiratory tract infections in line with the "common cold." However, SARS and MERS coronaviruses are much more deadly, being, upon their emergence into the human population, able to focus on pneumocytes (cells lining lung alveoli responsible for gas exchange), as well as bronchial epithelial cells and upper respiratory tract cells. Coronavirus uses its spike protein to mediate cell entry, whereafter the standard process is to engage in translation of viral proteins, and then trigger exocytosis. This basic process does not say much about mortality risk or other harm done--coronavirus is dynamic and can appear in a variety of forms, just like influenza.

The 2003 SARS outbreak was limited enough in scope that the efficacy of drug treatments at that time was inconclusive (Stockman et al., 2006). Finding treatment for MERS, originally described in 2012, also was even more limited by its scope (Momattin et al., 2019). As of February 2022, there have been only 2,585 laboratory-confirmed cases of MERS, though the case-fatality ratio of 34.4% highlights the disease's dangerousness (World Health Organization, 2022a). Meanwhile, COVID-19, far surpassing the number of cases required for sophisticated treatment protocols, has had its treatment options arguably limited by the diversity of response. This cornucopia includes vaccines, social distancing, drug regimens with varying efficacies and mechanisms of action, ventilation, and, particularly in situations involving mild or asymptomatic cases, "wait and see" attitudes that may relieve short-term burden on hospitals at the cost of long-term spread if isolation protocols are not followed.

RISK AND THE 1918 INFLUENZA PANDEMIC

The key to pandemic risk is that it comes from the unknown. Vaccines and treatments can be developed that drastically decrease harm in populations that have access, but these take time to develop. The efficacy of COVID-19 vaccines has peaked well above the typical efficacies for annual influenza vaccines. The mRNA-1273 vaccine manufactured by Moderna, recorded 94.1% efficacy in one major clinical trial, comparing cases in vaccinated individuals against cases expected if the individuals were not vaccinated (Baden et al., 2021). Meanwhile, seasonal influenza vaccine hovers around 50% using the same basic standard (Lewnard & Cobey, 2018). Average vaccine efficacy against hospitalization for the type A H1N1 influenza variant driving the 2009 pandemic was 61% (Lansbury et al., 2017).

While pandemics occur that overwhelm medical capacity, triage systems are put in place to determine the best way to apply limited critical care capacity (Downar et al., 2010). The particular triage system is shaped by both institutional and human response to the given pandemic. The human response to the influenza pandemic that started in 1918, also A/H1N1 (Krause et al., 2010), is clear when one considers a name it came to be called—"Spanish Flu." Because Spain's press freely reported on a disease that was rampant well beyond their borders, the flu became associated with Spain (Martini et al., 2019). Suppression of information worked well enough elsewhere that the following is an example report from a small area in the United States:

People are very anxious to know to what extent the Spanish Flu has gained a foothold in our country. The same question is asked a dozen times daily. There seems to be no satisfactory answer. The disease is not a reportable one and consequently does not figure on the records. It does not seem probable, however, that there is a large number of cases. Altogether, there may be less than 25 cases in the county. As the result of such quarantine measures as have been adopted, the spread of the disease should be arrested before long. It is perfectly thinkable, therefore, that in Montour County, Spanish Flu may not gain much of a foothold.

All are hoping for the best. The closing order, sweeping as it is, is being obeyed to the letter. It is especially hard on the schools—on the pupils, who will lose ground rapidly while the schools are closed, as well as the teachers, who will feel the effects of the forced idleness. Of the teachers employed yesterday, a few were already looking around for temporary employment as there is absolutely no telling when the schools may be reopened. Unless the epidemic spreads very rapidly in Danville, however, it would seem reasonable to suppose that 'in a couple of weeks' time the schools may be permitted to reopen. (Danville Morning News, 1918)

The influenza pandemic of 1918 took the lives of between 20 to 40 million people (Mills et al., 2004). The importance of quarantine is hard to overstate. In the South Pacific at the time, the islands of Samoa were split into two polities, one under the political control of New Zealand, and the other under the political control of the United States. In the case of the former, influenza ran rampant, but in the case of American Samoa, active quarantining significantly blunted the effect of the pandemic (Shanks & Brundage, 2013). However, the historical memory of the influenza pandemic is questionable, seemingly overshadowed by that of World War I. In some ways this is appropriate--World War I had a sequelae twenty years after its end, while the 1918 pandemic has not yet been followed by a similar event of greater magnitude.

What were, then, the consequences of the 1918 pandemic? The General Social Survey in the United States indicated that those who survived it had lower social trust, and passed it on to their descendants (Aassve et al., 2021). However, the negative effects of that pandemic on wages seem to have been large but short-term, and more significant in urban areas (Basco et al., 2021). In the influenza pandemic of 1957, people were scrambling to cope because of the difficulty of internalizing lessons learned from older collective experiences (Jackson, 2009).

The influenza type A viruses have been responsible for a number of pandemics: The subtype H1N1 caused the 1918 flu, H2N2 caused the 1957 "Asian" flu, and H3N2 caused the 1968 flu (de Jong et al., 1997). Beyond, humans are vulnerable to a number of zoonotic health threats (coming from other animals), including HIV/AIDS (human immunodeficiency virus/ acquired immunodeficiency syndrome) and SARS (Morse et al., 2012). Coronavirus can also come from other animals. The combination of potential threats with the difficulties in preparedness helps make pandemics very dangerous. Even seasonal flu in the United States causes tens of thousands of deaths annually, hundreds of thousands of hospitalizations, tens of millions of missed days of work and school, and hundreds of millions of days of illness, off of 25 to 50 million cases of influenza (Nichol & Treanor, 2006; Taubenberger & Morens, 2008).

Against a landscape where respiratory and other illnesses can cause so much devastation, vaccinations play a critical role. Vaccines are typically developed to spur the creation of antibodies, though methods like inducing cross-protective cell-mediated immunity have been the topic of research (Subbarao et al., 2006). Some of the experimentation that has been done includes comparing efficacy of mineral oil versus carbomer as a co-ingredient (Dürrwald et al., 2010).

The idea of "just the flu" is particularly salient in a world that now understands COVID-19, because community transmission of flu in a world open for business is an example of losses that people have historically accepted. The flu is not harmless. The flu kills, and coronavirus is by one study only 2.05 times as likely to cause pneumonia and 1.64 times as likely to cause death (Li et al., 2020).

COVID-19 RESPONSE

The response of the world to COVID-19 involves many pillars, all of which must be managed to deal with the pandemic effectively. Treatments and social guidelines are valuable. Citizen buy-in to behave in accordance with medical suggestions is also key. *Government* willingness and capacity to propagate the guidance of medical leaders is necessary as a third plank. Without each of these three aspects--medical treatments/recommendations, civilian buy-in, and government capacity--COVID-19 can proceed through a community with relatively little check. "Flattening the curve" through avoidance behavior is an excellent example of the social power against pandemics (Feng et al., 2020). There does seem to be a distinct need.

In the COVID-19 pandemic, healthcare workers are notably at risk from disease spread via aerosol (Wilson et al., 2020). Sharing the same space indoors is a major risk factor in COVID-19 spread (Allen & Marr, 2020). In one study, all known outbreaks involving three or more cases occurred indoors (Qian et al., 2020). The phrase "social distancing" has real relevance, and points to action that can save lives even if it reduces economic activity (Thunström et al., 2020). In situations without pharmaceutical interventions, which was the case everywhere in the early stages of the COVID-19 pandemic, arguably the only strategy against the pandemic was to reduce contact (Lewnard & Lo, 2020).

Neither the 1918 influenza pandemic, nor COVID-19, are singular events. Certainly each became prominent a hundred years from the other, but the science is clear that another pandemic with similar traits and capacities, or one even more deadly, is possible in the future. In the future, there may be new tools to deal with the threat, but the nature of the threat is likely to stay the same. Pandemics have huge and disproportionate impact. The elderly are particularly vulnerable (D'Adamo, 2020). Those who stay in long-term care facilities are vulnerable for reasons related to immune susceptibility and community transmission (Lai et al., 2020; Levitt & Ling, 2020). Those who need hemodialysis may also be especially vulnerable (Li & Xu, 2020).

A tool that will be in the toolbox for the future are the mRNA vaccines that have been deployed against COVID-19, one by the combination of effort from the companies Pfizer and BioNTech, and the other by Moderna (Lin et al., 2020). The idea is to sensitize the immune system by introducing, in the case of COVID, RNA that encodes for the viral spike protein of COVID, while not creating a case of the disease. These vaccines carry viral RNA using a lipid nanoparticle platform (Pacheco et al., 2020). To sensitize the body, two doses of either vaccine are part of the primary schedule (Livingston, 2021). Moderna has intended a booster shot for variants (Tanne, 2021), and Pfizer/BioNTech have signaled similar readiness (Burki, 2022). A combined trial of both mRNA vaccines has showed 94% efficacy at two doses for adults against hospitalization, though caution must be associated with this number, as COVID-19 continues to mutate and develop new variants (Tenforde et al., 2021).

The mRNA vaccines exist in a context, and are accompanied by a range of other vaccines expanding upon more traditional technologies. An alternative produced by Novavax sensitizes the adaptive immune system to the spike protein directly and showed two-dose efficacy against infection at 89.7% in a significant trial (Heath et al., 2021). The Novavax vaccine mechanism of action seems particularly competitive with the mRNA vaccines against coronavirus (Wadman, 2021). However, Novavax the company hit manufacturing issues when trying to produce their product at scale, leading to difficulties getting traction (Tinari & Riva, 2021).

While this chapter cannot provide an up-to-date picture of the state of vaccine approvals and efficacies, it can provide a view of how the landscape has shifted so far. Broadly, a number of private, public, academic, or non-profit organizations around the world have produced or have been developing vaccines (Le et al., 2020). In 2020, the count of developing vaccines included over a dozen in China, over a dozen in Europe, dozens in North America, and likely over a dozen in the rest of Asia and Australia. Kashte et al. (2021) indicated 232 vaccine candidates at the time of their writing, with 60 in clinical development and 9 approved under at least one country's Emergency Use Authorization (EUA). The 9 included the pair of mRNA vaccines, both approved under EUA in the United States (the Pfizer and BioNTech vaccine was also given EUA approval in Bahrain, Canada, Mexico, and the United Kingdom). Meanwhile, a non-replicating viral vector vaccine from the University of Oxford/AstraZeneca was listed by Kashte et al. as under EUA approval in the United Kingdom. Another viral vector vaccine, Sputnik V, and a peptide vaccine, EpiVacCorona, were given approval by the Russian government, while China gave approval to 3 inactivated vaccines (containing inactivated virus). One of this last group, from Beijing Institute of Biological Products/Sinopharm, was also given EUA in the United Arab Emirates. A slightly more recent study, from Ghiasi et al. (2021), published in June (the Kashte et al. paper was published in March) highlights just how many approvals happened in 3 months–AstraZeneca moved up to 65 approvals for emergency or conditional use, leading the pack, with Pfizer/BioNTech in an apparent second place at 58. The state of COVID vaccines is constantly developing, though the following two points may be likely to be consistently true into the future–first, vaccine availability will be dependent on region, and second, relevant guidance will continue to mature as data and options are clarified.

The efficacy of vaccines is contained by their context. As of July 2021, while 19 vaccines were approved for use by one or more countries, and over 3 billion doses were delivered worldwide, only 0.9% of individuals in low-income countries received a dose (Sharma et al., 2021). The developing booster shot recommendations exacerbate access disparity further (Burki, 2022). The mRNA vaccines involve frozen storage conditions that necessitate supply chain care, limiting their reach (Crommelin et al., 2021). Rare cases of anaphylaxis associated with the administration of mRNA vaccines in the United States–December 14 to December 23, 2020 reporting showing 11.1 per million after the first dose for Pfizer-BioNTech (Shimabukuro & Nair, 2021), and December 21, 2020 to January 10, 2021 reporting 2.1 per million after the first dose for Moderna (CDC COVID-19 Response Team & Food and Drug Administration, 2021)--highlight a concern for monitoring potential unknowns related to such treatment that has formal medical implications, despite no deaths being reported in these tranches (Shimabukuro et al., 2021). As both review of treatments and some uncertainty is tied to the medical research progress, any individual with anxiety about the *response* to COVID can find real medical information that can encourage a sense of nuance or hesitation, creating a space for COVID vaccine hesitancy even when COVID vaccines overall have been demonstrably effective. While vaccines are particularly valuable because they are preventative, other drugs like dexamethasone, remdesivir, and anticoagulants, as well as supportive care, have found their place in the constellation of medical responses to COVID-19 (van Eijk et al., 2021). It should not be forgotten that vaccines are far from the only response to COVID, even in places with ample supply.

In the face of techniques and treatments applicable to the COVID pandemic, which may be useful for future outbreaks of disease, engaging with the human element is important. Vaccine refusal activity with COVID began before a vaccine was publicly available, and some associated false claims about effects, for clear reasons, are focused on symptoms that have nothing to do with a vaccine (Stein et al., 2021). This sort of belief is associated with downplaying the threat of pandemic, and not taking preventative actions such as wearing a mask, in addition to not believing in the safety of a vaccine and not intending to get vaccinated (Romer & Jamieson, 2020). A study released in 2020 showed that 25% of people in the United States and 20% of Canadians did not intend to get vaccinated against COVID-19, a rate that would make it very difficult to achieve herd immunity and prevent community transmission of the virus (Taylor et al., 2020). Hesitancy to get the COVID vaccine seems to be a worldwide issue. Overall reasons vary from mistrust, to fear of side effects, efficacy, lack of information, conspiracy beliefs, and social influence (Bogart et al., 2020; Palamenghi et al., 2020; Roy et al., 2022). Research from Italy dating near the beginning of the pandemic makes stark that vaccine hesitancy is a significant factor in difficulties of blocking the spread of the disease (Palamenghi et al., 2020). Research on hesitancy to get vaccinated against COVID-19 in the United Kingdom suggests it is difficult to isolate the characteristics that make some merely uncertain about the vaccine, as opposed to unwilling (Paul et al., 2021).

Against this behavior is the fact that the long-term personal impacts of COVID-19 in survivors is, at the time of writing, partly or largely unknown. There is evidence of neurological sequelae (Fiani et al., 2020; Troyer et al., 2020) neuropsychiatric sequelae (Hao et al., 2020) respiratory and neurological sequelae (Wang et al., 2020), and respiratory and psychophysical sequelae (Bellan et al., 2021), though there is evidence against those with mild-to-moderate cases being at greater risk of developing pulmonary fibrosis (Rogliani et al., 2020). There are many possible psychiatric sequelae, including clinically significant depression, anxiety, symptoms of posttraumatic stress disorder (PTSD), suicidal ideation or behavior, and grief (Murtara et al., 2021). Symptom persistence after infection recovery, deemed "Long COVID," seems set to be a focus of etiological research for some time (Raveendran et al., 2021).

This book is inevitably a piece of history. At the time of the final revision of this text, in 2022, there seems to be a strong chance COVID-19 will circulate indefinitely. Therefore, understanding the relationship of COVID-19 to pandemics past and possible pandemics future is important. Even though this chapter cannot put COVID-19 in a retrospective context, a more limited conclusion can be put forward. Two major elements of COVID-19's arrival–social and symptomatic pressures–are shared with similar outbreaks. These are highly likely to be of continual import in epidemiological study as they combine to shape the scope of pandemics. As an example of a complex double bind, the risk of blaming foreigners, and the value of controlling access of people coming from another country, who may be infected, must both be addressed (Paul, 2020). Social distancing needs to be understood as a low-technology way of saving lives, despite its economic cost (Adolph et al., 2020) and mental health cost (Liu et al., 2020). The limitations of border and travel restrictions--unlikely to slow spread by more than three weeks---should be understood, as should the fact that household quarantines and reactive school closures may substantially reduce ultimate disease burden (Ferguson et al., 2006). The way household sanitation does and does not play a role, including the limits of worldwide access to clean water, also needs to be understood (Howard et al., 2020).

In the spirit of transparency, the COVID-19 pandemic was the impetus for this book, as it was surely the impetus for a great deal of other writings. Humans respond to the experiences they face, and try to make sense of them.

REFERENCES

Aassve, A., Alfani, G., Gandolfi, F., & Le Moglie, M. (2021). Epidemics and trust: The case of the Spanish flu. *Health Economics*, *30*(4), 840–857. doi:10.1002/hec.4218 PMID:33554412

Adolph, C., Amano, K., Bang-Jensen, B., Fullman, N., & Wilkerson, J. (2021). Pandemic politics: Timing state-level social distancing responses to COVID-19. *Journal of Health Politics, Policy and Law*, *46*(2), 211–233. doi:10.1215/03616878-8802162 PMID:32955556

Al-Muharrmi, Z. (2010). Understanding the Influenza A H1N1 2009 Pandemic. *Sultan Qaboos University Medical Journal*, *10*(2), 187–195. PMID:21509228

Allen, J. G., & Marr, L. C. (2020). Recognizing and controlling airborne transmission of SARS-CoV-2 in indoor environments. *Indoor Air*, *30*(4), 557–558. doi:10.1111/ina.12697 PMID:32557915

Baden, L. R., El Sahly, H. M., Essink, B., Kotloff, K., Frey, S., Novak, R., Diemert, D., Spector, S. A., Rouphael, N., Creech, C. B., McGettigan, J., Khetan, S., Segall, N., Solis, J., Brosz, A., Fierro, C., Schwartz, H., Neuzil, K., Corey, L., ... Zaks, T.COVE Study Group. (2021). Efficacy and Safety of the mRNA-1273 SARS-CoV-2 Vaccine. *The New England Journal of Medicine*, *384*(5), 403–416. doi:10.1056/NEJMoa2035389 PMID:33378609

Basco, S., Domènech, J., & Rosés, J. R. (2021). The redistributive effects of pandemics: Evidence on the Spanish flu. *World Development*, *141*, 105389. doi:10.1016/j.worlddev.2021.105389

Bellan, M., Soddu, D., Balbo, P. E., Baricich, A., Zeppegno, P., Avanzi, G. C., Baldon, G., Bartolomei, G., Battaglia, M., Battistini, S., Binda, V., Borg, M., Cantaluppi, V., Castello, L. M., Clivati, E., Cisari, C., Costanzo, M., Croce, A., Cuneo, D., ... Pirisi, M. (2021). Respiratory and psychophysical sequelae among patients with COVID-19 four months after hospital discharge. *JAMA Network Open*, *4*(1), e2036142–e2036142. doi:10.1001/jamanetworkopen.2020.36142 PMID:33502487

Bogart, L. M., Ojikutu, B. O., Tyagi, K., Klein, D. J., Mutchler, M. G., Dong, L., ... Kellman, S. (2021). COVID-19 related medical mistrust, health impacts, and potential vaccine hesitancy among Black Americans living with HIV. *Journal of Acquired Immune Deficiency Syndromes, 86*(2), 200. doi:10.1097/QAI.0000000000002570

Burki, T. K. (2022). Omicron variant and booster COVID-19 vaccines. *The Lancet. Respiratory Medicine*, *10*(2), e17. doi:10.1016/S2213-2600(21)00559-2 PMID:34929158

Castrucci, M. R., Donatelli, I., Sidoli, L., Barigazzi, G., Kawaoka, Y., & Webster, R. G. (1993). Genetic reassortment between avian and human influenza A viruses in Italian pigs. *Virology*, *193*(1), 503–506. doi:10.1006/viro.1993.1155 PMID:8438586

CDC COVID-19 Response Team and Food & Drug Administration. (2021). Allergic reactions including anaphylaxis after receipt of the first dose of Moderna COVID-19 vaccine—United States, December 21, 2020–January 10, 2021. *Morbidity and Mortality Weekly Report*, *70*(4), 125–129. doi:10.15585/mmwr.mm7004e1 PMID:33507892

Crommelin, D. J., Anchordoquy, T. J., Volkin, D. B., Jiskoot, W., & Mastrobattista, E. (2021). Addressing the cold reality of mRNA vaccine stability. *Journal of Pharmaceutical Sciences*, *110*(3), 997–1001. doi:10.1016/j.xphs.2020.12.006 PMID:33321139

D'Adamo, H., Yoshikawa, T., & Ouslander, J. G. (2020). Coronavirus disease 2019 in geriatrics and long-term care: The ABCDs of COVID-19. *Journal of the American Geriatrics Society*, *68*(5), 912–917. doi:10.1111/jgs.16445 PMID:32212386

D'Ascanio, M., Innammorato, M., Pasquariello, L., Pizzirusso, D., Guerrieri, G., Castelli, S., Pezzuto, A., De vitis, C., Anibaldi, P., Marcolongo, A., Mancini, R., Ricci, A., & Sciacchitano, S. (2021). Age is not the only risk factor in COVID-19: The role of comorbidities and of long staying in residential care homes. *BMC Geriatrics*, *21*(1), 1–10. doi:10.118612877-021-02013-3 PMID:33451296

Danville Morning News. (1918, October 8). *Spanish flu: Old newspapers offer insight into modern pandemic*. https://www.mymcpl.org/blogs/spanish-flu-old-newspapers-offer-insight-modern-pandemic

Dawson, W. K., Lazniewski, M., & Plewczynski, D. (2018). RNA structure interactions and ribonucleoprotein processes of the influenza A virus. *Briefings in Functional Genomics*, *17*(6), 402–414. doi:10.1093/bfgp/elx028 PMID:29040388

de Jong, J. D., Claas, E. C. J., Osterhaus, A. D., Webster, R. G., & Lim, W. L. (1997). A pandemic warning? *Nature*, *389*(6651), 554–554. doi:10.1038/39218 PMID:9335492

Downar, J., & Seccareccia, D. (2010). Palliating a pandemic: "all patients must be cared for. *Journal of Pain and Symptom Management*, *39*(2), 291–295. doi:10.1016/j.jpainsymman.2009.11.241 PMID:20152591

Dürrwald, R., Krumbholz, A., Baumgarte, S., Schlegel, M., Vahlenkamp, T. W., Selbitz, H. J., Wutzler, P., & Zell, R. (2010). Swine influenza A vaccines, pandemic (H1N1) 2009 virus, and cross-reactivity. *Emerging Infectious Diseases*, *16*(6), 1029–1030. doi:10.3201/eid1606.100138 PMID:20507767

Feng, Z., Glasser, J. W., & Hill, A. N. (2020). On the benefits of flattening the curve: A perspective. *Mathematical Biosciences*, *326*, 108389. doi:10.1016/j.mbs.2020.108389 PMID:32473161

Ferguson, N. M., Cummings, D. A., Fraser, C., Cajka, J. C., Cooley, P. C., & Burke, D. S. (2006). Strategies for mitigating an influenza pandemic. *Nature*, *442*(7101), 448–452. doi:10.1038/nature04795 PMID:16642006

Fiani, B., Covarrubias, C., Desai, A., Sekhon, M., & Jarrah, R. (2020). A contemporary review of neurological sequelae of COVID-19. *Frontiers in Neurology*, *11*, 640. doi:10.3389/fneur.2020.00640 PMID:32655489

Ghiasi, N., Valizadeh, R., Arabsorkhi, M., Hoseyni, T. S., Esfandiari, K., Sadighpour, T., & Jahantigh, H. R. (2021). Efficacy and side effects of Sputnik V, Sinopharm and AstraZeneca vaccines to stop COVID-19; a review and discussion. *Immunopathologia Persa*, *7*(2), e31–e31. doi:10.34172/ipp.2021.31

Hao, F., Tam, W., Hu, X., Tan, W., Jiang, L., Jiang, X., Zhang, L., Zhao, X., Zou, Y., Hu, Y., Luo, X., McIntyre, R. S., Quek, T., Tran, B. X., Zhang, Z., Pham, H. Q., Ho, C. S. H., & Ho, R. C. (2020). A quantitative and qualitative study on the neuropsychiatric sequelae of acutely ill COVID-19 inpatients in isolation facilities. *Translational Psychiatry*, *10*(1), 1–14. doi:10.103841398-020-01039-2 PMID:33077738

Heath, P. T., Galiza, E. P., Baxter, D. N., Boffito, M., Browne, D., Burns, F., Chadwick, D. R., Clark, R., Cosgrove, C., Galloway, J., Goodman, A. L., Heer, A., Higham, A., Iyengar, S., Jamal, A., Jeanes, C., Kalra, P. A., Kyriakidou, C., McAuley, D. F., ... Toback, S. (2021). Safety and efficacy of NVX-CoV2373 Covid-19 vaccine. *The New England Journal of Medicine*, *385*(13), 1172–1183. Advance online publication. doi:10.1056/NEJMoa2107659 PMID:34192426

Howard, G., Bartram, J., Brocklehurst, C., Colford, J. M. Jr, Costa, F., Cunliffe, D., Dreibelbis, R., Eisenberg, J. N. S., Evans, B., Girones, R., Hrudey, S., Willetts, J., & Wright, C. Y. (2020). COVID-19: urgent actions, critical reflections and future relevance of 'WaSH': lessons for the current and future pandemics. *Journal of Water and Health*, *18*(5), 613–630. doi:10.2166/wh.2020.162 PMID:33095188

Huang, H. C., Araz, O. M., Morton, D. P., Johnson, G. P., Damien, P., Clements, B., & Meyers, L. A. (2017). Stockpiling ventilators for influenza pandemics. *Emerging Infectious Diseases*, *23*(6), 914–921. doi:10.3201/eid2306.161417 PMID:28518041

Jackson, C. (2009). History lessons: The Asian flu pandemic. *The British Journal of General Practice*, *59*(565), 622–623. doi:10.3399/bjgp09X453882 PMID:22751248

Kashte, S., Gulbake, A., El-Amin, S. F. III, & Gupta, A. (2021). COVID-19 vaccines: Rapid development, implications, challenges and future prospects. *Human Cell*, *34*(3), 711–733. doi:10.100713577-021-00512-4 PMID:33677814

Krause, J. C., Tumpey, T. M., Huffman, C. J., McGraw, P. A., Pearce, M. B., Tsibane, T., Hai, R., Basler, C. F., & Crowe, J. E. Jr. (2010). Naturally occurring human monoclonal antibodies neutralize both 1918 and 2009 pandemic influenza A (H1N1) viruses. *Journal of Virology*, *84*(6), 3127–3130. doi:10.1128/JVI.02184-09 PMID:20042511

Kutter, J. S., Spronken, M. I., Fraaij, P. L., Fouchier, R. A., & Herfst, S. (2018). Transmission routes of respiratory viruses among humans. *Current Opinion in Virology*, *28*, 142–151. doi:10.1016/j.coviro.2018.01.001 PMID:29452994

Lai, C. C., Wang, J. H., Ko, W. C., Yen, M. Y., Lu, M. C., Lee, C. M., & Hsueh, P. R. (2020). COVID-19 in long-term care facilities: An upcoming threat that cannot be ignored. *Journal of Microbiology, Immunology, and Infection*, *53*(3), 444–446. doi:10.1016/j.jmii.2020.04.008 PMID:32303483

Lansbury, L. E., Smith, S., Beyer, W., Karamehic, E., Pasic-Juhas, E., Sikira, H., Mateus, A., Oshitani, H., Zhao, H., Beck, C. R., & Nguyen-Van-Tam, J. S. (2017). Effectiveness of 2009 pandemic influenza A (H1N1) vaccines: A systematic review and meta-analysis. *Vaccine*, *35*(16), 1996–2006. doi:10.1016/j.vaccine.2017.02.059 PMID:28302409

Le, T. T., Andreadakis, Z., Kumar, A., Román, R. G., Tollefsen, S., Saville, M., & Mayhew, S. (2020). The COVID-19 vaccine development landscape. *Nature Reviews. Drug Discovery*, *19*(5), 305–306. doi:10.1038/d41573-020-00073-5 PMID:32273591

Levitt, A. F., & Ling, S. M. (2020). COVID-19 in the long-term care setting: The CMS perspective. *Journal of the American Geriatrics Society*, *68*(7), 1366–1369. doi:10.1111/jgs.16562 PMID:32406084

Lewnard, J. A., & Cobey, S. (2018). Immune History and Influenza Vaccine Effectiveness. *Vaccines*, *6*(2), 28. doi:10.3390/vaccines6020028 PMID:29883414

Lewnard, J. A., & Lo, N. C. (2020). Scientific and ethical basis for social-distancing interventions against COVID-19. *The Lancet. Infectious Diseases*, *20*(6), 631–633. doi:10.1016/S1473-3099(20)30190-0 PMID:32213329

Li, D., Wolk, D. M., & Cantor, M. N. (2020). Comparing clinical characteristics of influenza and common coronavirus infections using electronic health records. *The Journal of Infectious Diseases*. Advance online publication. doi:10.1093/infdis/jiaa626

Li, J., & Xu, G. (2020). Lessons from the experience in Wuhan to reduce risk of COVID-19 infection in patients undergoing long-term hemodialysis. *Clinical Journal of the American Society of Nephrology; CJASN*, *15*(5), 717–719. doi:10.2215/CJN.03420320 PMID:32241778

Lin, C. J., Mecham, R. P., & Mann, D. L. (2020). RNA vaccines for COVID-19: Five things every cardiologist should know. *Basic to Translational Science.*, *5*(12), 1240–1243. doi:10.1016/j.jacbts.2020.11.006 PMID:33251385

Liu, J. J., Bao, Y., Huang, X., Shi, J., & Lu, L. (2020). Mental health considerations for children quarantined because of COVID-19. *The Lancet. Child & Adolescent Health*, *4*(5), 347–349. doi:10.1016/S2352-4642(20)30096-1 PMID:32224303

Livingston, E. H. (2021). Necessity of 2 doses of the Pfizer and Moderna COVID-19 vaccines. *Journal of the American Medical Association*, *325*(9), 898–898. doi:10.1001/jama.2021.1375 PMID:33533893

Martini, M., Gazzaniga, V., Bragazzi, N. L., & Barberis, I. (2019). The Spanish Influenza Pandemic: A lesson from history 100 years after 1918. *Journal of Preventive Medicine and Hygiene*, *60*(1), E64–E67. doi:10.15167/2421-4248/jpmh2019.60.1.1205 PMID:31041413

Mills, C. E., Robins, J. M., & Lipsitch, M. (2004). Transmissibility of 1918 pandemic influenza. *Nature*, *432*(7019), 904–906. doi:10.1038/nature03063 PMID:15602562

Moghadami, M. (2017). A narrative review of influenza: A seasonal and pandemic disease. *Iranian Journal of Medical Sciences*, *42*(1), 2–13. PMID:28293045

Momattin, H., Al-Ali, A. Y., & Al-Tawfiq, J. A. (2019). A Systematic Review of therapeutic agents for the treatment of the Middle East Respiratory Syndrome Coronavirus (MERS-CoV). *Travel Medicine and Infectious Disease*, *30*, 9–18. doi:10.1016/j.tmaid.2019.06.012 PMID:31252170

Morse, S. S., Mazet, J. A., Woolhouse, M., Parrish, C. R., Carroll, D., Karesh, W. B., Zambrana-Torrelio, C., Lipkin, W. I., & Daszak, P. (2012). Prediction and prevention of the next pandemic zoonosis. *Lancet*, *380*(9857), 1956–1965. doi:10.1016/S0140-6736(12)61684-5 PMID:23200504

Muralidar, S., Ambi, S. V., Sekaran, S., & Krishnan, U. M. (2020). The emergence of COVID-19 as a global pandemic: Understanding the epidemiology, immune response and potential therapeutic targets of SARS-CoV-2. *Biochimie*, *179*, 85–100. doi:10.1016/j.biochi.2020.09.018 PMID:32971147

Murata, S., Rezeppa, T., Thoma, B., Marengo, L., Krancevich, K., Chiyka, E., Hayes, B., Goodfriend, E., Deal, M., Zhong, Y., Brummit, B., Coury, T., Riston, S., Brent, D. A., & Melhem, N. M. (2021). The psychiatric sequelae of the COVID-19 pandemic in adolescents, adults, and health care workers. *Depression and Anxiety*, *38*(2), 233–246. doi:10.1002/da.23120 PMID:33368805

Nichol, K. L., & Treanor, J. J. (2006). Vaccines for seasonal and pandemic influenza. *The Journal of Infectious Diseases*, *194*(s2), S111–S118. doi:10.1086/507544 PMID:17163383

Nishiura, H. (2010). Case fatality ratio of pandemic influenza. *The Lancet. Infectious Diseases*, *10*(7), 443–444. doi:10.1016/S1473-3099(10)70120-1 PMID:20610325

Pacheco, T. J. A., da Silva, V. C. M., & de Souza, D. G. (2020). Nano COVID-19 Vaccines: The firsts RNA lipid nanoparticle vaccines being approved from history-Review. *Research. Social Development*, *9*(12), e20191211123–e20191211123. doi:10.33448/rsd-v9i12.11123

Palamenghi, L., Barello, S., Boccia, S., & Graffigna, G. (2020). Mistrust in biomedical research and vaccine hesitancy: The forefront challenge in the battle against COVID-19 in Italy. *European Journal of Epidemiology*, *35*(8), 785–788. doi:10.100710654-020-00675-8 PMID:32808095

Paul, E., Steptoe, A., & Fancourt, D. (2021). Attitudes towards vaccines and intention to vaccinate against COVID-19: Implications for public health communications. *The Lancet Regional Health-Europe*, *1*, 100012. doi:10.1016/j.lanepe.2020.100012 PMID:33954296

Paul, R. (2020). Europe's essential workers: Migration and pandemic politics in Central and Eastern Europe during COVID-19. *European Policy Analysis*, *6*(2), 238–263. doi:10.1002/epa2.1105 PMID:34616908

Petersen, E., Koopmans, M., Go, U., Hamer, D. H., Petrosillo, N., Castelli, F., Storgaard, M., Al Khalili, S., & Simonsen, L. (2020). Comparing SARS-CoV-2 with SARS-CoV and influenza pandemics. *The Lancet. Infectious Diseases*, *20*(9), e238–e244. doi:10.1016/S1473-3099(20)30484-9 PMID:32628905

Qian, H., Miao, T., Liu, L., Zheng, X., Luo, D., & Li, Y. (2021, May). (2020). Indoor transmission of SARS-CoV-2. *Indoor Air*, *31*(3), 639–645. Advance online publication. doi:10.1111/ina.12766 PMID:33131151

Raveendran, A. V., Jayadevan, R., & Sashidharan, S. (2021). Long COVID: An overview. *Diabetes & Metabolic Syndrome*, *15*(3), 869–875. doi:10.1016/j.dsx.2021.04.007 PMID:33892403

Robson, C., Baskar, S. R., Booy, R., Ferguson, P. E., Gilroy, N., Kok, J., ... Dwyer, D. (2019). Influenza: Overview on prevention and therapy. *Australian Prescriber*, *42*(2), 51–55. doi:10.18773/austprescr.2019.013 PMID:31048938

Rogliani, P., Calzetta, L., Coppola, A., Puxeddu, E., Sergiacomi, G., D'Amato, D., & Orlacchio, A. (2020). Are there pulmonary sequelae in patients recovering from COVID-19? *Respiratory Research*, *21*(1), 1–4. doi:10.118612931-020-01550-6 PMID:33126869

Romer, D., & Jamieson, K. H. (2020). Conspiracy theories as barriers to controlling the spread of COVID-19 in the U.S. *Social Science & Medicine, 263*, 113356. doi:10.1016/j.socscimed.2020.113356

Roy, D. N., Biswas, M., Islam, E., & Azam, M. S. (2022). Potential factors influencing COVID-19 vaccine acceptance and hesitancy: A systematic review. *PLoS One*, *17*(3), e0265496. doi:10.1371/journal.pone.0265496 PMID:35320309

Shanks, G. D., & Brundage, J. F. (2013). Pacific islands which escaped the 1918–1919 influenza pandemic and their subsequent mortality experiences. *Epidemiology and Infection*, *141*(2), 353–356. doi:10.1017/S0950268812000866 PMID:22564320

Sharma, K., Koirala, A., Nicolopoulos, K., Chiu, C., Wood, N., & Britton, P. N. (2021). Vaccines for COVID-19: Where do we stand in 2021? *Paediatric Respiratory Reviews*, *39*, 22–31. doi:10.1016/j.prrv.2021.07.001 PMID:34362666

Shimabukuro, T., & Nair, N. (2021). Allergic reactions including anaphylaxis after receipt of the first dose of Pfizer-BioNTech COVID-19 vaccine. *JAMA Insights*, *325*(8), 780–781. doi:10.1001/jama.2021.0600 PMID:33475702

Shimabukuro, T. T., Cole, M., & Su, J. R. (2021). Reports of anaphylaxis after receipt of mRNA COVID-19 vaccines in the US—December 14, 2020-January 18, 2021. *JAMA Insights*, *325*(11), 1101–1102. doi:10.1001/jama.2021.1967 PMID:33576785

Simonsen, L., Spreeuwenberg, P., Lustig, R., Taylor, R. J., Fleming, D. M., Kroneman, M., Van Kerkhove, M. D., Mounts, A. W., & Paget, W. J. (2013). Global mortality estimates for the 2009 Influenza Pandemic from the GLaMOR project: A modeling study. *PLoS Medicine*, *10*(11), e1001558. doi:10.1371/journal.pmed.1001558 PMID:24302890

Stein, R. A., Ometa, O., Pachtman Shetty, S., Katz, A., Popitiu, M. I., & Brotherton, R. (2021). Conspiracy theories in the era of COVID-19: A tale of two pandemics. *International Journal of Clinical Practice*, *75*(2), e13778. doi:10.1111/ijcp.13778 PMID:33480171

Stockman, L. J., Bellamy, R., & Garner, P. (2006). SARS: Systematic review of treatment effects. *PLoS Medicine*, *3*(9), e343. doi:10.1371/journal.pmed.0030343 PMID:16968120

Subbarao, K., Murphy, B. R., & Fauci, A. S. (2006). Development of effective vaccines against pandemic influenza. *Immunity*, *24*(1), 5–9. doi:10.1016/j.immuni.2005.12.005 PMID:16413916

Tanne, J. H. (2021). Covid-19: Moderna plans booster doses to counter variants. *BMJ (Clinical Research Ed.)*, *372*(232), n232. doi:10.1136/bmj.n232 PMID:33500251

Taubenberger, J. K., & Morens, D. M. (2006). 1918 Influenza: The mother of all pandemics. *Emerging Infectious Diseases*, *12*(1), 15–22. doi:10.3201/eid1209.05-0979 PMID:16494711

Taubenberger, J. K., & Morens, D. M. (2008). The pathology of influenza virus infections. *Annual Review of Pathology*, *3*(1), 499–522. doi:10.1146/annurev.pathmechdis.3.121806.154316 PMID:18039138

Taylor, S., Landry, C. A., Paluszek, M. M., Groenewoud, R., Rachor, G. S., & Asmundson, G. J. (2020). A proactive approach for managing COVID-19: The importance of understanding the motivational roots of vaccination hesitancy for SARS-CoV2. *Frontiers in Psychology*, *11*, 2890. doi:10.3389/fpsyg.2020.575950 PMID:33192883

Tenforde, M. W., Olson, S. M., Self, W. H., Talbot, H. K., Lindsell, C. J., Steingrub, J. S., Shapiro, N. I., Ginde, A. A., Douin, D. J., Prekker, M. E., Brown, S. M., Peltan, I. D., Gong, M. N., Mohamed, A., Khan, A., Exline, M. C., Files, D. C., Gibbs, K. W., Stubblefield, W. B., ... Zunie, T. (2021). Effectiveness of Pfizer-BioNTech and Moderna vaccines against COVID-19 among hospitalized adults aged ≥65 years— United States, January–March 2021. *Morbidity and Mortality Weekly Report*, *70*(18), 674–679. doi:10.15585/mmwr.mm7018e1 PMID:33956782

Thompson, W. W., Shay, D. K., Weintraub, E., Brammer, L., Cox, N., Anderson, L. J., & Fukuda, K. (2003). Mortality associated with influenza and respiratory syncytial virus in the United States. *Journal of the American Medical Association*, *289*(2), 179–186. doi:10.1001/jama.289.2.179 PMID:12517228

Thunström, L., Newbold, S. C., Finnoff, D., Ashworth, M., & Shogren, J. F. (2020). The benefits and costs of using social distancing to flatten the curve for COVID-19. *Journal of Benefit-Cost Analysis*, *11*(2), 179–195. doi:10.1017/bca.2020.12

Tinari, S., & Riva, C. (2021). Covid-19: Whatever happened to the Novavax vaccine? *BMJ (Clinical Research Ed.)*, *375*, n2965. Advance online publication. doi:10.1136/bmj.n2965 PMID:34880071

Troyer, E. A., Kohn, J. N., & Hong, S. (2020). Are we facing a crashing wave of neuropsychiatric sequelae of COVID-19? Neuropsychiatric symptoms and potential immunologic mechanisms. *Brain, Behavior, and Immunity*, *87*, 34–39. doi:10.1016/j.bbi.2020.04.027 PMID:32298803

V'kovski, P., Kratzel, A., Steiner, S., Stalder, H., & Thiel, V. (2021). Coronavirus biology and replication: Implications for SARS-CoV-2. *Nature Reviews. Microbiology*, *19*(3), 155–170. doi:10.103841579-020-00468-6 PMID:33116300

van Eijk, L. E., Binkhorst, M., Bourgonje, A. R., Offringa, A. K., Mulder, D. J., Bos, E. M., ... van Goor, H. (2021). COVID-19: Immunopathology, pathophysiological mechanisms, and treatment options. *The Journal of Pathology*, *254*(4), 307–331. doi:10.1002/path.5642 PMID:33586189

Wadman, M. (2021). The overlooked superpower of mRNA vaccines. *Science*, *373*(6554), 479. doi:10.1126cience.373.6554.479 PMID:34326217

Wang, F., Kream, R. M., & Stefano, G. B. (2020). Long-Term Respiratory and Neurological Sequelae of COVID-19. *Medical Science Monitor*, *26*, e928996. doi:10.12659/MSM.928996 PMID:33177481

Wang, M., & Veit, M. (2016). Hemagglutinin-esterase-fusion (HEF) protein of influenza C virus. *Protein & Cell*, *7*(1), 28–45. doi:10.100713238-015-0193-x PMID:26215728

Wilson, N. M., Norton, A., Young, F. P., & Collins, D. W. (2020). Airborne transmission of severe acute respiratory syndrome coronavirus-2 to healthcare workers: A narrative review. *Anaesthesia*, *75*(8), 1086–1095. doi:10.1111/anae.15093 PMID:32311771

World Health Organization. (2022a, February). *MERS situation update, February 2022*. World Health Organization. http://www.emro.who.int/health-topics/mers-cov/mers-outbreaks.html

World Health Organization. (2022b, April 8). *WHO Coronavirus (COVID-19) Dashboard*. World Health Organization. https://covid19.who.int/

Chapter 8
Profile:
Malaria

ABSTRACT

This chapter will focus on malaria, which John Whitfield, writing for Nature, starkly labeled as a disease that "may have killed half of all the people that ever lived." This statistic has been criticized directly, and an alternative value of between four to five percent put forward. However, it is stubbornly difficult to clearly disprove, in part because humanity evolved in regions of Africa where malaria was endemic. Malaria seems to have impacted human genetics, as resistance was selected for, and continues to be a blight on large populations that cannot avoid malaria-carrying mosquitos.

INTRODUCTION

Malaria is protean. Malaria stems from protozoan parasites in the *Plasmodium* genus (Tuteja, 2007). These protozoans travel via mosquitos to larger organisms, and the lack of efficacious malaria vaccines, coupled with drug-resistant protozoans, and insecticide-resistant mosquitoes, collectively point to a very dangerous disease. How dangerous? In contemporary times, each year, there are approximately half a billion cases and one million deaths (Eckhoff, 2011). When examined cumulatively, throughout history, malaria is believed to be the single most deadly infectious disease to have ever impacted humanity (Faure, 2014). The genome of *Plasmodium* species has been examined (Howick et al., 2019). *Plasmodium* appears to be particularly available to both

DOI: 10.4018/978-1-7998-8689-1.ch008

selection pressures and genetic drift, creating a situation of high availability to evolution (Chang et al., 2013). The malaria parasite *Plasmodium knowlesi* exists as a zoonosis, and so can use non-human primates to substitute for humans in the relevant part of its lifecycle (Escalante & Pacheco, 2019). Zoonotic diseases exist in animal reservoirs outside of the human population, creating a special difficulty when attempting to repress or eradicate them. In the specific case of malaria, the existence of malarial parasites that rely on primates but are not known to affect humans is evidence for an ancestral co-evolutionary relationship between humans and malaria that ties to early human development in Africa. Other evidence is the existence of various hemoglobin structure and production disorders, including α+-thalassemia and sickle cell trait, that seem to be prevalent in humans because they are associated with malarial resistance (Williams, et al., 2005).

PATHOGENS AND BURDEN

Six species of malaria parasites are known to infect humans (Milner, 2018). These are *Plasmodium falciparum*, *Plasmodium vivax*, *Plasmodium ovale wallickeri*, *Plasmodium ovale curtisi*, *Plasmodium malariae*, and *Plasmodium knowlesi*. These species have an involved lifecycle that can involve more than ten morphological states, not all of which contribute to the symptoms of malaria. However, the interaction of the malarial pathogen with the human body can create a wide variety of symptoms, including fever, anemia, and coma. It is critical in understanding the nature of the malarial pathogen to note that most reproduction cycles of *Plasmodium* do not cause fatal results. Note from the numbers above that it takes 500 cases of malaria to result in 1 death. This case fatality rate may seem limited, and is less than the case fatality rate of approximately 0.5% that is associated with the influenza pandemic H1N1 which spread globally in 2009 (Nishiura, 2010). However, because of the huge number of cases that occur in areas infested with malaria-carrying mosquitos, the overall population toll is quite severe. Malaria's burden is greatest on children under the age of 5 who live in Africa--this group comprised the majority of fatal cases in 2012 (World Health Organization, 2013). *Plasmodium falciparum*, being both widespread and the most severe malarial pathogen, was responsible for 91% of these deaths. However, Africa has a great number of different climates, and it is specifically in tropical regions that the mosquitos are able to live and spread their parasites to humans (Giribaldi et al., 2014).

In malarial anemia, mortality greatly increases when hemoglobin is below 3 g/dL (White, 2018). Antimalarial drugs can significantly reduce nationwide cases of anemia. Malaria can complicate pregnancy (Brabin, 1983). In 1995, countries that counted as having intensive endemic malaria had overall income levels only one third as high as countries that did not have such malaria (Gallup & Sachs, 2001). Malaria is associated with poverty, decreased fertility and population growth, and deficits in savings, investment, and worker productivity (Sachs & Malaney, 2002). Mechanisms by which some of this occurs include absenteeism, medical spending, and early mortality. Exposure to malaria *in utero* and postnatal is associated with notably decreased educational attainment levels, and increased poverty rates (Barreca, 2010). Severe malaria causes devastating personal and economic complications (Chima et al., 2003). An estimate of the cost of a single case of malaria computed by combining data from Rwanda, the Solenzo medical district of Burkina Faso, the Mayo-Kebbi district, Chad, and the city of Brazzaville in Congo is twelve days of productivity (Shephard et al., 1991). Malaria prevalence not only reduces the rates of improvement in agricultural development, it also can be spread by certain agricultural practices (Asenso-Okyere et al., 2010).

Malaria has extensively interacted with the human genetic code. People who do not deal with malaria directly pay the price for the way the human body adapted to deal with malaria, in the absence of modern healthcare. Recall the genetics discussed above–the sickle hemoglobin allele, which can cause a blood disorder, appears to have spread because of its protective effect against malaria (Piel et al., 2010). In terms of the process of malaria, the major parasite *Plasmodium falciparum* creates significant changes in host red blood cells (Mohandas & An, 2012). Adhesiveness and permeability increase, and the cells are prone to destruction because of these membrane changes. Genetically-induced modifications of the nature of human blood throw up barriers to the *Plasmodium* lifecycle, at the cost of creating harm to humans that persist even when malarial exposure may be generations in the past.

THE MALARIA INFECTION

An expanded description of infection by malaria goes like this:

A human is bitten by a female mosquito of the genus *Anopheles* (Mawson, 2013; Giribaldi et al., 2014). Only female mosquitos take blood meals, and can be vectors. *Plasmodium* parasites, in a form known as the sporozoite, enter the human bloodstream. The sporozoites make their way to liver cells, and reproduce asexually for a week to ten days. Then, as merozoites, a new form, the parasites leave the liver cells inside structures known on vesicles, and go on a long journey. They head through the heart to capillaries in the lungs, and when the vesicles disintegrate, the parasites reenter the bloodstream, then enter a new type of cell, the erythrocytes (red blood cells). These cells in turn break apart under the weight of the invasion, and more invasions of erythrocytes follow. Clinical symptoms of malaria, such as fever, occur at this point, and are associated with erythrocyte rupture. However, the fever is an immune response, and is peripheral to the lifecycle of the *Plasmodium* parasites, which continues apace. Some of the infected cells in the bloodstream host *Plasmodium* parasites that turn into sexual forms, called gametocytes. These gametocytes can then enter an *Anopheles* mosquito when that mosquito bites a host human. The malarial lifecycle is not quite done at this point, however. Malaria might be a disease that affects humans, but *Plasmodium* parasites are involved with mosquitos, too. Once in mosquitos, the gametocytes develop into mature gametes, then ookinetes, and then oocysts, which are nestled into the mid-gut wall of their host *Anopheles*, and grow thousands of sporozoites inside themselves. When sporozoites should be ready, the oocyst they are growing in breaks open, and then the sporozoites travel to the salivary glands of the host mosquito, in the form and place they need to be in to head into a human that the mosquito bites. This is the full lifecycle.

What is particularly notable about this lifecycle is how the symptoms of malaria infection are peripheral to the actual malarial parasite, *Plasmodium*. *Plasmodium* does not require the illness of the human host, and the illness of the human host does not necessarily help any part of the *Plasmodium* lifecycle. True, in order to reproduce in the manner described above, *Plasmodium* parasites require mosquitoes to bite humans, require liver cells to enter, and do explosive damage to erythrocytes, but cells in the human body die for many reasons. That the number of erythrocytes killed by the *Plasmodium* lifecycle triggers a reaction that risks the health and life of the host body is not particularly useful to *Plasmodium*. After all, a deceased human cannot produce or sustain the liver cells or erythrocytes involved in the *Plasmodium* lifecycle. However, the harm done to the human body by the *Plasmodium* infection does not prevent the lifecycle. A human can be sick and dying while mosquitos do their work.

Since malaria is transmitted through mosquito bite, and not through the air, despite its name, understanding the mosquito is critical to understanding the impact of the disease. Of the approximately 460 *Anopheles* mosquito species, 68 can transmit malaria (Giribaldi et al., 2014). Transmission rates appear at their maximum when a person receives 200 infective bites annually. Even though the bite is necessary to spread the disease, mosquitoes are difficult to contain, and so, while malaria spread is naturally contained to areas where *Anopheles* mosquitoes are present, within those areas, spread may not be.

MALARIA, TRANSPORT, VIOLENCE, AND HISTORY

Malaria was a relevant factor in both the First and Second World Wars. In World War I, more than 1.5 million soldiers were affected by malaria, with case fatalities ranging from 0.2% to 5.0% (Brabin, 2014). Major epidemics occurred in Italy, Macedonia, Palestine, and Mesopotamia, fueled by the population movements associated with the war. Outbreaks of malaria did not go unnoticed, and efforts at containment and mitigation were put in place, ranging from nets to application of the drug quinine, but knowledge the *Plasmodium* parasite at that time was more limited than it is today, and the intensity of prevention efforts varied at a local and even individual level. That population movements caused by war create new opportunities for malaria to spread is something of a theme.

In World War II, United States troops in the south and southwest Pacific used nets to prevent mosquito spread of malaria (Joy, 1999). Quinine, at that point well-known to be a treatment for malaria, was, in March 1942, suddenly made a much scarcer commodity when the Japanese invaded the Dutch East Indies, in what is now modern Indonesia (Worthen, 1996). The desire for resources that spurred the Japanese push south led to a situation where the Allies were now deprived of a relevant resource. The United States had stockpiled large amounts of quinine and the cinchona tree that helps produce it, but the requirements of the war theaters exceeded this stockpile. North Africa, the Pacific, Europe, and the area around Southeast Asia all had regions where malaria was present, and these were nearly the full list of regions that saw combat during the war. As a result, Allied scientists worked to develop substitutes to manage one of the many risks in the ongoing fighting (Bechtold et al., 2021; Worthen, 1996) The United States devoted substantial military research to try to find a good solution (Condon-Rall, 1994). While a synthetic called atabrine was deployed in time to make an impact on the war, one major side effect was causing skin to turn a yellow color, which was seized on by Japanese propaganda, as the Japanese had a military interest during the war in keeping the Allied forces as weak as possible (Ockenhouse, 2005). With the coloration effect of atabrine a useful hook to create noncompliance--rumors became rampant that the drug caused impotence--the U.S. military continued to work on alternatives. Eventually, more antimalarial drugs emerged--chloroquine, amodiaquine, primaquine, proguanil, and pyrimethamine.

Malaria may have had more influence on the course of wars than any other infectious disease, including inflicting casualties when Napoleon was defending at Walcheren, when the Union was attempting to take the Mississippi River during the American Civil War, when U.S. marines were present on Guadalchanal and Efate during the Second World War, and during strife in Liberia in 2003 (Ockenhouse et al., 2005). The displacements that occurred during World War Two in the Pacific increased the burden of malaria on native Melanesians (Bennett, 2006).

More broadly, malaria, like many diseases, was empowered by the spread of human interactions, in places like West Africa (Gale, 1982; Bond, 2018). However, humans have fought back. The way in which malaria acted as an additional player in the Second World War, in places like New Guinea, is one more indication of the complexity.

TREATMENTS

One of the major drugs discovered as effective against malaria is quinine, the properties of which were documented about 400 years ago by Jesuit priests (Achan et al., 2011). However, quinine has poor tolerability and it is hard to get recipients to follow complicated dosing rules.

Beyond quinine, artemisinin was found in the annals of traditional Chinese medicine as a drug with good treatment properties against malaria, following a research drive by the Chinese government that began in the late 1960s (Wang et al., 2019). Artemisinin and drug derivatives, called ARTs, kill parasites through protein damage, and by interfering with proteasome activity (Bridgeford et al., 2018) Malaria nets continue to be an important tool in the fight against the disease, particularly insecticide nets (Pryce et al., 2018), and notably in parts of Africa, including the Gambia, where malaria is widespread and children are susceptible (Killeen et al., 2007; Snow et al., 1988) In Benin, another part of West Africa, malaria nets are used to help in areas with emerging resistance (N'Guessan et al., 2007). The use of malaria nets for purposes other than keeping away mosquitos, like fishing, highlights the critical role of social context in fighting the disease in spaces where economics may also be a matter of life and death (Gettleman, 2015).

In the context of other major infectious diseases, like smallpox and plague, malaria seems to have persisted in a much more significant way into the modern day. Smallpox has been effectively eliminated via international effort at vaccination. Plague still circulates, but with modern antibiotic treatments, is much less threatening than in places and times when it could run over a quarter of a continent's population. Combined with the epidemic nature of plague's spread in the times of its greatest devastation, malaria is still endemic, which makes it less of a difference from normal, and thus less of a show for the headlines, but malaria is still a critical front on the battle to improve the human condition. In the early 1960s, malaria was almost ended in India, but shortages in the poisonous pesticide DDT helped it reemerge (Sharma, 1996). In Brazil, rapid settlement of the Amazon led to a rise in malaria cases, 83.7% from *Plasmodium vivax*, and 16.3% from *Plasmodium falciparum* (Oliveira-Ferreira et al., 2010) Malaria is still deadly in South America into the twenty-first century, with an apparent rise, commensurably, of glucose-6-phosphate dehydrogenase deficiency, a detrimental condition in non-malarial circumstances which is encouraged by mutation that seems to help humans resist malaria (Recht et al., 2017).

Into the future, control of the *Anopheles* mosquitoes that spread malaria will continue to be important in controlling the disease (Benelli & Beier, 2017). Malaria parasites can and do acquire artemisinin resistance through mutations in the Pfk13 gene (Zhu et al., 2018). Cambodia in 2008 through 2013 saw the spread of the multidrug resistant lineage of *Plasmodium falciparum*--KEL1/PLA1 (Hamilton et al., 2019). This resistance highlights the importance of finding new drugs to supplement the current standard of Artemisinin combination therapy (ACT), including drugs that target aspartic proteases (Favuzza et al., 2020). Meanwhile, mosquitoes that carry the malarial parasite can and do become resistant to insecticides as well, highlighting the importance of a multipronged strategy (Antonio-Nkondjio et al., 2017). Using gene drives, which spread a trait throughout a population, would unleash a powerfully dangerous tool that might weaken or reduce the numbers of malaria-carrying mosquitos (Hoermann et al., 2021; Hammond et al., 2017). However, work still needs to be done to develop this tool, and clarify its ethical implications.

REFERENCES

Achan, J., Talisuna, A. O., Erhart, A., Yeka, A., Tibenderana, J. K., Baliraine, F. N., Rosenthal, P. J., & D'Alessandro, U. (2011). Quinine, an old anti-malarial drug in a modern world: Role in the treatment of malaria. *Malaria Journal, 10*(1), 1–12. doi:10.1186/1475-2875-10-144 PMID:21609473

Antonio-Nkondjio, C., Sonhafouo-Chiana, N., Ngadjeu, C. S., Doumbe-Belisse, P., Talipouo, A., Djamouko-Djonkam, L., Kopya, E., Bamou, R., Awono-Ambene, P., & Wondji, C. S. (2017). Review of the evolution of insecticide resistance in main malaria vectors in Cameroon from 1990 to 2017. *Parasites & Vectors, 10*(1), 1–14. doi:10.118613071-017-2417-9 PMID:29017590

Asenso-Okyere, K., Asante, F. A., Tarekegn, J., & Andam, K. S. (2011). A review of the economic impact of malaria in agricultural development. *Agricultural Economics, 42*(3), 293–304. doi:10.1111/j.1574-0862.2010.00515.x

Barreca, A. I. (2010). The long-term economic impact of in utero and postnatal exposure to malaria. *The Journal of Human Resources, 45*(4), 865–892. doi:10.3368/jhr.45.4.865

Bechtold, H. D., Cruz, A. T., & Kaziny, B. D. (2021). From World War II to COVID-19: A Historical Perspective on the American Medical Supply Chain. *Disaster Medicine and Public Health Preparedness, 1-4*, 1–2. Advance online publication. doi:10.1017/dmp.2021.94 PMID:33762064

Benelli, G., & Beier, J. C. (2017). Current vector control challenges in the fight against malaria. *Acta Tropica, 174*, 91–96. doi:10.1016/j.actatropica.2017.06.028 PMID:28684267

Bennett, J. A. (2006). Malaria, medicine, and Melanesians: Contested hybrid spaces in World War II. *Health and History, 8*(1), 27–55. doi:10.1353/hah.2006.0017

Bond, G. (2018). "Love Him and Let Him Go": The American Colonization Society's James Brown—Pioneering African-American apothecary in the United States and Liberia, 1802-1853, Part II—Liberia. *Pharmacy in History, 60*(4), 124–141. doi:10.26506/pharmhist.60.4.0124

Brabin, B. J. (1983). An analysis of malaria in pregnancy in Africa. *Bulletin of the World Health Organization, 61*(6), 1005–1016. PMID:6370484

Brabin, B. J. (2014). Malaria's contribution to World War One - the unexpected adversary. *Malaria Journal, 13*(1), 497. doi:10.1186/1475-2875-13-497 PMID:25515618

Bridgford, J. L., Xie, S. C., Cobbold, S. A., Pasaje, C. F. A., Herrmann, S., Yang, T., Gillett, D. L., Dick, L. R., Ralph, S. A., Dogovski, C., Spillman, N. J., & Tilley, L. (2018). Artemisinin kills malaria parasites by damaging proteins and inhibiting the proteasome. *Nature Communications, 9*(1), 1–9. doi:10.103841467-018-06221-1 PMID:30228310

Chang, H. H., Moss, E. L., Park, D. J., Ndiaye, D., Mboup, S., Volkman, S. K., Sabeti, P. C., Wirth, D. F., Neafsey, D. E., & Hartl, D. L. (2013). Malaria life cycle intensifies both natural selection and random genetic drift. *Proceedings of the National Academy of Sciences of the United States of America, 110*(50), 20129–20134. doi:10.1073/pnas.1319857110 PMID:24259712

Chima, R. I., Goodman, C. A., & Mills, A. (2003). The economic impact of malaria in Africa: A critical review of the evidence. *Health Policy (Amsterdam), 63*(1), 17–36. doi:10.1016/S0168-8510(02)00036-2 PMID:12468115

Condon-Rall, M. E. (1994). The Army's war against malaria: Collaboration in drug research during World War II. *Armed Forces and Society, 21*(1), 129–143. doi:10.1177/0095327X9402100108

DeMichele. (2016, December 7). *Malaria killed half the people who have ever lived. Fact/Myth.* http://factmyth.com/factoids/malaria-killed-half-the-people-who-have-ever-lived/

Eckhoff, P. A. (2011). A malaria transmission-directed model of mosquito life cycle and ecology. *Malaria Journal, 10*(1), 1–17. doi:10.1186/1475-2875-10-303 PMID:21999664

Escalante, A. A., & Pacheco, M. A. (2019). Malaria Molecular Epidemiology: An Evolutionary Genetics Perspective. *Microbiology Spectrum, 7*(4), doi:10.1128/microbiolspec.AME-0010-2019

Faure, E. (2014). Malarial pathocoenosis: Beneficial and deleterious interactions between malaria and other human diseases. *Frontiers in Physiology, 5*, 441. doi:10.3389/fphys.2014.00441 PMID:25484866

Favuzza, P., de Lera Ruiz, M., Thompson, J. K., Triglia, T., Ngo, A., Steel, R. W., Vavrek, M., Christensen, J., Healer, J., Boyce, C., Guo, Z., Hu, M., Khan, T., Murgolo, N., Zhao, L., Penington, J. S., Reaksudsan, K., Jarman, K., Dietrich, M. H., ... Cowman, A. F. (2020). Dual plasmepsin-targeting antimalarial agents disrupt multiple stages of the malaria parasite life cycle. *Cell Host & Microbe*, *27*(4), 642–658. doi:10.1016/j.chom.2020.02.005 PMID:32109369

Gale, T. (1982). Hygeia and Empire: The Impact of Disease on the Coming of Colonial Rule in British West Africa. *Transafrican Journal of History, 11*, 80-91. https://www.jstor.org/stable/24328534

Gallup, J. L., & Sachs, J. D. (2001). The economic burden of malaria. *The American Journal of Tropical Medicine and Hygiene*, *64*(1), 85–96. doi:10.4269/ajtmh.2001.64.85 PMID:11425181

Gettleman, J. (2015, January 24). *Meant to keep malaria out, mosquito nets are used to haul fish in*. https://www.nytimes.com/2015/01/25/world/africa/mosquito-nets-for-malaria-spawn-new-epidemic-overfishing.html

Giribaldi, G., D'Alessandro, S., Prato, M., & Basilico, N. (2014). Etiopathogenesis and pathophysiology of malaria. *Human and Mosquito Lysozymes: Old Molecules for New Approaches Against Malaria*, 1–18. doi:10.1007/978-3-319-09432-8_1

Hamilton, W. L., Amato, R., van der Pluijm, R. W., Jacob, C. G., Quang, H. H., Thuy-Nhien, N. T., Hien, T. T., Hongvanthong, B., Chindavongsa, K., Mayxay, M., Huy, R., Leang, R., Huch, C., Dysoley, L., Amaratunga, C., Suon, S., Fairhurst, R. M., Tripura, R., Peto, T. J., ... Miotto, O. (2019). Evolution and expansion of multidrug-resistant malaria in southeast Asia: A genomic epidemiology study. *The Lancet. Infectious Diseases*, *19*(9), 943–951. doi:10.1016/S1473-3099(19)30392-5 PMID:31345709

Hammond, A. M., Kyrou, K., Bruttini, M., North, A., Galizi, R., Karlsson, X., ... Nolan, T. (2017). The creation and selection of mutations resistant to a gene drive over multiple generations in the malaria mosquito. *PLoS Genetics, 13*(10). doi:10.1371/journal.pgen.1007039

Hoermann, A., Tapanelli, S., Capriotti, P., Del Corsano, G., Masters, E. K., Habtewold, T., Christophides, G. K., & Windbichler, N. (2021). Converting endogenous genes of the malaria mosquito into simple non-autonomous gene drives for population replacement. *eLife*, *10*, e58791. doi:10.7554/eLife.58791 PMID:33845943

Howick, V. M., Russell, A. J., Andrews, T., Heaton, H., Reid, A. J., Natarajan, K., Butungi, H., Metcalf, T., Verzier, L. H., Rayner, J. C., Berriman, M., Herren, J. K., Billker, O., Hemberg, M., Talman, A. M., & Lawniczak, M. K. (2019). The Malaria Cell Atlas: Single parasite transcriptomes across the complete Plasmodium life cycle. *Science*, *365*(6455), eaaw2619. Advance online publication. doi:10.1126cience.aaw2619 PMID:31439762

Joy, R. J. (1999). Malaria in American troops in the south and southwest Pacific in World War II. *Medical History*, *43*(2), 192–207. doi:10.1017/S002572730006508X PMID:10885139

Killeen, G. F., Smith, T. A., Ferguson, H. M., Mshinda, H., Abdulla, S., Lengeler, C., & Kachur, S. P. (2007). Preventing childhood malaria in Africa by protecting adults from mosquitoes with insecticide-treated nets. *PLoS Medicine*, *4*(7), e229. doi:10.1371/journal.pmed.0040229 PMID:17608562

Mawson, A. R. (2013). The pathogenesis of malaria: A new perspective. *Pathogens and Global Health*, *107*(3), 122–129. doi:10.1179/2047773213Y.0000000084 PMID:23683366

Milner, D. A. Jr. (2018). Malaria pathogenesis. *Cold Spring Harbor Perspectives in Medicine*, *8*(1), a025569. doi:10.1101/cshperspect.a025569 PMID:28533315

Mohandas, N., & An, X. (2012). Malaria and human red blood cells. *Medical Microbiology and Immunology*, *201*(4), 593–598. doi:10.100700430-012-0272-z PMID:22965173

N'Guessan, R., Corbel, V., Akogbéto, M., & Rowland, M. (2007). Reduced efficacy of insecticide-treated nets and indoor residual spraying for malaria control in pyrethroid resistance area, Benin. *Emerging Infectious Diseases*, *13*(2), 199–206. doi:10.3201/eid1302.060631 PMID:17479880

Nishiura, H. (2010). Case fatality ratio of pandemic influenza. *The Lancet. Infectious Diseases*, *10*(7), 443–444. doi:10.1016/S1473-3099(10)70120-1 PMID:20610325

Ockenhouse, C. F., Magill, A., Smith, D., & Milhous, W. (2005). History of US military contributions to the study of malaria. *Military Medicine*, *170*(4S), 12–16. doi:10.7205/MILMED.170.4S.12 PMID:15916279

Oliveira-Ferreira, J., Lacerda, M. V., Brasil, P., Ladislau, J. L., Tauil, P. L., & Daniel-Ribeiro, C. T. (2010). Malaria in Brazil: An overview. *Malaria Journal*, *9*(1), 1–15. doi:10.1186/1475-2875-9-115 PMID:20433744

Piel, F. B., Patil, A. P., Howes, R. E., Nyangiri, O. A., Gething, P. W., Williams, T. N., Weatherall, D. J., & Hay, S. I. (2010). Global distribution of the sickle cell gene and geographical confirmation of the malaria hypothesis. *Nature Communications*, *1*(1), 1–7. doi:10.1038/ncomms1104 PMID:21045822

Pomeroy, R. (2019, October 3). *Has malaria really killed half of everyone who ever lived?* RealClearScience. https://www.realclearscience.com/blog/2019/10/03/has_malaria_really_killed_half_of_everyone_who_ever_lived.html

Pryce, J., Richardson, M., & Lengeler, C. (2018). Insecticide-treated nets for preventing malaria. *Cochrane Database of Systematic Reviews*, (11). Advance online publication. doi:10.1002/14651858.CD000363.pub3 PMID:30398672

Recht, J., Siqueira, A. M., Monteiro, W. M., Herrera, S. M., Herrera, S., & Lacerda, M. V. (2017). Malaria in Brazil, Colombia, Peru and Venezuela: Current challenges in malaria control and elimination. *Malaria Journal*, *16*(1), 1–18. doi:10.118612936-017-1925-6 PMID:28676055

Roy, K. K. (2017). Targeting the active sites of malarial proteases for antimalarial drug discovery: Approaches, progress and challenges. *International Journal of Antimicrobial Agents*, *50*(3), 287–302. doi:10.1016/j.ijantimicag.2017.04.006 PMID:28668681

Sachs, J., & Malaney, P. (2002). The economic and social burden of malaria. *Nature*, *415*(6872), 680–685. doi:10.1038/415680a PMID:11832956

Sharma, V. P. (1996). Re-emergence of malaria in India. *The Indian Journal of Medical Research*, *103*, 26–45. PMID:8926025

Shepard, D. S., Ettling, M. B., Brinkmann, U., & Sauerborn, R. (1991). The economic cost of malaria in Africa. [*Tropical Medicine and Parasitology*, *42*(3), 199–203. PMID:1801147

Snow, R. W., Lindsay, S. W., Hayes, R. J., & Greenwood, B. M. (1988). Permethrin-treated bed nets (mosquito nets) prevent malaria in Gambian children. *Transactions of the Royal Society of Tropical Medicine and Hygiene*, *82*(6), 838–842. doi:10.1016/0035-9203(88)90011-9 PMID:2908286

Tuteja, R. (2007). Malaria– an overview. *The FEBS Journal*, *274*(18), 4670–4679. doi:10.1111/j.1742-4658.2007.05997.x PMID:17824953

Wang, J., Xu, C., Wong, Y. K., Li, Y., Liao, F., Jiang, T., & Tu, Y. (2019). Artemisinin, the magic drug discovered from traditional Chinese medicine. *Engineering*, *5*(1), 32–39. doi:10.1016/j.eng.2018.11.011

White, N. J. (2018). Anaemia and malaria. *Malaria Journal*, *17*(1), 1–17. doi:10.118612936-018-2509-9 PMID:30340592

Whitfield, J. (2002, October 3). Portrait of a serial killer: A round up of the history and biology of the malaria parasite. *Nature*. https://www.nature.com/news/2002/021001/full/news021001-6.html doi:10.1038/news021001-6

Williams, T. N., Mwangi, T. W., Wambua, S., Peto, T. E., Weatherall, D. J., Gupta, S., Recker, M., Penman, B. S., Uyoga, S., Macharia, A., Mwacharo, J. K., Snow, R. W., & Marsh, K. (2005). Negative epistasis between the malaria-protective effects of α+-thalassemia and the sickle cell trait. *Nature Genetics*, *37*(11), 1253–1257. doi:10.1038/ng1660 PMID:16227994

World Health Organization. (2013). *World Malaria Report: 2013*. WHO library cataloguing-in-publication data. http://apps.who.int/iris/bitstream/10665/97008/1/9789241564694_eng.pdf

Worthen, D. B. (1996). The national quinine pool: When quinine went to war. *Pharmacy in History*, *38*(3), 143–147. https://www.jstor.org/stable/41111763 PMID:11618891

Zhu, L., Tripathi, J., Rocamora, F. M., Miotto, O., van der Pluijm, R., Voss, T. S., Mok, S., Kwiatkowski, D. P., Nosten, F., Day, N. P. J., White, N. J., Dondorp, A. M., & Bozdech, Z. (2018). The origins of malaria artemisinin resistance defined by a genetic and transcriptomic background. *Nature Communications*, *9*(1), 1–13. doi:10.103841467-018-07588-x PMID:30514877

Chapter 9
Profile:
Tuberculosis

ABSTRACT

Tuberculosis, once commonly called consumption, may have killed one in seven people who ever lived. Tuberculosis is driven by a bacterial pathogen that largely transmits by air. The disease itself is notable for extended chronic cases featuring long periods of quiescence, where the pathogen is blockaded in granulomas established with the aid of the human immune system. While reactivation is rare, the sheer number of individuals who are infected with this disease worldwide—about two billion people—means that even this rareness is enough to cause an immense human toll. Because of the chronic nature of tuberculosis, those who have weakened immune systems for any reason are at particular risk of an adverse outcome.

INTRODUCTION

Tuberculosis is linked to the pathogen *Mycobacterium tuberculosis* (Adigun & Signh, 2020). While the disease concentrates its effect on the lungs, it can spread across the various organ systems of the body, and has been responsible for significant mortality in the human population since ancient times, with signs of infection found on remains thousands of years old. *M. tuberculosis* does not have a known reservoir outside of circulation in humans. However, it has an effective pattern of infiltration. In a standard pattern, *M. tuberculosis* spreads to humans via aerosol, entering the lungs and being ingested by

DOI: 10.4018/978-1-7998-8689-1.ch009

alveolar macrophages (Ehlers & Schaible, 2013). These macrophages are unable to destroy the bacteria, and, by being enveloped, the bacteria are safe from many common immune responses. This leads to a system of intracellular infection, replication, and spread. An additional complication comes in the form of a peculiar intermediate stage common during a tuberculosis infection. This involves the formation of quiescent granulomas--aggregates of immune cells surrounding the pathogen--that are formed by a sort of stalemate of *M. tuberculosis* survival and reproduction efforts, and the human immune response. On the one hand, pathogen bacilli only reactivate in about 10% of latent cases (Silva Miranda et al., 2012). On the other hand, *M. tuberculosis* are able to leverage granuloma formation enough to take advantage of how necrotizing granulomas migrate into bronchial cavities, so that, upon disease reactivation, the bacteria will be that much more able to carry on their lifecycle (Ehlers & Schaible, 2013). Réactivation becomes more likely under a wide variety of stressors, including high risk factors like human immunodeficiency virus, organ transplantation, silicosis, tumor necrosis factor-alpha blockers, close contact with individuals who have pulmonary tuberculosis, and kidney dialysis, as well as smoking and being underweight (Ai et al., 2016). Contemporary reactivation rates in data collected in the United States for reactivation of latent tuberculosis infection are estimated at 0.084 cases per 100 person-years (Shea et al., 2014). The standard model of tuberculosis transmission is through the respiratory tract, where a host releases contagious bacili through a mechanism such as coughing (Turner et al., 2017).

TRANSMISSION, BURDEN, AND TREATMENT

How does tuberculosis transmit? Tuberculosis is an urban disease that spreads effectively in crowded conditions (Riberio et al., 2015). Individuals who have active laryngeal or pulmonary tuberculosis transmit aerosols through coughing, singing, shouting, sneezing, or other active airway uses that push respiratory secretions (Churchyard et al., 2017). Despite the variety of developments in medicine that have occurred throughout the intertwined history of tuberculosis and the human species, distancing and ventilation measures in all their forms are still some of the most powerful tools available to decrease disease incidence. In an oddly concrete sense, the disease cannot transmit in the presence of "fresh air," if fresh air is defined as air without the presence of *M. tuberculosis* pathogen or aerosol. In sufficient conditions, tuberculosis transmission is stymied by the presence of ultraviolet light, which has a germicidal quality (Mamahlodi, 2019).

What does tuberculosis burden actually look like? Around 5,000 tuberculosis cases occur daily, 95% of which occur in countries classified as low- or middle income (Abdulkader et al., 2019). The pathogen behind tuberculosis is constantly changing, and does not exist in a vacuum. Drug-resistant tuberculosis is becoming increasingly relevant, and HIV increases disease burden associated with tuberculosis. Ethiopia is a country with a high burden of tuberculosis and multidrug resistant tuberculosis. In a recent study of tuberculosis and treatment in Northern Ethiopia presented by Abdulkader et al., 12.7% of those who received treatment were classified as cured, 4.1% died, and 76.7% concluded with a status of "treatment complete," emphasizing the difficulties in eradicating tuberculosis from the body, as well as the ways it can go dormant. In this research, 18.8% of patients had HIV/tuberculosis co-infection, compared to the national average at the same time of 10.7%. While the HIV/tuberculosis co-infection rate seen in the study was high for Ethiopia overall, it is less than parts of Ethiopia and other countries, such as Cameroon, which are attempting to manage tuberculosis. The key idea here is that HIV infection weakens the immune system, both through depletion of $CD4^{+}$ T cells and collateral effects (Esmail et al., 2018).

What tuberculosis treatments exist? There are a variety of different complex drug cocktails that have been developed or are in use, issued daily at different levels depending on whether treatment is in an intensive phase, or a maintenance phase (Rabahi et al., 2017). Major drugs that can be included in the cocktail include rifampin, isoniazid, and pyrazinamide, and this particular triple, known as the RHZ regimen, was developed in the 1970s. In 2009, Brazil began to use fixed-dose combination tablets, and added the drug ethambutol to the cocktail. This change was motivated by an increase in primary resistance to isoniazid from 4.4% to 6.0%. For patients with meningitis due to tuberculosis, treatment is different, and commonly includes the oral corticosteroid prednisone, or the IV corticosteroid dexamethasone. The expanded RHZE cocktail is known and used outside of Brazil as well, including in the United States (Olson et al., 2019).

HISTORY AND TUBERCULOSIS

While the future of tuberculosis likely involves continuing efforts at improving treatment and eradication efforts, the past of tuberculosis connects with history in meaningful ways. With almost two billion humans infected in *M. tuberculosis* estimated worldwide, how could it not (Barberis et al., 2017)? Tuberculosis appears to have co-evolved with humanity in Africa. It was present in Egypt, and mummies dating to 2400 BCE have skeletal deformities typical of tuberculosis, while old Egyptian art shows signs of tuberculosis-characteristic abnormalities like Pott's lesions. This indicates tuberculosis that has penetrated bone (Garg & Somvanshi, 2011). Writings about tuberculosis exist in Indian literature 3,300 years ago, and in Chinese literature 2,300 years ago (Barberis et al., 2017). The ancient Hebrew word *schachepheth* in Leviticus and Deuteronomy appears to describe tuberculosis. In Ancient Greece, the word appears to be Phthisis, which was described, clearly by its lung lesions, by the famous physician Hippocrates, who noted how its burden seemed to lie particularly on young adults. Research on tuberculosis in civilizations influenced by the Greek tradition did not stop after his death--other famous authors who wrote about this disease were Galen and Avicenna. By the time of the Middle Ages in Europe, a well-known form of tuberculosis was described as scrofula, which affected cervical lymph nodes, and was also called, in England and France, "king's evil." While Galen recommended fresh air, along with milk and sea voyages, as a treatment for tuberculosis--seeming equivalent to the idea of rest and relaxation--while Avicenna understood tuberculosis' contagious nature, scrofula was commonly considered to be curable by the touch of a monarch.

The idea that a powerful leader could cure a disease has a great deal of implications for the way humans understand history and power, and the fact that this treatment does not make sense by the standards of allopathic medicine should not interference with an understanding of why it could be believed, and how his belief could be propagated. If powerful leaders could fix or solve other ills, why not scrofula, or tuberculosis? Besides, tuberculosis had a way of being chronic but not always symptomatic, leaving opportunity for confusion for why a case had gone away. To make the story even clearer, consider reporting by William of Malesbury, a 12th century English historian who reported that treatments complementary to a direct "king's touch" could include visits to royal tombs or use of a coin as a talisman (Barberis et al., 2017). Two of these options would give those with tuberculosis a chance to attempt a royal cure, while helpfully preventing the actual monarch from being at risk of acquiring the disease from the petitioner.

This apparent false direction in the treatment of tuberculosis seems, however, to have been advanced at the same time that more allopathic-style understandings of the disease were also being propagated (Barberis et al., 2017). Guy de Chauliac, a French surgeon active around the time of the Black Death, considered an appropriate response to scrofula to be excision of the scrofulous gland itself. While this treatment may not be up to modern allopathic standards, in modern times, surgical interventions for peripheral lymph node tuberculosis can be a treatment of last resort for lymph nodes about to burst and antibiotics are insufficient (Lekhbal et al., 2020; Subrahmanyam, 1993).

As research, treatments, and cases of tuberculosis continued, so naturally did conversations surrounding the disease. Another term for tuberculosis used in the 1700s was 'consumption' (Barberis et al., 2017). In Western Europe in the 1700s, mortality from tuberculosis was as high as 900 per 100,000, even higher in the young. By around 1800, another particular name for tuberculosis was the "Captain of All These Men of Death," as tuberculosis increased to be so prevalent in Europe and North America as to have apparently been the cause of one in four deaths. In the mid-1800s, the actual term tuberculosis was coined by Johann Lukas Schönlein, to displace consumption and phthisis. In that century, there was still great concern about tuberculosis' exact etiology. Into modern times, tuberculosis developed or maintained a stigmatic reputation as a disease of the dirty (Juniarti & Evans, 2011). Was it an infectious disease, as it was commonly considered in Southern Europe? Hereditary, as was a common belief in Northern Europe? Or was it a form of cancer? Scientific thinking did not lead immediately to full answers, as is clear when looking at the way back to systematic individuals like Hippocrates, Galen, and Ibn Sina.

A breakthrough came when Robert Koch was able to identify the bacillus at play, stain it with methylene blue, and use the bacterium to reproduce the disease in laboratory animals (Barberis et al., 2017). These results were presented to Berlin's Society of Physiology in 1882, providing more definitive answers to the mysteries of tuberculosis than had been available previously. Thereafter, skin tests, and drugs like streptomycin and then the RHZE cocktail were able to be developed and delivered.

To give a better sense of the burden of tuberculosis, it is worth making note of some of the famous people who died due to this condition. Andrew Jackson, seventh president of the United States, famous for his military victories and role in facilitating Native American expulsions from lands whites wished to occupy, appears to have died from tuberculosis in 1845. A wide variety of famous writers died from tuberculosis, including Jane Austen, sisters in prolific Brontë family, John Keats, Elizabeth Browning, Anton Chekov, Henry David Thoureau, and *1984* writer George Orwell, as well as the absurdists Albert Camus and Franz Kafka (Walters, 2017). By about 1800, tuberculosis is presumed to have killed around one out of seven people who ever lived. In Victorian Britain of the 1800s, tuberculosis reached such a peculiar part of the zeitgeist that symptomatic pallor and thinness were seen as signs of beauty among women (Roberts, 2020). Even at the more recent year of 1948, Muhammad Ali Jinnah, considered to be the founder of Pakistan, died from a complication of tuberculosis, a disease he carefully hid from his political opponents to help ensure the creation of his country (Collins & Lapierre, 1975, pp. 110–111).

What happened? Why did tuberculosis seem to rise to such a crescendo just before breakthroughs made by Robert Koch and others, and then, at least in certain important ways, start to become more manageable worldwide? It is reasonable to believe that the early phases of industrialization, as embodied by urban poverty, overcrowding, and the transportation networks that enable these tied the world increasingly together, contributed to an explosion of tuberculosis cases, while, as decades passed, improved understandings of the disease's nature lead to better treatments, hygiene, and the understanding of the importance of isolation of cases. The development of efficacious tuberculin testing, starting in the late nineteenth century with the help of the work of Robert Koch, likely also helped a great deal (Goldstein et al., 2002).

TUBERCULOSIS AND THE CONCEPT OF MODERNITY

As with many diseases, the relationship of tuberculosis with what is commonly thought of as modernity was not a simple pattern of increasing technological sophistication leading to improvements in outcomes. Certain hallmarks of modernity could increase the prevalence of the disease, and understanding who this is still true helps in understanding more about the places where it is still a common and heavy burden. Recall that level of development plays a role in the presence of disease, and notably, the story is not that less development strictly equates to more disease. Rather, it seems as if the process of "developing"--industrial concentration and networking outstripping hygiene--has a great deal to do with transmission.

The idea of partial modernity sustaining tuberculosis is not simple speculation. Newly effective transportation networks need not be linked to parallel developments in public health. There is evidence that the presence of modern public forms of transportation in South Africa, particularly minibus taxis, play an important role in spreading the disease (Andrews et al., 2013). Buses again were found as a particular risk factor in tuberculosis in Lima, Peru (Horna-Campos et al., 2007; Zamudio et al., 2015). City buses were seen as a risk factor in data from around the United States city of Houston (Feske et al., 2011). A metaanalysis clearly identified potential risk surrounding buses and trains, even if with the lack of concrete certainty that often characterizes ongoing research (Edelson & Phypers, 2011).

Despite the association of certain forms of modern transit that put individuals in close proximity with potential rises in cases of tuberculosis, it is also important to think of disease burden in terms of a broader spectrum of risk factors. There does not appear to have been a single intervention that brought tuberculosis cases to more manageable levels in certain regions. Rather, it perhaps can be said that there was a general "de-vulnerabilizing" impetus on a number of metrics that improved health in general, as well as specifically pertaining to tuberculosis. Remember that almost a fifth of cases in the Northern Ethiopian tuberculosis study cited above involved HIV occurring along with tuberculosis. Tuberculosis is a disease that can be suppressed in granulomas, but *M. tuberculosis* can escape granulomas, and it seems more likely to do so when the patient is in a state of vulnerability.

Work by Chan et al., shows that malnourished mice had weakened immune reactions in the context of tuberculosis infection, including weakened granulomatous reactions (1996). Notably, and as an interesting reinforcement of Galen's suggestion of a comfortable environment as a treatment for tuberculosis, the mice in question could have tuberculosis cases on an apparently progressively fatal course reversed by the restoration of a full protein diet (2% protein to 20% protein).

The idea of undernutrition as contributing to the burden of tuberculosis is borne out by more than just work with mice. Around 800 million individuals in the world are chronically undernourished, overwhelmingly (98%) in low- and middle-income countries, and it is apparent that the undernutrition in general weakens immune response to tuberculosis, promotes higher incidence of the disease, and worsens disease outcomes (Sinha et al., 2019). Stress itself may directly weaken immune response, which is particularly relevant to outcomes in a disease like tuberculosis, where, without treatment, in order to remain asymptomatic, patients need the granulomas encasing *M. tuberculosis* to be able to hold (Lerner, 1996). Elevated tuberculosis prevalence rates have been noted in refugee populations (Kimbrough et al., 2012). Illicit drug use is a risk factor for tuberculosis (Deiss et al., 2009).

Tuberculosis spreads and is limited in cycles of infection, transmission, and control, as do other infectious diseases (Gambhir et al., 2007). However, too much oversimplification may obscure the fact that each step of disease pathogen, and each step of responders, is mediated through specific factors. Stress, proximity to contagious individuals due to transportation, and weakened immune response do not combine to provide a complete picture of tuberculosis, but the mentioned elements do contribute to its burden on the global human population. Social factors and general immune factors naturally must interact with the specific nature of the bacterium *M. tuberculosis* itself, and effective treatments require an understanding of specific ways *M. tuberculosis* interacts with the human body, as well as specific points in its reproduction, self-maintenance, and general lifecycle that may be particularly suitable to be targeted by drugs or other interventions. However, tuberculosis does exist in a macro-context that goes beyond drug interventions and allied treatments. There is increasing awareness that *Mycobacterium bovis*, which is most commonly found in cattle and similar animals, also lays a tuberculosis burden on humans (Olea-Popelka et al., 2017). The ongoing fight to control the disease involves integration of all factors.

REFERENCES

Abdulkader, M., van Aken, I., Niguse, S., Hailekiros, H., & Spigt, M. (2019). Treatment outcomes and their trend among tuberculosis patients treated at peripheral health settings of Northern Ethiopia between 2009 and 2014: A registry-based retrospective analysis. *BMC Research Notes*, *12*(1), 786. doi:10.118613104-019-4824-9 PMID:31791388

Adigun, R., & Singh, R. (2020). *Tuberculosis, StatPearls. (2021 Jan-)*. StatPearls Publishing. https://www.ncbi.nlm.nih.gov/books/NBK441916/

Ai, J. W., Ruan, Q. L., Liu, Q. H., & Zhang, W. H. (2016). Updates on the risk factors for latent tuberculosis reactivation and their managements. *Emerging Microbes & Infections*, *5*(2), e10. doi:10.1038/emi.2016.10 PMID:26839146

Andrews, J. R., Morrow, C., & Wood, R. (2013). Modeling the role of public transportation in sustaining tuberculosis transmission in South Africa. *American Journal of Epidemiology*, *177*(6), 556–561. doi:10.1093/aje/kws331 PMID:23423215

Barberis, I., Bragazzi, N. L., Galluzzo, L., & Martini, M. (2017). The history of tuberculosis: From the first historical records to the isolation of Koch's bacillus. *Journal of Preventive Medicine and Hygiene*, *58*(1), E9–E12. PMID:28515626

Chan, J., Tian, Y., Tanaka, K. E., Tsang, M. S., Yu, K., Salgame, P., Carroll, D., Kress, Y., Teitelbaum, R., & Bloom, B. R. (1996). Effects of protein calorie malnutrition on tuberculosis in mice. *Proceedings of the National Academy of Sciences of the United States of America*, *93*(25), 14857–14861. doi:10.1073/pnas.93.25.14857 PMID:8962145

Churchyard, G., Kim, P., Shah, N. S., Rustomjee, R., Gandhi, N., Mathema, B., Dowdy, D., Kasmar, A., & Cardenas, V. (2017). What we know about tuberculosis transmission: An overview. *The Journal of Infectious Diseases*, *216*(suppl_6), S629–S635. doi:10.1093/infdis/jix362 PMID:29112747

Collins, L., & Lapierre, D. (1975). *Freedom at midnight*. Academic Press.

Deiss, R. G., Rodwell, T. C., & Garfein, R. S. (2009). Tuberculosis and illicit drug use: Review and update. *Clinical Infectious Diseases*, *48*(1), 72–82. doi:10.1086/594126 PMID:19046064

Edelson, P. J., & Phypers, M. (2011). TB transmission on public transportation: A review of published studies and recommendations for contact tracing. *Travel Medicine and Infectious Disease*, *9*(1), 27–31. doi:10.1016/j.tmaid.2010.11.001 PMID:21167784

Ehlers, S., & Schaible, U. E. (2013). The granuloma in tuberculosis: Dynamics of a host-pathogen collusion. *Frontiers in Immunology*, *3*, 411. doi:10.3389/fimmu.2012.00411 PMID:23308075

Esmail, H., Riou, C., du Bruyn, E., Lai, R. P. J., Harley, Y. X., Meintjes, G., Wilkinson, K. A., & Wilkinson, R. J. (2018). The immune response to Mycobacterium tuberculosis in HIV-1-coinfected persons. *Annual Review of Immunology*, *36*(1), 603–638. doi:10.1146/annurev-immunol-042617-053420 PMID:29490165

Feske, M. L., Teeter, L. D., Musser, J. M., & Graviss, E. A. (2011). Giving TB wheels: Public transportation as a risk factor for tuberculosis transmission. *Tuberculosis (Edinburgh, Scotland)*, *91*, S16–S23. doi:10.1016/j.tube.2011.10.005 PMID:22088323

Gambhir, M., Basáñez, M. G., Turner, F., Kumaresan, J., & Grassly, N. C. (2007). Trachoma: Transmission, infection, and control. *The Lancet. Infectious Diseases*, *7*(6), 420–427. doi:10.1016/S1473-3099(07)70137-8 PMID:17521595

Garg, R. K., & Somvanshi, D. S. (2011). Spinal tuberculosis: A review. *The Journal of Spinal Cord Medicine*, *34*(5), 440–454. doi:10.1179/2045772311Y.0000000023 PMID:22118251

Goldstein, E. J., Lee, E., & Holzman, R. S. (2002). Evolution and current use of the tuberculin test. *Clinical Infectious Diseases*, *34*(3), 365–370. doi:10.1086/338149 PMID:11774084

Horna-Campos, O. J., Sánchez-Pérez, H. J., Sánchez, I., Bedoya, A., & Martín, M. (2007). Public transportation and pulmonary tuberculosis, Lima, Peru. *Emerging Infectious Diseases*, *13*(10), 1491–1493. doi:10.3201/eid1310.060793 PMID:18257992

Juniarti, N., & Evans, D. (2011). A qualitative review: The stigma of tuberculosis. *Journal of Clinical Nursing*, *20*(13-14), 1961–1970. doi:10.1111/j.1365-2702.2010.03516.x PMID:21040040

Kimbrough, W., Saliba, V., Dahab, M., Haskew, C., & Checchi, F. (2012). The burden of tuberculosis in crisis-affected populations: A systematic review. *The Lancet. Infectious Diseases*, *12*(12), 950–965. doi:10.1016/S1473-3099(12)70225-6 PMID:23174381

Lekhbal, A., Chaker, K., Halily, S., Abada, R. L., Rouadi, S., Roubal, M., & Mahtar, M. (2020). Treatment of cervical lymph node tuberculosis: When surgery should be performed? A retrospective cohort study. *Annals of Medicine and Surgery (London)*, *55*, 159–163. doi:10.1016/j.amsu.2020.05.006 PMID:32489658

Lerner, B. H. (1996). Can stress cause disease? Revisiting the tuberculosis research of Thomas Holmes, 1949-1961. *Annals of Internal Medicine*, *124*(7), 673–680. doi:10.7326/0003-4819-124-7-199604010-00008 PMID:8607596

Mamahlodi, M. T. (2019). Potential benefits and harms of the use of UV radiation in transmission of tuberculosis in South African health facilities. *Journal of Public Health in Africa*, *10*(1), 742. doi:10.4081/jphia.2019.742 PMID:31285811

Olea-Popelka, F., Muwonge, A., Perera, A., Dean, A. S., Mumford, E., Erlacher-Vindel, E., Forcella, S., Silk, B. J., Ditiu, L., El Idrissi, A., Raviglione, M., Cosivi, O., LoBue, P., & Fujiwara, P. I. (2017). Zoonotic tuberculosis in human beings caused by Mycobacterium bovis—A call for action. *The Lancet. Infectious Diseases*, *17*(1), e21–e25. doi:10.1016/S1473-3099(16)30139-6 PMID:27697390

Olson, G., Nathavitharana, R. R., & Lederer, P. A. (2019). Diagnostic delays and treatment complications for patients with isoniazid-resistant tuberculosis: A case report and review of the literature. *Open Forum Infectious Diseases*, *6*(6), ofz222. Advance online publication. doi:10.1093/ofid/ofz222 PMID:31211162

Rabahi, M. F., Silva Júnior, J., Ferreira, A., Tannus-Silva, D., & Conde, M. B. (2017). Tuberculosis treatment. *Jornal Brasileiro de Pneumologia: Publicacao Oficial da Sociedade Brasileira de Pneumologia e Tisilogia*, *43*(6), 472–486. doi:10.1590/S1806-37562016000000388

Remini, R. V. (1980). The final days and hours in the life of General Andrew Jackson. *Tennessee Historical Quarterly*, *39*(2), 167–177. https://www.jstor.org/stable/42626070 PMID:11636099

Ribeiro, F. K. C., Pan, W., Bertolde, A., Vinhas, S. A., Peres, R. L., Riley, L., Palaci, M., & Maciel, E. L. (2015). Genotypic and spatial analysis of Mycobacterium tuberculosis transmission in a high-incidence urban setting. *Clinical Infectious Diseases*, *61*(5), 758–766. doi:10.1093/cid/civ365 PMID:25948063

Roberts, C. (2020). Fashionable but debilitating diseases: Tuberculosis past and present. In S. Sheridan & L. Gregoricka (Eds.), *Purposeful pain* (pp. 21–38). doi:10.1007/978-3-030-32181-9_2

Shea, K. M., Kammerer, J. S., Winston, C. A., Navin, T. R., & Horsburgh, C. R. Jr. (2014). Estimated rate of reactivation of latent tuberculosis infection in the United States, overall and by population subgroup. *American Journal of Epidemiology*, *179*(2), 216–225. doi:10.1093/aje/kwt246 PMID:24142915

Silva Miranda, M., Breiman, A., Allain, S., Deknuydt, F., & Altare, F. (2012). The tuberculous granuloma: An unsuccessful host defence mechanism providing a safety shelter for the bacteria? *Clinical & Developmental Immunology*, *139127*, 1–14. Advance online publication. doi:10.1155/2012/139127 PMID:22811737

Sinha, P., Davis, J., Saag, L., Wanke, C., Salgame, P., Mesick, J., Horsburgh, C. R. Jr, & Hochberg, N. S. (2019). Undernutrition and Tuberculosis: Public Health Implications. *The Journal of Infectious Diseases*, *219*(9), 1356–1363. doi:10.1093/infdis/jiy675 PMID:30476125

Springer, Cham. doi:10.1007/978-3-030-32181-9_2

Subrahmanyam, M. (1993). Role of surgery and chemotherapy for peripheral lymph node tuberculosis. *Journal of British Surgery*, *80*(12), 1547–1548. doi:10.1002/bjs.1800801218 PMID:8298921

Turner, R. D., Chiu, C., Churchyard, G. J., Esmail, H., Lewinsohn, D. M., Gandhi, N. R., & Fennelly, K. P. (2017). Tuberculosis infectiousness and host susceptibility. *The Journal of Infectious Diseases*, *216*(suppl_6), S636–S643. doi:10.1093/infdis/jix361 PMID:29112746

Waters, D. D. (2017). The rise and fall of tuberculosis and atherosclerosis: First there is a mountain…. *The Canadian Journal of Cardiology*, *33*(3), 295–297. doi:10.1016/j.cjca.2016.11.012 PMID:28081868

Zamudio, C., Krapp, F., Choi, H. W., Shah, L., Ciampi, A., Gotuzzo, E., Heymann, J., Seas, C., & Brewer, T. F. (2015). Public transportation and tuberculosis transmission in a high incidence setting. *PLoS One*, *10*(2), e0115230. doi:10.1371/journal.pone.0115230 PMID:25706530

Chapter 10
Profile:
Smallpox

ABSTRACT

This chapter will deal with smallpox, a disease which, in addition to playing a critical role in the history of the development of vaccination, also may have killed 300 million people in the 20th century alone, three times the estimated loss in that period from armed conflict. Smallpox is perhaps more emblematic than any other disease that was brought under control by science. This means understanding smallpox helps to clarify human disease response past and present. However, smallpox is a deadly disease in its own right, outside of context, and this fact drives all responses to it.

INTRODUCTION

Smallpox has a long history of being extremely deadly, with its more deadly pathogen, Variola major, killing as many as 30% of those infected (Voigt et al., 2016), or, in the twentieth century, 300 to 500 million alone (Alcamí, 2020). The practice of inoculation, ancient, stands as one of the clearest examples in medical science of the long social fight against smallpox and infectious disease in general. Smallpox historically was a particularly human disease with no external animal reservoir (Belongia & Naleway, 2003). Despite its enormous impact on history and susceptible individuals, smallpox is considered to have been eradicated in the 1970s thanks to vaccination, a more efficient tool than inoculation in preventing the disease.

DOI: 10.4018/978-1-7998-8689-1.ch010

Smallpox probably arose around 3,000 to 6,000 years ago (Geddes, 2006). Variola virus, the causative agent of smallpox has been seen in humans for over 2,000 years (Li et al., 2007). Smallpox appears to have arisen by variola virus transferring to humans through another animal, possibly via a camel population that migrated to Africa (Babkin & Babkina, 2015; Bray & Buller, 2004). Smallpox may be notably vulnerable through this origin. The possible high fidelity of variola's DNA polymerase made the virus retain characteristics of its brethren outside of our species--replicative fidelity--which allowed for vaccination containing a related virus, vaccina, to provide protection against smallpox, and, as another quirk of the virus' nature, transfer long-term immunity. As a complication caused by these kind of close associations, PCR assays intended to detect Variola may not classify between the major and minor strains, though melt curves or more targeted assays can make a distinction (Loveless et al., 2009). The mortality of Variola minor is less than 1% (Voigt et al., 2016).

NATURE AND PROGRESSION

The smallpox virus is in the poxvirus family (Simonsen & Snowden, 2020). As a poxvirus, its genome is made of double-stranded DNA. Poxviruses are able to replicate in the cytoplasm because they carry within their virion the necessary enzymatic machinery to initiate and then carry out the process. Normally, viral smallpox is approximately between 300 and 350 nm long. Unlike plague, smallpox has no animal reservoir, and unlike plague and malaria, it does not use insects as a form of transport from one human host to the next. Instead, smallpox transits via airborne respiratory droplets, or direct contact with a contaminated surface. In the airborne form of transmission, infectivity persists along with lesions (abnormal tissue) in the oropharynx (the space around the back of the tongue, tonsils, and soft palate). While these lesions may be well placed to spread the virus, the virus can be expected to spread well outside the oropharynx after entering the body. The virus engages in replication in regional lymph nodes, and viremia (the presence of virus in the blood) can be expected on day 3 or day 4 after infection. At this point, the virus does not show clinical symptoms, but does propagate to bone marrow, spleen, and further lymph nodes. Upon day 8 to day 12 after infection, there is additional viremia, along with fever and symptomatic infection. The virus concentrates in mucosa of the oropharynx, as well as blood vessels in the dermis. This consequence to the dermis leads to rash, as well as a direct-contact method of spreading the virus. It is not enough that breath becomes infectious--with the virus so near the surface all over the body, touch is a meaningful vector of spread, too.

The rash, one of the hallmarks of smallpox, has a characteristic progression (Simonsen & Snowden, 2020). Lesions on the skin progress through phases together, from macules (distinct discolored areas less than a centimeter wide), into papules (a raised area of the skin, still less than one centimeter wide, that is normally inflamed, but not pus-producing), then vesicles (fluid-filled sacs visible on the surface of the skin), then pustules (sacs filled with pus), and finally crust (arising when the pustule breaks, and its contents dry). Crusts may seem to be a more resolved form of symptom, but crusts themselves can contain viral particles. In any case, the lesions progress from each step to the next in about 48 hours, with complete crusting across the body finished in 2 to 3 weeks after the onset of the rash. In contract, in chickenpox, a rash with a similar general progression is less coordinated in its phases across the body (Pergam, 2009).

TREATMENTS AND RESPONSE

As stated, treatments against smallpox have been around for an extremely long time, historically. Variolation, or the deliberate application of pustule smallpox to a healthy individual, in the hopes of triggering a more mild form of the disease, while still granting adaptive immunity, has been described in texts as old as 1500 BCE (Simonsen & Snowden, 2020). In China, a smallpox inoculation or variolation technique developed that involved blowing a combination of plant material and intentionally-aged smallpox crust up a patient's nasal mucosa (Milton, 2012). The Reverend Cotton Mather, who experienced a smallpox outbreak in Boston on the British North American colonial seaboard in 1721, became an advocate for inoculation after learning about the practice from Onesimus, a person from Africa Mather had held as a slave (Best et al., 2004; Hansen, 2002). George Washington mandated variolation of nonimmune soldiers and fresh recruits under his command in 1777, potentially the first ever military preventive care measure of its type (Geppert & Paul, 2019). As prior to the inoculation effort, 90% of Continental Army casualties were from infectious disease, and substantially from smallpox, the relevance of this work is hard to refute. While variolation is genuine infection, and has the risk of creating severe symptoms, as well as spreading the virus, a famous contribution to fighting the disease came with a 1798 publication by Edward Jenner. Jenner, building on the context of preemptive work against smallpox, publicized the finding that infection by the mild cowpox virus created immunity against smallpox without the risks of even a mild direct infection. This was vaccination, so named after the Latin word for "cow." For somewhat mysterious reasons, as smallpox vaccination began to take hold around the world, the substance of the vaccination had shifted by the end of the nineteenth century to the vaccinia virus (Jacobs et al., 2009). However, the vaccinia virus is able to do the job of vaccination just like cowpox can. The World Health Organization launched a major push to eradicate smallpox in 1959 (Voigt et al., 2016). Because smallpox is unable to hide in nonhuman populations, worldwide efforts towards vaccination led to the year 1977 and Somalia, the year and place of the last-known naturally-occurring case of smallpox (Simonsen & Snowden, 2020). In 1980, the World Health Assembly certified that smallpox had been eradicated globally.

Unfortunately, smallpox is still of clinical relevance because of the ongoing existence of stored samples, and the impossible-to-eliminate chance of natural reemergence (Simonsen & Snowden, 2020). The vaccinia virus vaccine was such a powerful tool for the medical profession because smallpox itself is so deadly, but it does come with a number of significant side effects. These include a generalized or progressive case of vaccinia itself, or postvaccinal encephalitis. These side effects are more reasonable to expect the public to undergo if smallpox is present in community transmission. Along with the eradication of smallpox in the wild, vaccination against smallpox gradually discontinued (Melamed et al., 2018). This means that more and more people are born without the expectation of being vaccinated against smallpox, leading to a worldwide vulnerability. It is notable that the United States military still persists in a program of smallpox vaccination for its members (Kramer, 2018), but discontinuing general use of the vaccine does carry the benefit of preventing inadvertent vaccinia disease outbreak transmission (Neff et al., 2002). The possible severe or fatal complications of traditional smallpox vaccination, while nowhere near common enough to eliminate the strong benefit of vaccination in an environment where smallpox is in the wild, are more common than with other types of vaccination, and serve as components of the broader cost-benefit analysis that has led to the current degree of smallpox vaccination desistance. Research to find an alternative is still important and active. In 2018, tecovirimat was approved in the United States as the first antiviral therapy for smallpox (Simonsen & Snowden, 2020).

The danger of smallpox, combined with its inability to hide in nonhuman populations, or animal reservoirs, led to the disease's apparent eradication outside of labs by 1980, as the push towards worldwide vaccination became powerful and organized. By 1984, two of the last four countries known to have engaged in smallpox research, Great Britain and South Africa, had given up their programs, setting the context for the only two smallpox-containing labs approved by the WHO to exist into the present day: the Centers for Disease Control and Prevention in Atlanta in the United States, and the State Research Center of Virology and Biotechnology in Koltsovo, Russia (NCEZID & DHCPP, 2021). However, the legacy of the virus is important to understand, because of how it has shaped human history.

HISTORY

Smallpox was clearly described in China at least as early as the fifteenth century, and seems to have been an endemic childhood disease in China of the Song Dynasty era of the tenth century (Leung, 2011). This is merely a sample of the viruses' spread. The fact that smallpox ravaged the indigenous population of the Americas exists in the context of the disease's spread and lethality. Settlers who came to the Americas, and their descendants, could be vulnerable, but the lack of an *endemic* context among Native Americans meant that disease burden was not disproportionately weighing on innocent and economically less-productive children, but rather on indigenous populations as a whole--there was a great deal of death among Native Americans during colonization, and the sudden and widespread death of adults could not help but impact indigenous societies (Duffy, 1951).

As an example of what a smallpox wave could do to immunologically naive populations, consider the smallpox epidemic of 1781 to 1782 in the Hudson Bay region of modern Canada. Estimates of mortality in the indigenous population range from under 20% to over 50% (Carlos & Lewis, 2012). Native American customs and health practices were able to adapt to moderate the effects of the disease, and leadership figures were able to show efficacy and retain their power, but this blunting of impact could only do so much when smallpox unchecked caused such great danger (Kelton, 2004). This vulnerability could be, and was, exploited in horrific ways. In North America of the eighteenth century, smallpox was used by British military decision makers as a biological warfare agent in their conflict with Native American groups (Fenn, 2000). In one well-known example, the besieged

British garrison at Fort Pitt seems to have spread contaminated cloth to Native Americans during a 1763 parlay, weaponizing an outbreak within the fort to disastrous effect.

The physical impact of smallpox contributed to its experience. Smallpox is systematically characterized by skin lesions (Martin, 2002). This, and possible scarring, may have helped smallpox be characterized as a demonic affliction in Edo Japan (Rotermund & Tyler, 2001). Smallpox even has been evident in a sixteenth century Italian mummy (Marennikova et al., 1990). Smallpox was a fearsome presence in seventeenth century Europe (Langer, 1976). George Washington himself had a smallpox scar, which was far from uncommon in his day and age (Schwartz, 2010). In the era before smallpox was publicly eradicated, signs of smallpox scarring on a person were a very real indicator of their virility, since they survived a deadly infection (Kerr, 2021). This was similar to how, in Victorian Britain, tuberculosis pallor could be seen as beautiful (Roberts, 2020).

Against smallpox, the resilience of populations in the era before mass vaccination is striking. In England, isolation and cancelation of public events helped to control the disease, even before the inoculations that picked up steam in the eighteenth century (Davenport et al., 2018). And then, in the eighteenth century, as stated above, George Washington had the Continental Army inoculated as a group (Hasselgren, 2020).

The virus variola was not isolated until the 1940s, but the work against it began far earlier than that (Pajer et al., 2017). One of the most important details in understanding that history of the response to smallpox is understanding how vaccination spread across the world.

Popularization of effective treatments against smallpox are tied to a physician named Edward Jenner. Jenner's name is very associated with the smallpox vaccine, but the late eighteenth century included a flowering of knowledge about vaccination, and another figure who deserves credit for practicing and evangelizing vaccination is Benjamin Jesty, a farmer (Hammarsten et al., 1979). Vaccination with cowpox occurred in England more than twenty years before Jenner became active on the topic (Gross & Sepkowitz, 1998). Further, all this work was based on research from places like Turkey that had already established less-effective-but-still-valuable inoculation, among other treatments. The dawn of vaccination was an inflection point and not a complete disruption from the past. One ethically problematic aspect of this bridge came when Lady Mary Wortly Montagu, wife of the British ambassador to Constantinople, who, in 1718, well before Jenner, attempted to convince the Prince of Wales to inoculate his children--the Prince was convinced after the successful inoculation of six orphan children first (Lakhani, 1992).

Nevertheless, Jenner's epoch represents a meaningful disruption. Vaccination was safer than inoculation. Work was done to spread the rare cowpox, valuable for vaccination (Rusnock, 2009). Vaccinations in Spain began in a documented fashion in December 1800 (Torrijos & Tuells, 2019), and then the Spanish royal philanthropic expedition spread vaccination to Spanish territories across the New World and Asia (Franco-Paredes et al., 2005). This massive immunization campaign, the first of its kind, lasted from 1803 to 1813 (Mark & Rigau-Pérez, 2009). The freedom from smallpox that it heralded was known in Guatemala in advance of the expedition actually arriving (Few, 2010).

This theme of vaccinations pushing against smallpox contextualized the history of the disease in the nineteenth century. Just because vaccines existed did not mean the protection of vaccinations were everywhere. For example, in 1816, twenty-one-year-old King Girvana of Nepal died of smallpox (Reddy, 2018). But programs of vaccination did continue to spread, and flourished in the United States in the early nineteenth century (Esparza, 2020). During the American Civil War (1861-1865), smallpox vaccination was a required Union protocol for soldier recruits, and this was also true in the Confederacy (Duggan et al., 2020). In the United States in 1870, Henry Austin Martin introduced the concept of an animal vaccine farm (Esparza et al., 2020). These places, often established by doctors for profit, first were devoted to producing smallpox vaccine, but then branched out to preventatives of diphtheria, and antitoxins.

Unfortunately, in the Pacific in the nineteenth century, certain drives linked to efficiency crystallized in a way that was very bad for the locals. As Pacific islands became more interconnected with the rest of the world, the Marquesas were devastated by smallpox in addition to tuberculosis, typhoid, and influenza (Martin & Combes, 1996). There was a smallpox epidemic in Hawaii in 1853 (Hammond, 2017). Polynesian population decreased significantly (Judd, 1997). Easter Island acquired smallpox through kidnaped islander men who were returned, who had spent too long in the wrong place in the outside world (Métraux, 1937). The population of the island of Rapa collapsed via smallpox or dysentery in 1864 after a return of population from Peru (Hurles et al., 2003). It is hard to overplay these events--the same sort of immunologically naive horror that was experienced in the Americas was playing out again, and smallpox was a great culprit, and one great tool that could have mitigated the death--vaccination, was not available in time.

However, in some ways this is the beginning of the end of the modern story. Smallpox could be horrific in places where it was not contained, but into the twentieth century, it was increasingly contained. So much so that there is value in discussing the effects of treatment. Smallpox vaccination is quite effective. In a study of long-term immunity, over 90% of subjects vaccinated between 25 and 75 years earlier retained substantial immune response to the vaccinia virus (Hammarlund et al., 2003). Antibody responses remained stable, while T-cell responses had a half life of around 8 to 15 years. While vaccine protection seems to be more linked to T-cells than antibody-producing B-cells (Gordon et al., 2011), suggesting a nuance in what the standard vaccine actually does, the overall picture here seems good. Vaccination, administered appropriately, can provide a benefit while being less dangerous than variolation (variolation is direct exposure to matter from smallpox patients in the hope of mild infection). In China there were recorded smallpox outbreaks from variolation as late as 1962 to 1965 (Jiang et al., 1988).

By 1962, in North America, the disease was already considered to be enough of a thing of the past that there was a scare that year when signs of smallpox arrived in New York and Toronto (Jarvis, 2007). Worldwide eradication proceeded into the 1970s, and was accomplished by the end of the decade (Belongia & Naleway, 2006; Fenner, 1982).

With the end of smallpox in the wild, an important question was the ongoing application of vaccines when there was no more threat. The risk-reward being negative, desistance of smallpox vaccination has occurred. Smallpox vaccinations do come with risk, particularly to infants--fatalities are rare but not unheard of, as the vaccina underlying the vaccine is capable of becoming symptomatic (Belongia & Naleway, 2003; Kempe, 1960). Particular risks range from eczema (Vora et al., 2008) and spread of poxvirus into the wild (Damaso et al., 2000). These risks may easily make sense in an environment where smallpox is already prevalent and deadly, but when it is no longer realistic to contract smallpox, the risk-reward changes. Even in the 1970s, when smallpox was not quite publicly eradicated, the dozens of foreign-travel-related cases that spread in Western countries that had, by their assets, already largely eliminated home-originated outbreaks, were not considered to be enough to create a situation where child vaccination was moral imperative (Mack, 1972).

SMALLPOX'S PRESENCE TODAY

Today, smallpox is mostly a thing of the past, but it might not stay a thing of the past, and the lessons learned from eradication play a role in why. During the global eradication campaign, finding the financing was difficult, even though, from an essentially financial standpoint, benefits of eradication would come four-hundred-fold (Barrett, 2007). This means that any recurrence of smallpox would likely face a new era of coordination issues. If smallpox returns, its R_0, or reproduction number, of 3.5 to 6, suggests that about that many people would catch the virus from a single infected individual, leading to a vast outbreak in a newly immunologically-naive younger population--herd immunity had greatly diminished now that vaccination is no longer a standard practice (Gani & Leach, 2001).

If smallpox returns, it will likely be because of a human mistake. Whether that mistake is due to mismanagement at a lab, or the accidental unleashing of smallpox from some hidden corner of the world, or bioterrorism, the concern is salient regardless (Halloran et al., 2002; Henderson et al., 1999). Past records suggest that a median of 2,155 smallpox vaccine doses per case need to be administered to halt an outbreak (Meltzer et al., 2001). Smallpox might be the first human disease that humans have eradicated, but the World Health Organization-spearheaded success has left humanity with a restored vulnerability (Olson & Shchelkunov, 2017), even if the a current cost-benefit analysis of widespread smallpox vaccination suggests the risks outweigh the benefits. The fact that, historically, people have resorted to racism to try to find an outlet of their feelings about infectious disease, in outbreaks ranging from smallpox to the coronavirus, points out the heavy lift that prevention strategists must face when attempting public communication strategies (Heinrich, 2020). Research also indicates that some first responders might not attend to duties in the face of a smallpox epidemic, potentially for reasons tied to fear of vaccination (Mackler et al., 2007).

Modeling of potential smallpox outbreaks in Sydney, Australia, and New York City, United States, shows that the highest infection rates would likely occur in persons between infancy and 19 years of age, while the highest death rates would occur in those older than 45 (MacIntyre et al., 2018). This is despite the fact that smallpox vaccination was common in New York until 1980--this model considered residual protection from old immunizations to be relatively low. Smallpox disease burden, as with much disease burden, is distributed unequally, even when it is not actually present in the wild.

REFERENCES

Alcamí, A. (2020). Was smallpox a widespread mild disease? *Science*, *369*(6502), 376–377. doi:10.1126cience.abd1214 PMID:32703866

Babkin, I. V., & Babkina, I. N. (2015). The origin of the variola virus. *Viruses*, *7*(3), 1100–1112. doi:10.3390/v7031100 PMID:25763864

Barrett, S. (2007). The smallpox eradication game. *Public Choice*, *130*(1), 179–207. doi:10.100711127-006-9079-z

Belongia, E. A., & Naleway, A. L. (2003). Smallpox vaccine: The good, the bad, and the ugly. *Clinical Medicine & Research*, *1*(2), 87–92. doi:10.3121/cmr.1.2.87 PMID:15931293

Best, M., Neuhauser, D., & Slavin, L. (2004). "Cotton Mather, you dog, dam you! I'l inoculate you with this; with a pox to you": Smallpox inoculation, Boston, 1721. *BMJ Quality & Safety*, *13*(1), 82–83. doi:10.1136/qshc.2003.008797 PMID:14757807

Bray, M., & Buller, M. (2004). Looking back at smallpox. *Clinical Infectious Diseases*, *38*(6), 882–889. doi:10.1086/381976 PMID:14999635

Carlos, A. M., & Lewis, F. D. (2012). Smallpox and Native American mortality: The 1780s epidemic in the Hudson Bay region. *Explorations in Economic History*, *49*(3), 277–290. doi:10.1016/j.eeh.2012.04.003

Damaso, C. R., Esposito, J. J., Condit, R. C., & Moussatché, N. (2000). An emergent poxvirus from humans and cattle in Rio de Janeiro State: Cantagalo virus may derive from Brazilian smallpox vaccine. *Virology*, *277*(2), 439–449. doi:10.1006/viro.2000.0603 PMID:11080491

Davenport, R. J., Satchell, M., & Shaw-Taylor, L. M. W. (2018). The geography of smallpox in England before vaccination: A conundrum resolved. *Social Science & Medicine*, *206*, 75–85. doi:10.1016/j.socscimed.2018.04.019 PMID:29684651

Duffy, J. (1951). Smallpox and the Indians in the American colonies. *Bulletin of the History of Medicine*, *25*(4), 324–341. https://www.jstor.org/stable/44443622 PMID:14859018

Duggan, A. T., Klunk, J., Porter, A. F., Dhody, A. N., Hicks, R., Smith, G. L., Humphreys, M., McCollum, A. M., Davidson, W. B., Wilkins, K., Li, Y., Burke, A., Polasky, H., Flanders, L., Poinar, D., Raphenya, A. R., Lau, T. T. Y., Alcock, B., McArthur, A. G., ... Poinar, H. N. (2020). The origins and genomic diversity of American Civil War Era smallpox vaccine strains. *Genome Biology*, *21*(1), 1–11. doi:10.118613059-020-02079-z PMID:32684155

Esparza, J. (2020). Three different paths to introduce the smallpox vaccine in early 19th century United States. *Vaccine*, *38*(12), 2741–2745. doi:10.1016/j.vaccine.2020.01.077 PMID:32057569

Esparza, J., Lederman, S., Nitsche, A., & Damaso, C. R. (2020). Early smallpox vaccine manufacturing in the United States: Introduction of the "animal vaccine" in 1870, establishment of "vaccine farms", and the beginnings of the vaccine industry. *Vaccine*, *38*(30), 4773–4779. doi:10.1016/j.vaccine.2020.05.037 PMID:32473878

Fenn, E. A. (2000). Biological warfare in eighteenth-century North America: Beyond Jeffery Amherst. *The Journal of American History*, *86*(4), 1552–1580. doi:10.2307/2567577 PMID:18271127

Fenner, F. (1982). Global eradication of smallpox. *Reviews of Infectious Diseases*, *4*(5), 916–930. doi:10.1093/clinids/4.5.916 PMID:6293036

Few, M. (2010). Circulating smallpox knowledge: Guatemalan doctors, Maya Indians and designing Spain's smallpox vaccination expedition, 1780-1803. *British Journal for the History of Science*, *43*(4), 519–537. doi:10.1017/S000708741000124X PMID:21553626

Franco-Paredes, C., Lammoglia, L., & Santos-Preciado, J. I. (2005). The Spanish royal philanthropic expedition to bring smallpox vaccination to the New World and Asia in the 19th century. *Clinical Infectious Diseases*, *41*(9), 1285–1289. doi:10.1086/496930 PMID:16206103

Gani, R., & Leach, S. (2001). Transmission potential of smallpox in contemporary populations. *Nature*, *414*(6865), 748–751. doi:10.1038/414748a PMID:11742399

Geddes, A. M. (2006). The history of smallpox. *Clinics in Dermatology*, *24*(3), 152–157. doi:10.1016/j.clindermatol.2005.11.009 PMID:16714195

Geppert, C. M., & Paul, R. A. (2019). The shot that won the Revolutionary War and is still reverberating. *Federal Practitioner*, *36*(7), 298–299. PMID:31384117

Gordon, S. N., Cecchinato, V., Andresen, V., Heraud, J. M., Hryniewicz, A., Parks, R. W., Venzon, D., Chung, H., Karpova, T., McNally, J., Silvera, P., Reimann, K. A., Matsui, H., Kanehara, T., Shinmura, Y., Yokote, H., & Franchini, G. (2011). Smallpox vaccine safety is dependent on T cells and not B cells. *The Journal of Infectious Diseases*, *203*(8), 1043–1053. doi:10.1093/infdis/jiq162 PMID:21450994

Gross, C. P., & Sepkowitz, K. A. (1998). The myth of the medical breakthrough: Smallpox, vaccination, and Jenner reconsidered. *International Journal of Infectious Diseases*, *3*(1), 54–60. doi:10.1016/S1201-9712(98)90096-0 PMID:9831677

Halloran, M. E., Longini, I. M. Jr, Nizam, A., & Yang, Y. (2002). Containing bioterrorist smallpox. *Science*, *298*(5597), 1428–1432. doi:10.1126cience.1074674 PMID:12434061

Hammarlund, E., Lewis, M. W., Hansen, S. G., Strelow, L. I., Nelson, J. A., Sexton, G. J., Hanifin, J. M., & Slifka, M. K. (2003). Duration of antiviral immunity after smallpox vaccination. *Nature Medicine*, *9*(9), 1131–1137. doi:10.1038/nm917 PMID:12925846

Hammarsten, J. F., Tattersall, W., & Hammarsten, J. E. (1979). Who discovered smallpox vaccination? Edward Jenner or Benjamin Jesty? *Transactions of the American Clinical and Climatological Association*, *90*, 44–55. PMID:390826

Hammond, J. J. (2017). The Mormon Hawaiian Mission and the Smallpox Epidemic of 1853. *The John Whitmer Historical Association Journal, 37*(1), 117-131. https://www.jstor.org/stable/26316895

Hansen, A. C. (2002). African Americans in medicine. *Journal of the National Medical Association*, *94*(4), 266–271. PMID:11991340

Hasselgren, P. O. (2020). The smallpox epidemics in America in the 1700s and the role of the surgeons: Lessons to be learned during the global outbreak of COVID-19. *World Journal of Surgery*, *44*(9), 2837–2841. doi:10.100700268-020-05670-4 PMID:32623571

Heinrich, A. L. (2020). *Before coronavirus, China was falsely blamed for spreading smallpox. Racism played a role then, too*. The Conversation.

Henderson, D. A., Inglesby, T. V., Bartlett, J. G., Ascher, M. S., Eitzen, E., Jahrling, P. B., Hauer, J., Layton, M., McDade, J., Osterholm, M. T., O'Toole, T., Parker, G., Perl, T., Russell, P. K., & Tonat, K.for the Working Group on Civilian Biodefense. (1999). Smallpox as a biological weapon: Medical and public health management. *Journal of the American Medical Association*, *281*(22), 2127–2137. doi:10.1001/jama.281.22.2127 PMID:10367824

Hurles, M. E., Maund, E., Nicholson, J., Bosch, E., Renfrew, C., Sykes, B. C., & Jobling, M. A. (2003). Native American Y chromosomes in Polynesia: The genetic impact of the Polynesian slave trade. *American Journal of Human Genetics*, *72*(5), 1282–1287. doi:10.1086/374827 PMID:12644966

Jacobs, B. L., Langland, J. O., Kibler, K. V., Denzler, K. L., White, S. D., Holechek, S. A., Wong, S., Huynh, T., & Baskin, C. R. (2009). Vaccinia virus vaccines: Past, present and future. *Antiviral Research*, *84*(1), 1–13. doi:10.1016/j.antiviral.2009.06.006 PMID:19563829

Jarvis, E. (2007). A contagious journey within a culture of complacency: The smallpox scare of 1962 in New York and Toronto. *Canadian Bulletin of Medical History*, *24*(2), 343–366. doi:10.3138/cbmh.24.2.343 PMID:18447310

Jiang, Y., Ma, J., Xiahou, G., & Henderson, D. A. (1988). Outbreaks of smallpox due to variolation in China, 1962–1965. *American Journal of Epidemiology*, *128*(1), 39–45. doi:10.1093/oxfordjournals.aje.a114956 PMID:2837897

Judd, C. S. (1977). Depopulation in Polynesia. *Bulletin of the History of Medicine*, *51*(4), 585–593. https://www.jstor.org/stable/44450469 PMID:343845

Kelton, P. (2004). Avoiding the smallpox spirits: Colonial epidemics and Southeastern Indian survival. *Ethnohistory (Columbus, Ohio)*, *51*(1), 45–71. doi:10.1215/00141801-51-1-45

Kempe, C. H. (1960). Studies on smallpox and complications of smallpox vaccination: E. Mead Johnson Award address. *Pediatrics*, *26*(2), 176–189. doi:10.1542/peds.26.2.176 PMID:14408455

Kerr, M. N. (2021, January 21). *Wearable immunity: Beauty lessons from the pockmarking era*. Nursing Clio. https://nursingclio.org/2021/01/21/wearable-immunity-beauty-lessons-from-the-pockmarking-era

Kramer, T. R. (2018). Post-Smallpox Vaccination Skin Eruption in a Marine. *Military Medicine*, *183*(9-10), e649–e653. doi:10.1093/milmed/usx133 PMID:29546340

Lakhani, S. (1992). Early clinical pathologists: Edward Jenner (1749-1823). *Journal of Clinical Pathology*, *45*(9), 756–758. doi:10.1136/jcp.45.9.756 PMID:1401201

Langer, W. L. (1976). Immunization against smallpox before Jenner. *Scientific American*, *234*(1), 112–117. doi:10.1038cientificamerican0176-112 PMID:766184

Leung, A. K. C. (2011). "Variolation" and vaccination in late imperial China, Ca 1570–1911. In History of Vaccine Development (pp. 5-12). Springer.

Li, Y., Carroll, D. S., Gardner, S. N., Walsh, M. C., Vitalis, E. A., & Damon, I. K. (2007). On the origin of smallpox: Correlating variola phylogenics with historical smallpox records. *Proceedings of the National Academy of Sciences of the United States of America*, *104*(40), 15787–15792. doi:10.1073/pnas.0609268104 PMID:17901212

Loveless, B. M., Mucker, E. M., Hartmann, C., Craw, P. D., Huggins, J., & Kulesh, D. A. (2009). Differentiation of Variola major and Variola minor variants by MGB-Eclipse probe melt curves and genotyping analysis. *Molecular and Cellular Probes*, *23*(3-4), 166–170. doi:10.1016/j.mcp.2009.03.002 PMID:19345728

MacIntyre, C. R., Costantino, V., Chen, X., Segelov, E., Chughtai, A. A., Kelleher, A., Kunasekaran, M., & Lane, J. M. (2018). Influence of population immunosuppression and past vaccination on smallpox reemergence. *Emerging Infectious Diseases*, *24*(4), 646–653. doi:10.3201/eid2404.171233 PMID:29553311

Mack, T. M. (1972). Smallpox in Europe, 1950–1971. *The Journal of Infectious Diseases*, *125*(2), 161–169. doi:10.1093/infdis/125.2.161 PMID:5007552

Mackler, N., Wilkerson, W., & Cinti, S. (2007). Will first-responders show up for work during a pandemic? Lessons from a smallpox vaccination survey of paramedics. *Disaster Management & Response*, *5*(2), 45–48. doi:10.1016/j.dmr.2007.02.002 PMID:17517362

Marennikova, S. S., Shelukhina, E. M., Zhukova, O. A., Yanova, N. N., & Loparev, V. N. (1990). Smallpox diagnosed 400 years later: Results of skin lesions examination of 16th century Italian mummy. *Journal of Hygiene, Epidemiology, Microbiology, and Immunology*, *34*(2), 227–231. PMID:2212645

Mark, C., & Rigau-Pérez, J. G. (2009). The world's first immunization campaign: The Spanish Smallpox Vaccine Expedition, 1803–1813. *Bulletin of the History of Medicine*, *83*(1), 63–94. doi:10.1353/bhm.0.0173 PMID:19329842

Martin, D. B. (2002). The cause of death in smallpox: An examination of the pathology record. *Military Medicine*, *167*(7), 546–551. doi:10.1093/milmed/167.7.546 PMID:12125845

Martin, P. M., & Combes, C. (1996). Emerging infectious diseases and the depopulation of French Polynesia in the 19th century. *Emerging Infectious Diseases*, *2*(4), 359–361. doi:10.3201/eid0204.960416 PMID:8969256

Melamed, S., Israely, T., & Paran, N. (2018). Challenges and achievements in prevention and treatment of smallpox. *Vaccines*, *6*(1), 8. doi:10.3390/vaccines6010008 PMID:29382130

Meltzer, M. I., Damon, I., LeDuc, J. W., & Millar, J. D. (2001). Modeling potential responses to smallpox as a bioterrorist weapon. *Emerging Infectious Diseases*, *7*(6), 959–969. doi:10.3201/eid0706.010607 PMID:11747722

Métraux, A. (1937). The kings of Easter Island: Kingship. *The Journal of the Polynesian Society, 46*(182), 41-62. https://www.jstor.org/stable/20702667

Milton, D. M. (2012). What was the primary mode of smallpox transmission? Implications for biodefense. *Frontiers in Cellular and Infection Microbiology*, *2*, 150. doi:10.3389/fcimb.2012.00150 PMID:23226686

NCEZID (Centers for Disease Control and Prevention, National Center for Emerging and Zoonotic Infectious Diseases) & DHCPP (Division of High-Consequence Pathogens and Pathology). (2021, February 20). *History of Smallpox.* Centers for Disease Control and Prevention. https://www.cdc.gov/smallpox/history/history.html

Neff, J. M., Lane, J. M., Fulginiti, V. A., & Henderson, D. A. (2002). Contact vaccinia—Transmission of vaccinia from smallpox vaccination. *Journal of the American Medical Association, 288*(15), 1901–1905. doi:10.1001/jama.288.15.1901 PMID:12377090

Olson, V. A., & Shchelkunov, S. N. (2017). Are we prepared in case of a possible smallpox-like disease emergence? *Viruses, 9*(9), 242. doi:10.3390/v9090242 PMID:32962316

Pajer, P., Dresler, J., Kabíckova, H., Písa, L., Aganov, P., Fucik, K., Elleder, D., Hron, T., Kuzelka, V., Velemínsky, P., Klimentova, J., Fucikova, A., Pejchal, J., Hrabakova, R., Benes, V., Rausch, T., Dundr, P., Pilin, A., Cabala, R., ... Meyer, H. (2017). Characterization of two historic smallpox specimens from a Czech museum. *Viruses, 9*(8), 200. doi:10.3390/v9080200 PMID:28749451

Pergam, S. A., Limaye, A. P., & AST Infectious Diseases Community of Practice. (2009). Varicella zoster virus (VZV) in solid organ transplant recipients. *American Journal of Transplantation: Official Journal of the American Society of Transplantation and the American Society of Transplant Surgeons, 9*(Suppl 4), S108–S115. doi:10.1111/j.1600-6143.2009.02901.x

Reddy, K. R. (2018). Is smallpox dead? (The story of highly contagious and most feared disease). *Journal of Gandaki Medical College-Nepal, 11*(1). Advance online publication. doi:10.3126/jgmcn.v11i1.20784

Roberts, C. (2020). Fashionable but debilitating diseases: Tuberculosis past and present. In S. Sheridan & L. Gregoricka (Eds.), *Purposeful pain* (pp. 21–38). Springer. doi:10.1007/978-3-030-32181-9_2

Rotermund, H. O., & Tyler, R. (2001). Demonic affliction or contagious disease? Changing perceptions of smallpox in the late Edo period. *Japanese Journal of Religious Studies*, 373–398. doi:10.18874/jjrs.28.3-4.2001.373-398

Rusnock, A. (2009). Catching cowpox: The early spread of smallpox vaccination, 1798–1810. *Bulletin of the History of Medicine, 83*(1), 17–36. doi:10.1353/bhm.0.0160 PMID:19329840

Schwartz, J. H. (2010). Getting to know George Washington. *Western Pennsylvania History*, 52-62.

Simonsen, K. A., & Snowden, J. (2020). *Smallpox, StatPearls. (2021 Jan-)*. StatPearls Publishing. https://www.ncbi.nlm.nih.gov/books/NBK470418/

Torrijos, J. L. D., & Tuells, J. (2019). The beginnings of smallpox vaccination in Spain seen through the correspondence of Ignacio María Ruiz de Luzuriaga (1801–1802). *Vaccine*, *37*(32), 4651–4657. doi:10.1016/j.vaccine.2019.05.088 PMID:31262586

Voigt, E. A., Kennedy, R. B., & Poland, G. A. (2016). Defending against smallpox: A focus on vaccines. *Expert Review of Vaccines*, *15*(9), 1197–1211. doi:10.1080/14760584.2016.1175305 PMID:27049653

Vora, S., Damon, I., Fulginiti, V., Weber, S. G., Kahana, M., Stein, S. L., ... Marcinak, J. (2008). Severe eczema vaccinatum in a household contact of a smallpox vaccinee. *Clinical Infectious Diseases, 46*(10), 1555-1561. doi:10.1086/587668

World Health Organization. (2011). *Bugs, drugs and smoke: Stories from public health*. World Health Organization. https://www.who.int/about/history/publications/public_health_stories/en/

Chapter 11
Profile:
Plague

ABSTRACT

This chapter focuses on plague, which as the Black Death began in the 1300s, possibly killing one third of the people of Europe, as well as vast numbers farther east. Plague is less relevant today than in the past because of the use of antibiotics, but the shifting relation of plague with human society, driven by human capacity, should serve as a recapitulation of the central ideas of this book. Simultaneously, a disease capable of creating pandemic, a disease that can be limited by medicine, and a disease that can be deadly in modern times to those who contract it, plague, along with its animal reservoirs, shows how disease flexibility interacts with human ingenuity.

INTRODUCTION

Plague has high lethality, and is caused by *Yersinia pestis*, which is a zoonotic Gram stain negative bacterium (Gage et al., 2005). The zoonotic, or nonhuman-animal-spread part of the disease is important (Perry & Fetherston, 1997). Zoonoses can lurk in animal reservoirs before returning to human populations. Plague has been present in humans for more than 5,000 years, and, in three major pandemics, killed as much as 60% of people who lived in the Eastern Hemisphere (Morozova et al., 2020) The first of these three pandemics is Plague of Justinian, which spread through the Sassanian Empire (centered in modern Iran) and the Mediterranean Sea from 541-544 CE, with aftershocks

DOI: 10.4018/978-1-7998-8689-1.ch011

lasting until about 750 CE. Next was the Black Death, which revealed itself in Europe in 1347-1351 and had follow-up waves into the 1700s. Finally, the Third Plague Pandemic emerged in China in 1855, and lasted through the twentieth century. Plague is still active in the world, but, thanks to modern healthcare, not as dangerous as it has been in previous centuries. Since as recently as 2000, there have been over 20 plague outbreaks, including one in 2017 in Madagascar. Archaeologically-discovered plague might date to the Bronze Age in Eurasia (Drancourt & Raoult, 2016), and even previous to the three epidemics mentioned above, there was the Antonine Plague in the Roman Empire in the era of Marcus Aurelius (Duncan-Jones, 1996), but plague demonstrates meaningful continuity to the present day.

The importance of plague's zoonotic aspect should not be forgotten in understanding its longevity. The Plague of Justinian and the Black Death appear to have been independent transitions of *Yersinia pestis* lineages in rodent populations (Wagner et al., 2014). Modern DNA analysis is clear in tying the pathogen in the Justinian outbreak to the later outbreaks (Harbeck et al., 2013).

DISEASE PROGRESSION AND TYPES

The progression of a *Yersinia pestis* inside the human body is also important to understand (Demeure et al., 2019). *Y. pestis*, and thus plague, can pass via the bite of a flea, or respiratory droplets. In both of those vectors, immune response is typically initially absent, as *Y. pestis* has some ability to evade the mechanics of innate immunity. One key is understanding the degree of *Y. pestis*' robustness. It does trigger the innate immune response, and is commonly phagocytosed, or swallowed, by both neutrophils and macrophages. However, once inside these immune cells, *Y. pestis* can survive. Despite being a bacterium, its evolutionary profile allows it to exist within larger cells. In both neutrophils and macrophages, *Y. pestis* can not only survive, but replicate. In general, *Y. pestis* is able to exploit the human immune and lymphatic systems.

Early infection in the bubonic or flea-carried variant of plague is characterized by the migration of the bacterium from the flea's injection site to lymph nodes, which does not require the bacterium being swallowed by phagocytes like macrophages or neutrophils (Demeure et al.., 2019). Lymphatic flow itself is enough to provide transport, though the ability for *Y. pestis* to subsist inside phagocytes is clearly not a limitation. Once in lymph nodes,

Y. pestis is associated with cell death. The mechanism of this is a subject of research. However, because *Y. pestis* has the advantage of being able to live inside immune cells that it kills, it is in a position to have more access to the mechanisms by which cells can destroy themselves and their peers.

In other words, *Y. pestis* appears to be able to include necroptosis (Arifuzzaman et al., 2018). Necroptosis is a form of regulated necrosis, or cell death (Dhuriya & Sharma, 2018). There are multiple methods for cells in the human body to contribute to their own destruction. Necroptosis is one of them. This form of destruction is mediated by specific signals with a cell, which *Y. pestis* can trigger (Arifuzzaman et al., 2018). *Y. pestis* seems to be able to interact with this mechanism of cellular death by Yersinia outer protein J (YopJ). Cellular chemical signaling involves a complex system of molecular regulation, and YopJ can downregulate a suppressor of cell death programs that are receptor-interacting protein kinase 1 (RIPK1) mediated. A decent metaphor for this appears to be a car break. If the suppressor is removed like a foot from the break, via YopJ, necroptosis may commence. The destruction of immune cells leads to bacterial release, which naturally creates more opportunity for phagocytes to uptake the same line of *Y. pestis* bacteria that just proceeded in hijacking cellular mechanisms (Demeure et al., 2019). How this process is highly dangerous to a human host seems very clear from this standpoint--cascading immune cell death in lymph nodes is not consistent with normal functioning.

While *Y. pestis*' destruction of immune functioning has thus far been described in the context of a flea-driven or bubonic model, bubonic plague (buboes refer to inflamed lymph nodes) is not the only form (Demeure et al., 2019). Pneumonic plague, which travels via aerosol, naturally has *Y. pestis* enter, focus on, and target the lungs. In pneumonic plague, as in bubonic, *Y. pestis* can inhabit phagocytes, and a disease progression seems to first target resident alveolar macrophages, then neutrophils. Early inflammation appears to be blocked by activation of IL-1RA, the IL-1 receptor antagonist, which can be thought to characterize the early pre-inflammatory phase of the disease (Sivaraman et al., 2015). After this phase, pneumonic plague becomes highly inflammatory, and is recorded as 100% fatal, though antibiotic treatment is effective in the pre-inflammatory phase. Given the complex interaction of intercellular signaling, *Y. pestis*' usage of IL-1RA does not mean that the immune system did not attempt to respond to infection in its initial stages. Research suggests that IL-1β/IL-18 activation occurs at least 30 hours before other inflammation indicators, for pneumonic plague. However IL-1RA *physically* blocks binding sites that other members of the IL-1 family can use to promote the inflammatory response (Dayer et al., 2017).

One important detail here is the complicated interaction *Y. pestis* has with the immune system. It is not that *Y. pestis* needs to completely evade the host immune system--it has already been established that *Y. pestis* can leverage immune and lymphatic responses to achieve reproductive goals. It is rather that *Y. pestis* seems to want to facilitate an optimal immune response for its needs, with the implication being that too much inflammatory response too early would not be optimal for reproduction. Another important detail is how this state of affairs came about. It is very easy when describing immune or pathogenic behavior to resort to statements that imply intentionality. This need not be full anthropomorphization, merely an appreciation that the specific mechanisms by which *Y. pestis* attempts to regulate the human immune response are the product of a great deal of evolutionary interaction, mediated by the random genetic fluctuations that are the necessary substrate upon which natural selection works. The ways *Y. pestis* evades and modifies the human immune response may not be perfect even from a goal of *Y. pestis* reproduction and survival, but are undeniably effective.

In any case, after initial interactions with the immune system, pneumonic plague leads to death, and, in recorded history, has been more deadly than any other disease from a bacterial pathogen (Anderson et al., 2009). Death occurs with congestion of the lower respiratory tract, severe hemorrhage, and edema secondary to a vast increase in the colonizing *Y. pestis* population. Bacteria can leave the lungs and cause systemic infections with systemic hemorrhage, and treatment that begins more than 12 hours after the onset of fever is, at the onset of the twenty-first century, not considered to be effective.

After discussing some of the patterns associated with bubonic and pneumonic plague, it is worth discussing the third major type--septicemic, or bloodborne. The vector of septicemic plague is associated with animal contact, but, in contrast with bubonic plague, which is closely associated with the lymph nodes, and pneumonic plague, which is more closely associated with the lungs, septicemic plague is more generalized and is difficult to diagnose. Septicemic plague can be a complication of pneumonic or bubonic plague (Centers for Disease Control and Prevention, 2018). In this fashion, it occurs through bites of an infected animal, like a flea, or some other method of skin breakage allowing for *Y. pestis* to enter the body. These are theoretically identical vectors to those that can introduce bubonic plague (recall that pneumonic plague, involving *Y. pestis* dwelling in the lungs is aerosolized). However, in septicemic plague by itself, infection does not result in the characteristic swelling of lymph glands (the buboes).

In order to understand septicemic plague better, as well as plague in general, and how it persists to the modern day, a particular case of septicemic plague will be discussed.

CASE STUDY: CALIFORNIA

This case occurred in rural California in the United States, where plague is known to be endemic in the local rodent population (Margolis, 2008). It is notable for the difficulties in diagnosis that are characteristic of septicemic plague. A 79-year-old woman who lived alone was brought to a local hospital upon a neighbor's discovery of her altered mental status. Her home contained evidence of mouse and wood rat droppings, and appeared neglected. Her initial diagnosis was community-acquired pneumonia, which led to treatment with ceftriaxone, ampicillin/sulbactam, and levofloxacin. This led to decrease in fever and improvement in mentation. However, at 48 hours after admission, renal failure had notably worsened, and acidosis and thrombocytopenia emerged. The woman was transferred to the hospital's academic center, and developed the need for intubation and hemodynamic support. A new diagnosis of thrombotic thrombocytopenic purpura was considered. This diagnosis, in layman's terms, contains terms that refer to clotting, low blood platelet count, and the bursting of small blood vessels (Knöbl, 2018).

In the case, progression continued with plaques of necrotic skin on the chest and upper extremities (Margolis, 2008). Multiple toes suffered from gangrene. Histopathology showed no visible organisms. However, the admission urine culture returned with signs of *Pseudomonas aeruginosa*, which led to an antibiotic change to meropenem and gentamicin. *Pseudomonas aeruginosa* is a common cause of hospital-acquired pneumonia, and is known to leave the lung and cause bacteremia (i.e., as bacteria, it enters the blood) (Berube et al., 2016). The Gram stain status of the microbiota in question proved difficult to categorize, initially recorded with "gram-positive rods," on Day 4 of hospital admission, but then "gram-negative rod" on Day 6 (Margolis, 2008). Vitek automated biochemical isolate analysis returned with indications of *Y. pestis*, the ultimate diagnosis, but the same day as the Vitek work, a comparable analysis using an API product suggested that the disease culprit was *Escherichia coli* or a *Proteus* bacteria species. Subculture work began, and on day 9 *Y. pestis* was suggested by analytical profile index biochemical testing. Outreach to the San Diego County Public Health Laboratory gave additional confirmation by identifying *Y. pestis* from isolate using direct fluorescence antibody testing and polymerase chain reaction testing.

In an interesting example of what was possibly an excess of pattern recognition, on the evening of the identification, a nurse reported seeing live fleas in the patient's bed (Margolis, 2008). This resulted in moving the patient and sealing and fumigating the room, though the intruders in question were eventually classified as fruit flies. Unfortunately, after 10 days of treatment for *Y. pestis*, the patient, who was anuric, elected against renal replacement therapy, leading to death from uremia, as proper blood filtration could not take place.

Because plague is zoonotic and can inhabit animals other than humans, fieldwork was conducted around the patient's home with this property of *Y. pestis* in mind (Margolis, 2008). The patient had two dogs, and, after testing, one was determined to show *Y. pestis* at a titer of 1:64. This means that 64 parts of a diluent solution had to be merged with one part of the test-positive blood sample before the *Y. pestis* became undetectable. Two of three *Spermophilus beecheyi*, or California ground squirrels, that were found on the patient's land, showed *Y. pestis* titers at 1:2,048. A *S. beecheyi* carcass and rabbit hind leg also tested positive, as did five flea pools from rodents that themselves tested both positive and negative.

What kind of conclusions can be drawn from this case study? First, it is a clear example that plague, despite being famous historically, is still present in the modern world, if rarely enough that it took some work to determine the appropriate diagnosis. The case shows how a variety of social, procedural and contextual factors contributed to the poor outcome. The isolation of the patient, the age of the patient, and the limitations in testing likely all contributed to a worsening situation. Finally, the way the case is reported, it was the patient's personal choice that led proximately to the fatal result, though the patient was likely motivated by significant and highly relevant quality of life concerns. Even for a disease like septicemic plague, social and historical factors are highly relevant. The fact that *Y. pestis* survived in a local animal population is yet another factor that was critical to the outcome, but was not strictly tied to in-hospital intervention.

More context on modern cases of plague: In a survey of 762 published cases of treated plague that collected reports from 1937 to 2019, the following statistical summary can be gleaned (Nelson et al., 2020). Overall case fatality rate was 20%. For primary types of cases, 63% were bubonic, 21% were pneumonic, and 5% were septicemic. The case fatality rates for these respective groups were 17%, 27%, and 38%, which, especially in the context of pneumonic plague's much higher fatality rate if left untreated, shows the power of antimicrobial treatments. Of significant drugs administered to patients, tetracycline was associated with the lowest case fatality rate, being associated with 10% case fatality rates when it was administered. Without antimicrobial treatment, as stated, the case fatality rate for pneumonic cases is effectively full as is septicaemic, while, for the bubonic variant, the case fatality rate is between 40% and 70% (Stenseth et al., 2008).

PLAGUE AS A ZOONOSIS

So far, this chapter has provided a review of the nature of plague and its progression. The fact that plague is a zoonosis, existing in animals outside of the human species, is an important part of its character, and deserves to be discussed in further detail. The range of mammal species that can be infected by plague includes rodents, but also includes cats, dogs, rabbits, and camels, in addition to humans (Zeppelini et al., 2016). Indeed, over 200 mammal species are known to be susceptible to *Y. pestis* infection. Rats from the Eastern Hemisphere are thought to have been instrumental in spreading plague all over the world. However, fleas are known to be key as a direct transmission vector.

Because of the wide range of hosts in which *Y. pestis* can survive, a wide range of sylvatic, or wild, reservoir systems have been evidenced, where *Y. pestis* can circulate without needing to come into contact with humans (Zeppelini et al., 2016). Humans are but one of the many species that can contribute to cycles of *Y. pestis* survival. These ecological systems are key to the survival of *Y. pestis*, but are under-characterized, with much of the existing literature focusing on North American environments that only contribute to an estimated 1.2% of human cases of plague worldwide. While the complexity of the reservoir systems likely contributes to our lack of understanding, the mere fact of existence of these reservoir systems itself seems likely to have prevented plague from becoming as controlled as smallpox. This is problematic because the enormous lethality rates of *Y. pestis* in humans suggests that plague epidemics in humans are, from an evolutionary standpoint, quite possibly more of a byproduct of *Y. pestis* survival and circulation in other species, rather than something that really needs humans to survive. From case fatality rates alone, malaria, another zoonosis that has caused enormous death and suffering in the human population over time, has, compared to plague, been able to come to more of an endemic accommodation with the human species than plague has. Plague fatality rates can be dozens of times higher.

In any event, understanding the existence of plague reservoir systems is a key component in understanding the basic nature of *Y. pestis*, and plague, and while there is much work to be done, much work has been done. Zeppelini et al. (2016) compare four models of sylvatic reservoirs. The first, based on the traditional line of research that emphasizes the importance of rodent assemblages, emphasizes that rodent populations, active continuously around the year, allow for *Y. pestis*' continued circulation. The second model focuses on species that handle *Y. pestis* infections as chronic, animals that go so far as to present with granuloma-like lesions reminiscent of the way human immune systems manage chronic cases of tuberculosis. In an animal that does not experience plague or *Y. pestis* as an acute condition, the concern of how the disease can avoid killing hosts before it spreads becomes matched with a clear solution. The third model returns to a traditional organism associated with plague, and places primary emphasis on fleas. In this model, fleas are more than just vectors of transmission between mammals, but rather a full reservoir themselves, as multiple flea species can survive as many as 558 days with no feeding, and a complete blockage induced by *Y. pestis.*

What is a blockage? In the context of infection by *Y. pestis*, it is structural change the bacterium can induce on the flea, similar but possibly even more dramatic than the ways *Y. pestis* can hide inside human phagocytes and manipulate the human immune response. That is, *Y. pestis* can form a biofilm that blockades the flea's gut, at the cost of harming the flea's life expectancy (Gandon et al., 2019). More specifically, the block prevents the blood meal of a biting flea from reaching the midgut. Stuck, the blood meal mingles with adjacent *Y. pestis* and then is regurgitated, contaminated. The flea, which tried to feed, has, because of the biofilm, primarily succeeded in spreading its very affliction to another animal. The biofilm itself consists of *Y. pestis* meshed in an extracellular matrix of products synthesized by the *Yersinia hms* gene (Hinnebusch & Erickson, 2008). How much the life expectancy of the flea is actually harmed by the biofilm, and its implication, is clearly a point of contention here. One possible understanding of the blockade mechanism was presented over a hundred years ago by the scholar A. W. Bacot (1915), who suggested that incomplete blockages were ideal for the spread of infection. This has the advantage of intuition--a digestive tract mass that makes it more difficult for the flea to feed, but does not completely prevent it, may encourage more effort to feed, provide enough return for the flea to make the feeding efforts seem worthwhile, and, in the process of 'sloshing,' provide plenty of exposure between the *Y. petsis* biomass a the larger mammal from which the flea is trying to take a blood meal. All of this is, of course, something of a digression from Zeppelini et al.'s list of sylvantic reservoir models.

The fourth of the four reservoir models (Zeppelini et al., 2016) delves further into unfamiliar ecology, and posits that *Y. pestis* survives in the long-term by contaminating soil, to act as a parasite for soil Protozoa, plant tissues, or simply exist in a nonculturable state. To employ a comparison that does not exactly match *Y. pestis*' lifecycle, but does clarify the significance of pathogen soil saturation to human infection, dormancy is a fairly common pattern among human pathogens (Coussens & Daines, 2016). Gram-positive bacteria like *Bacillus anthracis* (causing anthrax), and a set of *Clostridium* genus, the species *tetani* (causing tetanus), *botulinum* (causing botulism) and *difficile* (causing colitis induced by antibiotic treatment), all can form spores in conditions that are not favorable to growth and reproduction.

Regardless of which model best reflects *Y. pestis*' normal behavior, the point is clear--*Y. pestis* is especially dangerous because it does not need humans to survive. Where did it come from?

EVOLUTION

When did *Y. pestis* first develop can serve as an anchor to start answering the question of where. Based on genetic similarities, it is believed that *Y. pestis* only emerged as a distinct lineage of bacteria between 3,000 and 6,000 years ago (Hinnebusch et al.,, 2016). At that point it seems to have spun off from a more consistent lineage that today is *Yersinia pseudotuberculosis*. *Y. pseudotuberculosis* is similar to *Y. pestis* in that it is a generalist, and can survive in a wide variety of environments and animals. Where it differs is in the nature of the infection it causes. *Y. pseudotuberculosis* is enteric, and its lifecycle involves fecal-oral transmission. *Y. pseudotuberculosis* infections are generally mild and self-limiting. Understanding how something like *Y. pseudotuberculosis* could turn into something like *Y. pestis*, seems like, and is, a challenge, but the relative youth of *Y. pestis*, combined with the survival of *Y. pseudotuberculosis* to the present day, gives special opportunity for paleogenomic techniques to track its spread. In a convergence of disciplines, once a gravesite suspected to be the resting place of individuals who died from *Y. pestis* is discovered, skeletal tissue like dental pulp and bone can be subjected to PCR (polymerase chain reaction) amplification to detect ancient *Y. pestis* DNA that presumably was involved in their deaths.

Now that there is some sense of how the narrative of *Y. pestis*' evolution might be unveiled, it is worth discussing findings. *Y. pestis* is believed to have emerged in central Asia (Hinnebusch et al., 2016). What the emergence meant, specifically, can be framed in terms of fleas. *Y. pseudotuberculosis* is capable of infecting fleas, and on initial infection, it triggers an acute toxic response. Death within 24 hours is fairly common (Erikson et al., 2007). If the flea survives this period, the center of infection moves to the flea hindgut (Hinnebusch et al., 2016). One of the innovations of *Y. pestis* is that it does not, upon entry, cause a drastic acute rise in flea mortality. Rather, it festers towards the front. The biofilm, or mass of *Y. pestis*, described earlier, forms in the midgut and proventriculus. This change is rather subtle from a certain point of view. Both *Yersinia* variants were originally enteric, and both substantially still are, but while *Y. pseudotuberculosis* is 'content' to remain in the flea gut, *Y. pestis* establishes itself in a way to use the flea gut as a launch pad. By establishing itself close to the location of any future bites, *Y. pestis* can pass itself along with the bite. This change seems to be at the core of the evolution.

HUMANS AND SPREAD

Once plague, in a given epidemic, reached a space where it transferred among human populations, a new question is the ways in which human individuals may or may not have been the main agents of transfer. There is evidence to suggest that while rodents may have, through human history, been an important plague *reservoir*, actual transfers during the Black Death were helped by nonhuman animals, but those animals were more likely to be fleas and lice (Dean et al., 2018). Networks and patterns of human and animal interaction are valuable in understanding the precise patterns of the Black Death--its spread was facilitated by migratory and travel patterns in general (Gómez & Verdú, 2017). As confusion on this issue is cleared up, one discovery is that distinct *Yersinia pestis* lineages collectively caused the Black Death, as well--the emergence of the disease into human populations seems to have occurred a number of times that do not match the discrete pandemic instances of human history (Haensch et al., 2010).

There are other patterns, or lack of patterns that can be associated with the Black Death too. To give a scattered sample: Sexual intercourse did not seem to have an impact on fatality rates of Londoners during the Black Death--this does not seem to have been a vector (DeWitte, 2009). The Black Death quite possibly was not meaningfully present in the Yuan Dynasty of China in the fourteenth century, or the Delhi Sultanate, meaning transportation patterns did not carry plague across all of Eurasia (Sussman, 2011).

To get a better sense of how the Black Death was thought of it its own time, here is a selection from a report put together by the Paris Medical Facility:

Seeing things which cannot be explained, even by the most gifted intellects, initially stirs the human mind to amazement; but after marvelling, the prudent soul next yields to its desire for understanding and, anxious for its own perfection, strives with all its might to discover the causes of the amazing events. For there is within the human mind an innate desire to seize on goodness and truth. As the Philosopher makes plain, all things seek for the good and want to understand.

…

We say that the distant and first cause of this pestilence was and is the configuration of the heavens. In 1345, at one hour after noon on 20 March, there was a major conjunction of three planets in Aquarius. This conjunction, along with other earlier conjunctions and eclipses, by causing a deadly corruption of the air around us, signifies mortality and famine – and also other things about which we will not speak here because they are not relevant. Aristotle testifies that this is the case in his book Concerning the causes of the properties of the elements, in which he says that mortality of races and the depopulation of kingdoms occur at the conjunction of Saturn and Jupiter, for great events then arise,their nature depending on the trigon in which the conjunction occurs.

…

Although major pestilential illnesses can be caused by the corruption of water or food, as happens at times of famine and infertility, yet we still regard illnesses proceeding from the corruption of the air as much more dangerous. This is because bad air is more noxious than food or drink in that it can penetrate quickly to the heart and lungs to do its damage. We believe that the present epidemic or plague has arisen from corrupt air in its substance, and has not changed in its attributes. By which we wish it be understood that air, being pure and clear by nature, can only become putrid or corrupt by being mixed with something else, that is to say, with evil vapours. What happened was that the many vapours which had been corrupted at the time of the conjunction were drawn up from the earth and water, and were then mixed with the air and spread abroad by frequent gusts of wind in the wild southerly, gales, and because of these alien vapours which they carried the winds corrupted the air in its substance, and are still doing so. (Paris Medical Facility, 1348)

So what can really be said about the Black Death? The Black Death changed society in the Italian city of Sienna (Bowsky, 1964). The Black Death was the antecedent of modern plague (Spyrou et al., 2016). Rats may have been too scarce to really spread Black Death (Davis, 1986). The tremendous toll of the Black Death had an impact on people's psyches (Lerner, 1981). The Black Death is the focus here because it is a particularly well-known spread of plague, but what connects it to the next part of the story of plague is the human element.

During the Black Death, the elderly and those exposed to physiological stressors were most susceptible (DeWitte, 2014). The disease was not indiscriminate. It targeted the frail (DeWitte & Wood, 2008). The push to understand plague led to the development of a hypothesis where there is a genetic relationship between plague and human immunodeficiency virus susceptibility, but this is tenuous (Cohn & Weaver, 2006).

Here is a powerful example of a human response to a London outbreak of plague in the seventeenth century:

Now shops are shut in, people rare and very few that walk about, in so much that the grass begins to spring up in some places, and a deep silence almost in every place, especially within the walls; no ratling Coaches, no prancing Horses, no calling in Customers, nor offering Wares; no London cries sounding in the ears; if any voice be heard, it is the groans of dying perions, breathing forth their last, and the funeral knells of them that are ready to be carried to their graves. Now shutting up of visited houses (there being so many) is at an end, and most of the well are mingled among the sick which otherwise would have got no help. Now in some places where the people did generally stay; not one house in an [sic] hundred but is infected; and in many houses half the family is swept away; in some the whole, from the eldest to the youngest; few escape with the death of but one or two: never did so many husbands and wives die together; never did so many parents carry their children with them to the grave, and go together into the same house under earth; who had lived together in the same house upon it. Now the nights are too short to bury the dead, the whole day though at so great a length is hardly sufficient to light the dead that fall therein into their beds. (Vincent, 1678, pp. 36-37)

As with other diseases, humanity came to better understand plague into the nineteenth century, with a plague outbreak in 1894 in Hong Kong being a key catalyst (Echenberg, 2002). At the center of this period of discovery was Alexandre Yersin, a French scientist who became renowned for work he did introducing rubber and quinine to Vietnam (Hawgood, 2008; Solomon, 1995, Nguyen-Viet, 2013).

Before proceeding with what Yersin did, it is worth exploring the context of the Third Plague Pandemic, which Yersin interacted with around China. In China, plague seems to proceed along different patterns; in the south, plague is more intense in times of less wetness, whereas in the north, plague is more intense with wetness (Xu et al., 2011). Intensity is speculated as being mediated through rodent activity in both areas. Flood events, meanwhile, have also been linked to the Third Plague Pandemic increasing its speed of spread in China, possibly, again, through its effects on rodents (Xu et al., 2014).

In order to understand what Alexandre Yersin was doing in Hong Kong in 1894, it may be best to hear from him in his own words (Lebreton-Mansuy, 2014):

Dear Mum,

I'm sure you must be a little anxious to receive this letter, knowing I'm in a place one wouldn't exactly describe as a tourist destination!

After spending a few days in the hotel, I had a straw hut built next to the hospital for plague victims and moved in with my personal belongings and laboratory equipment.

It wasn't at all straightforward and if I hadn't had the luck to meet a kindly Catholic missionary,who agreed to accompany me everywhere and act as my interpreter, I don't know how I would have got by! The missionary's name is Father Vigano. He has been living in Hong Kong for 30 years, so he knows everybody.

I've already been able to study a dozen cases and it wasn't difficult to identify the microbe that multiplies in the bubo, the lymph nodes, the spleen, etc.It looks like a little stick, longer than it is wide, and which is difficult to stain.

It kills mice and guinea pigs, which all display the lesions characteristic of the plague. It's always there; in my mind, there is no doubt.

Along with this letter I am sending a number of small sealed tubes containing pulp from plague buboes to the Institut Pasteur. The disease can then be studied in Paris. My experiments here are very limited because my laboratory is extremely poorly set up. (Lebreton-Mansuy, 2014)

Thusly, with effort, plague was identified. In 1910 to 1911, there was an international effort to combat an outbreak of plague in Manchuria (Knab, 2011). There is still some controversy about how linked the Third Plague Pandemic's *Yersinia pestis* was to the causative agent of the Black Death, but the answer may ultimately be a matter of different strains (Cohn, 2002). With greater hygiene and sanitation, the Third Plague Pandemic's spread in Europe was brought to a close in the 1940s, and greatly curtailed overall (Bramanti et al., 2019). The Third Pandemic certainly never was able to obtain the same scale of impact as the Black Death. However, the story of plague goes beyond Europe, so it is important to point out that plague lingered in Africa before the Third Pandemic, and, into the modern period, there were outbreaks in places like Madagascar (Neerinckx et al., 2010).

To close, the threats of plague into the future are impacted by modern science, and the nature of plague reservoirs. Hygiene and understanding of pathology might curb its spread, but this same understanding raises fears it might one day become a bioweapon (Inglesby, et al., 2000). Human development, as ever, can spread disease as well as it can spread people. For example, in China, surveillance from 2000 to 2015 suggests a specific recent plague outbreak was tied to construction of a reservoir on the Nanpan River, which appeared to displace infected rodents and fleas towards humans (Wang et al., 2017). It is important, in understanding the future of plague, the power of its zoonotic element. In China in 2016, septicemic (bloodborne) plague emerged in the province of Yunnan via dead house rat (Shi et al., 2018) Meanwhile, in the southwest United States, where plague has become endemic among woodrat populations, this species seems to experience periodic die-offs, but enough woodrats survive to maintain the reservoir (Kosoy et al., 2017). The most deadly outbreaks of plague have been well in the past, but the disease persists into a modern context.

REFERENCES

Anderson, D. M., Ciletti, N. A., Lee-Lewis, H., Elli, D., Segal, J., DeBord, K. L., Overheim, K. A., Tretiakova, M., Brubaker, R. R., & Schneewind, O. (2009). Pneumonic plague pathogenesis and immunity in Brown Norway rats. *American Journal of Pathology, 174*(3), 910–921. doi:10.2353/ajpath.2009.071168 PMID:19164505

Anisimov, A. P., & Amoako, K. K. (2006). Treatment of plague: Promising alternatives to antibiotics. *Journal of Medical Microbiology, 55*(11), 1461–1475. doi:10.1099/jmm.0.46697-0 PMID:17030904

Arifuzzaman, M., Ang, W., Choi, H. W., Nilles, M. L., St John, A. L., & Abraham, S. N. (2018). Necroptosis of infiltrated macrophages drives *Yersinia pestis* dispersal within buboes. *JCI Insight, 3*(18), e122188. doi:10.1172/jci.insight.122188 PMID:30232285

Bacot A. W. (1915). LXXXI. Further notes on the mechanism of the transmission of plague by fleas. *The Journal of Hygiene, 14*(Suppl), 774–776.3.

Berube, B. J., Rangel, S. M., & Hauser, A. R. (2016). Pseudomonas aeruginosa: Breaking down barriers. *Current Genetics, 62*(1), 109–113. doi:10.100700294-015-0522-x PMID:26407972

Bowsky, W. M. (1964). The impact of the Black Death upon Sienese government and society. *Speculum, 39*(1), 1–34. doi:10.2307/2850126 PMID:19588595

Bramanti, B., Dean, K. R., & Walløe, L., & Chr. Stenseth, N. (2019). The third plague pandemic in Europe. *Proceedings of the Royal Society B, 286*(1901), 20182429. 10.1098/rspb.2018.2429

Centers for Disease Control and Prevention. (2018, April 4). *Facts About Pneumonic Plague*. https://emergency.cdc.gov/agent/plague/factsheet.asp

Cohn, S. K. Jr. (2002). The Black Death: End of a paradigm. *The American Historical Review, 107*(3), 703–738. doi:10.1086/532493 PMID:12132537

Cohn, S. K. Jr, & Weaver, L. T. (2006). The Black Death and AIDS: CCR5-Δ32 in genetics and history. *Journal of the Association of Physicians, 99*(8), 497–503. doi:10.1093/qjmed/hcl076 PMID:16880184

Coussens, N. P., & Daines, D. A. (2016). Wake me when it's over–bacterial toxin–antitoxin proteins and induced dormancy. *Experimental Biology and Medicine*, *241*(12), 1332–1342. doi:10.1177/1535370216651938 PMID:27216598

Davis, D. E. (1986). The scarcity of rats and the Black Death: An ecological history. *The Journal of Interdisciplinary History*, *16*(3), 455–470. doi:10.2307/204499

Dayer, J. M., Oliviero, F., & Punzi, L. (2017). A brief history of IL-1 and IL-1 Ra in rheumatology. *Frontiers in Pharmacology*, *8*, 293. doi:10.3389/fphar.2017.00293 PMID:28588495

Dean, K. R., Krauer, F., Walløe, L., Lingjærde, O. C., Bramanti, B., Stenseth, N. C., & Schmid, B. V. (2018). Human ectoparasites and the spread of plague in Europe during the Second Pandemic. *Proceedings of the National Academy of Sciences of the United States of America*, *115*(6), 1304–1309. doi:10.1073/pnas.1715640115 PMID:29339508

Demeure, C. E., Dussurget, O., Mas Fiol, G., Le Guern, A. S., Savin, C., & Pizarro-Cerdá, J. (2019). *Yersinia pestis* and plague: An updated view on evolution, virulence determinants, immune subversion, vaccination, and diagnostics. *Genes and Immunity*, *20*(5), 357–370. doi:10.103841435-019-0065-0 PMID:30940874

DeWitte, S. N. (2009). The effect of sex on risk of mortality during the Black Death in London, AD 1349–1350. *American Journal of Physical Anthropology*, *139*(2), 222–234. doi:10.1002/ajpa.20974 PMID:19140182

DeWitte, S. N. (2014). Mortality risk and survival in the aftermath of the medieval Black Death. *PLoS One*, *9*(5), e96513. doi:10.1371/journal.pone.0096513 PMID:24806459

DeWitte, S. N., & Wood, J. W. (2008). Selectivity of Black Death mortality with respect to preexisting health. *Proceedings of the National Academy of Sciences of the United States of America*, *105*(5), 1436–1441. doi:10.1073/pnas.0705460105 PMID:18227518

Dhuriya, Y. K., & Sharma, D. (2018). Necroptosis: A regulated inflammatory mode of cell death. *Journal of Neuroinflammation*, *15*(1), 1–9. doi:10.118612974-018-1235-0 PMID:29980212

Drancourt, M., & Raoult, D. (2016). Molecular history of plague. *Clinical Microbiology and Infection, 22*(11), 911–915. doi:10.1016/j.cmi.2016.08.031 PMID:27615720

Duncan-Jones, R. P. (1996). The impact of the Antonine Plague. *Journal of Roman Archaeology, 9*, 108–136. doi:10.1017/S1047759400016524

Echenberg, M. (2002). Pestis redux: The initial years of the Third Bubonic Plague Pandemic, 1894-1901. *Journal of World History, 13*(2), 429–449. doi:10.1353/jwh.2002.0033 PMID:20712094

Erickson, D. L., Waterfield, N. R., Vadyvaloo, V., Long, D., Fischer, E. R., Ffrench-Constant, R., & Hinnebusch, B. J. (2007). Acute oral toxicity of *Yersinia pseudotuberculosis* to fleas: Implications for the evolution of vector-borne transmission of plague. *Cellular Microbiology, 9*(11), 2658–2666. doi:10.1111/j.1462-5822.2007.00986.x PMID:17587333

Gage, K. L., & Kosoy, M. Y. (2005). Natural history of plague: Perspectives from more than a century of research. *Annual Review of Entomology, 50*(1), 505–528. doi:10.1146/annurev.ento.50.071803.130337 PMID:15471529

Gandon, S., Heitzmann, L., & Sebbane, F. (2019). To block or not to block: The adaptive manipulation of plague transmission. *Evolution Letters, 3*(2), 152–161. doi:10.1002/evl3.111 PMID:31161047

Gómez, J. M., & Verdú, M. (2017). Network theory may explain the vulnerability of medieval human settlements to the Black Death pandemic. *Scientific Reports, 7*(1), 1–7. doi:10.1038rep43467 PMID:28262733

Haensch, S., Bianucci, R., Signoli, M., Rajerison, M., Schultz, M., Kacki, S., Vermunt, M., Weston, D. A., Hurst, D., Achtman, M., Carniel, E., & Bramanti, B. (2010). Distinct clones of *Yersinia pestis* caused the Black Death. *PLoS Pathogens, 6*(10), e1001134. doi:10.1371/journal.ppat.1001134 PMID:20949072

Harbeck, M., Seifert, L., Hänsch, S., Wagner, D. M., Birdsell, D., Parise, K. L., Wiechmann, I., Grupe, G., Thomas, A., Keim, P., Zöller, L., Bramanti, B., Riehm, J. M., & Scholz, H. C. (2013). *Yersinia pestis* DNA from skeletal remains from the 6th century AD reveals insights into Justinianic Plague. *PLoS Pathogens, 9*(5), e1003349. doi:10.1371/journal.ppat.1003349 PMID:23658525

Hawgood, B. J. (2008). Alexandre Yersin (1863–1943): Discoverer of the plague bacillus, explorer and agronomist. *Journal of Medical Biography*, *16*(3), 167–172. doi:10.1258/jmb.2007.007017 PMID:18653838

Hinnebusch, B. J., Chouikha, I., & Sun, Y. C. (2016). Ecological opportunity, evolution, and the emergence of flea-borne plague. *Infection and Immunity*, *84*(7), 1932–1940. doi:10.1128/IAI.00188-16 PMID:27160296

Hinnebusch, B. J., & Erickson, D. L. (2008). *Yersinia pestis* biofilm in the flea vector and its role in the transmission of plague. *Current Topics in Microbiology and Immunology*, *322*, 229–248. doi:10.1007/978-3-540-75418-3_11 PMID:18453279

Inglesby, T. V., Dennis, D. T., Henderson, D. A., Bartlett, J. G., Ascher, M. S., Eitzen, E., Fine, A. D., Friedlander, A. M., Hauer, J., Koerner, J. F., Layton, M., McDade, J., Osterholm, M. T., O'Toole, T., Parker, G., Perl, T. M., Russell, P. K., Schoch-Spana, M., & Tonat, K.Working Group on Civilian Biodefense. (2000). Plague as a biological weapon: Medical and public health management. *Journal of the American Medical Association*, *283*(17), 2281–2290. doi:10.1001/jama.283.17.2281 PMID:10807389

Knab, C. (2011). Plague times: Scientific internationalism and the Manchurian Plague of 1910/1911. *Itinerario*, *35*(3), 87–105. doi:10.1017/S0165115312000083

Knöbl, P. (2018). Thrombotic thrombocytopenic purpura. *Memo*, *11*(3), 220–226. doi:10.100712254-018-0429-6 PMID:30220931

Kosoy, M., Reynolds, P., Bai, Y., Sheff, K., Enscore, R. E., Montenieri, J., Ettestad, P., & Gage, K. (2017). Small-scale die-offs in woodrats support long-term maintenance of plague in the US southwest. *Vector Borne and Zoonotic Diseases (Larchmont, N.Y.)*, *17*(9), 635–644. doi:10.1089/vbz.2017.2142 PMID:28792853

Lebreton-Mansuy, A. (2014). *The discovery of the plague bacillus in Hong Kong, 1894* (H. Tomlinson, Trans.). http://www.bibnum.education.fr/sites/default/files/yersin-analysis-28.pdf

Lerner, R. E. (1981). The Black Death and Western European eschatological mentalities. *The American Historical Review*, *86*(3), 533–552. doi:10.2307/1860369 PMID:11611758

Margolis, D. A., Burns, J., Reed, S. L., Ginsberg, M. M., O'Grady, T. C., & Vinetz, J. M. (2008). Septicemic plague in a community hospital in California. *The American Journal of Tropical Medicine and Hygiene*, *78*(6), 868–871. doi:10.4269/ajtmh.2008.78.868 PMID:18541761

Morozova, I., Kasianov, A., Bruskin, S., Neukamm, J., Molak, M., Batieva, E., ... Schuenemann, V. J. (2020). New ancient Eastern European *Yersinia pestis* genomes illuminate the dispersal of plague in Europe. *Philosophical Transactions of the Royal Society B, 375*(1812), 20190569. doi:10.1098/rstb.2019.0569

Neerinckx, S., Bertherat, E., & Leirs, H. (2010). Human plague occurrences in Africa: An overview from 1877 to 2008. *Transactions of the Royal Society of Tropical Medicine and Hygiene*, *104*(2), 97–103. doi:10.1016/j.trstmh.2009.07.028 PMID:19716148

Nelson, C. A., Fleck-Derderian, S., Cooley, K. M., Meaney-Delman, D., Becksted, H. A., Russell, Z., Renaud, B., Bertherat, E., & Mead, P. S. (2020). Antimicrobial treatment of human plague: A systematic review of the literature on individual cases, 1937–2019. *Clinical Infectious Diseases*, *70*(Supplement_1), S3–S10. doi:10.1093/cid/ciz1226 PMID:32435802

Nguyen-Viet, H. (2013). What have we learned from Dr. Alexandre Yersin? *Y te Công Cong*, *28*, 79–82. https://hdl.handle.net/10568/33893

Pamuk, Ş. (2007). The Black Death and the origins of the 'Great Divergence' across Europe, 1300–1600. *European Review of Economic History*, *11*(3), 289–317. doi:10.1017/S1361491607002031

Paris Medical Faculty. (1348). *The Report of the Paris Medical Faculty*. University of Wisconsin-Milwaukee. https://sites.uwm.edu/carlin/the-report-of-the-paris-medical-faculty-october-1348/

Perry, R. D., & Fetherston, J. D. (1997). *Yersinia pestis*—Etiologic agent of plague. *Clinical Microbiology Reviews*, *10*(1), 35–66. doi:10.1128/CMR.10.1.35 PMID:8993858

Shi, L., Yang, G., Zhang, Z., Xia, L., Liang, Y., Tan, H., He, J., Xu, J., Song, Z., Li, W., & Wang, P. (2018). Reemergence of human plague in Yunnan, China in 2016. *PLoS One*, *13*(6), e0198067. doi:10.1371/journal.pone.0198067 PMID:29897940

Sivaraman, V., Pechous, R. D., Stasulli, N. M., Eichelberger, K. R., Miao, E. A., & Goldman, W. E. (2015). Yersinia pestis activates both IL-1β and IL-1 receptor antagonist to modulate lung inflammation during pneumonic plague. *PLoS Pathogens*, *11*(3), e1004688. doi:10.1371/journal.ppat.1004688 PMID:25781467

Solomon, T. (1995). Alexandre Yersin and the plague bacillus. *The Journal of Tropical Medicine and Hygiene*, *98*(3), 209–212. PMID:7783282

Spyrou, M. A., Tukhbatova, R. I., Feldman, M., Drath, J., Kacki, S., de Heredia, J. B., ... Krause, J. (2016). Historical *Y. pestis* genomes reveal the European Black Death as the source of ancient and modern plague pandemics. *Cell Host & Microbe*, *19*(6), 874–881. doi:10.1016/j.chom.2016.05.012 PMID:27281573

Stenseth, N. C., Atshabar, B. B., Begon, M., Belmain, S. R., Bertherat, E., Carniel, E., Gage, K. L., Leirs, H., & Rahalison, L. (2008). Plague: Past, present, and future. *PLoS Medicine*, *5*(1), e3. doi:10.1371/journal.pmed.0050003 PMID:18198939

Sussman, G. D. (2011). Was the Black Death in India and China? *Bulletin of the History of Medicine*, *85*(3), 319–355. doi:10.1353/bhm.2011.0054 PMID:22080795

Vincent, T. (1678). *God's Terrible Voice in the City*. Early English Books. https://quod.lib.umich.edu/e/eebo/A64990.0001.001?rgn=main;view=full text

Wagner, D. M., Klunk, J., Harbeck, M., Devault, A., Waglechner, N., Sahl, J. W., Enk, J., Birdsell, D. N., Kuch, M., Lumibao, C., Poinar, D., Pearson, T., Fourment, M., Golding, B., Riehm, J. M., Earn, D. J. D., DeWitte, S., Rouillard, J.-M., Grupe, G., ... Poinar, H. (2014). *Yersinia pestis* and the Plague of Justinian 541–543 AD: A genomic analysis. *The Lancet. Infectious Diseases*, *14*(4), 319–326. doi:10.1016/S1473-3099(13)70323-2 PMID:24480148

Wang, X., Wei, X., Song, Z., Wang, M., Xi, J., Liang, J., Liang, Y., Duan, R., Tian, K., Zhao, Y., Tang, G., You, L., Yang, G., Liu, X., Chen, Y., Zeng, J., Wu, S., Luo, S., Qin, G., ... Jing, H. (2017). Mechanism study on a plague outbreak driven by the construction of a large reservoir in southwest China (surveillance from 2000-2015). *PLoS Neglected Tropical Diseases*, *11*(3), e0005425. doi:10.1371/journal.pntd.0005425 PMID:28257423

Xu, L., Liu, Q., Stige, L. C., Ari, T. B., Fang, X., Chan, K. S., ... Zhang, Z. (2011). Nonlinear effect of climate on plague during the Third Pandemic in China. *Proceedings of the National Academy of Sciences of the United States of America, 108*(25), 10214–10219. doi:10.1073/pnas.1019486108 PMID:21646523

Xu, L., Stige, L. C., Kausrud, K. L., Ben Ari, T., Wang, S., Fang, X., . . . Zhang, Z. (2014). Wet climate and transportation routes accelerate spread of human plague. *Proceedings of the Royal Society B: Biological Sciences, 281*(1780), 20133159. 10.1098/rspb.2013.3159

Zeppelini, C. G., de Almeida, A. M., & Cordeiro-Estrela, P. (2016). Zoonoses As ecological entities: A case review of plague. *PLoS Neglected Tropical Diseases, 10*(10), e0004949. doi:10.1371/journal.pntd.0004949 PMID:27711205

Chapter 12
The Relationship Between Vulnerable Populations and the Stigma of Bearing Infectious Disease

ABSTRACT

In this chapter, the text pivots, dropping its focus on the biology of pathogens, as well as events that affected history and politics in any elite sense. Instead, this chapter examines the way infectious disease relates to the common idea of the subaltern. How are those with infectious disease treated? How has cleanliness, and fear of infection, been used to maintain distinctions between social classes? These sorts of questions form the backbone for an investigation of infectious disease that is different from the more top-down style used earlier in the book but may be no less critical to understanding infectious disease's impact on human society.

INTRODUCTION

One of the consequences of infectious disease being a perceived phenomenon, and one that is mediated through human sense experience, is that infectious disease is seen through human assumptions and conceits. Anthropomorphization, for example, is a well-known fallacy that features finding humanlike behavior in places where there is no human behavior to

DOI: 10.4018/978-1-7998-8689-1.ch012

be found (Coffey, 1992). Objects of anthropomorphization include animals (De Waal, 1999), robots (Duffy, 2003), and really every non-human domain imaginable, including clouds (Boyer, 1996). Anthropomorphization certainly also extends to infectious disease. Problematic ways of characterizing infectious disease have already been discussed. This chapter's focus is slightly different, on the situation when infectious disease is associated with real people, who, in important, significant, and meaningful ways, do not deserve responsibility for the weight of the blame placed on them. Infectious disease is, beyond its biological weight, a social stigma, and stigmas both have origin in some perceived cause, and, necessarily, effect how observers see the individual or individuals bearing the stigma.

HIV

A particularly modern example is HIV (human immunodeficiency virus). HIV-1, the predominant version, is a particularly pernicious virus because, while it transmits through the body fluid contact that can occur during intimacy, the birth of a child, or percutaneous drug use, as opposed to via air droplets (Shaw & Hunter, 2012), it also targets cells of the immune system to achieve its lifecycle, particularly $CD4^+$ T cells (Finzi et al., 1999). If left unchecked, by weakening the immune system, HIV can create acquired autoimmune deficiency syndrome, where acute opportunistic infections can overwhelm a body deprived of the tools that would otherwise be able to fight their underlying pathogens off (Zolopa et al., 2009). While untreated, individuals with HIV have a life expectancy of between eight and ten years (Porter et al., 1999; Sabin, 2013). With antiretroviral treatments, the gap can drop to eight years *short* of the life expectancy associated with those without HIV (Marcus et al., 2016). The work done to improve outcomes for individuals with HIV is tied to the enormous amount of attention placed on this uniquely frightening sexually transmitted infection (Carmona-Gutierrez et al., 2016). While the advent of successful antiretrovirals has done much to make the disease be and seem more manageable, the real link between HIV to sexual activity--even if sexual activity is not the only way to acquire HIV--has helped to create a cultural perception, from some corners, of those with HIV, that goes well beyond the confines of the condition (Colvin, 2014; Jefferies et al., 2015). The stigma associated with HIV has ranged from assignment of divine judgement as a cause of the condition (Parsons, 2019), to placement of blood donation restrictions on a group labeled 'men who have sex with men' (MSM) (Galarneau, 2010).

As the example of blood donation restrictions suggest, there is a tension between the awareness that HIV is a disease that requires a response, and difficulties in figuring out exactly what that response should be, especially for the billions of people who are not involved in creating antiretroviral treatments. Social responses are valuable in containing infectious disease, from isolation and contact tracing, notably useful in certain areas that successfully contained COVID-19 spread (Kretzschmar et al., 2021), to the impulse towards nursing and offering of relief that has helped establish a whole profession (Meehan, 2012). However, in a pattern with some similarities to how the human immune system can overreact, or react to stimuli that would not cause problems on their own, human social systems can overreact. This is stigma.

STIGMA

Stigma, as a formal concept, has a murky definition that seems somewhat befitting of the concept itself (Link & Phelan, 2001). One way to tie the varied definitions together is to place emphasis on both an 'exclusionary' subconcept, and an "explanation" subconcept. In other words, those bearing stigma must be socially punished for some identifiable cause. Punishments can include reduced access to housing, food, and medical care, through either formal or informal means. The subconcepts of "exclusion" and "explanation" can have varying degrees of linkage, from a presentation of stigma which frames human nature as naturally excluding those who present in fashions that are contrary to prevailing norms, to a presentation of stigma that meaningfully separates an explanatory attribute from a stereotype that embodies some degree of exclusion. Beyond this dyad, separating out the concepts of labeling, stereotyping and discrimination is valuable to explain the mechanism of social action in the context of stigma. In labeling, a trait or traits is identified. In stereotyping, assumptions about the bearer of the trait or traits are placed, which in a mental fashion separate out the bearer of the trait or traits from receiving nuanced examination. Finally, in discrimination, behavior is enacted by the stereotyper, using the stereotype to justify certain behavior.

What is striking about the description just provided of "active stigma" is that it is very close to the idea of heuristics. Heuristics are essentially decision-making processes that ignore some of the available information so to make a decision more efficiently (Gigerenzer & Gaissmaier, 2011). It is hard to think of any decision-making process that is not tied to this idea of a heuristic. What would it mean to make a decision based on *all* available information? Even someone who makes an effort to spend days, weeks, or years researching a question must at some point stop their research and decide that they have obtained enough grounding, if they have interest in making a decision. Despite actual definitions of stigma often not having a prominent moral component, when the term is used in practice, a moral component easily creeps in, and can frame stigma as something that must necessarily be diminished (Yang et al., 2007). This usage of the term stigma, is, indeed, largely the one employed by the present chapter, but to understand how simplifications about other humans can result in overreach, or inappropriate judgements, it seems valuable to put some emphasis on how stigma is not necessarily negative in all contexts.

For an example that is not intended by the author to be praiseworthy, but rather an example of complexity, return to the men who have sex with men category, and the idea of risk categories. Separate from the example, it makes sense that certain individuals whose blood would be harmful should not be able to donate. Beginning to reintroduce ethical complexity, the idea of coming up with rules that help determine whether a blood donor is likely to be safe also seems appropriate, given that decision-making processes must exist. The trouble comes when one of these categories is recent male-on-male sexual activity, which has been associated with higher-than normal risk of acquiring HIV (Zhang & Chu, 2005). Despite the fact that the exculsionary category in question is "men who have sex with men," and not gay men, or homosexual men, leaving the door open to those who identify as gay but do not engage in sex acts, as well as gay women, who, at least biologically, are less likely to engage in penetrative sex, "men who have sex with men" is still a category that is very closely linked to a specific group with a history of being discriminated against, raising the question about whether using the 'men who have sex with men' category is appropriate. It seems an open question whether stigma contributes more to infectious disease, or vice versa.

In other words, discrimination can cause real harm, and infectious disease can cause real harm. How can discrimination be used in its 'choosing-between-options' sense, rather than its 'inappropriate-negative-treatment' sense, to make the best choices in the space surrounding infectious disease? It is not clear there is a good answer to this question. Slipping into stereotypes is something of a natural process (Nelson et al., 1996). Stereotypes can be defined simply as categorical social information. Since human brains are associative, and link new information to old information as new connections form, it is possibly physically impossible to expect humans to place information about new individuals in their existing headspace without leaning to some degree on prior ideas about the way human beings behave, and thus resorting to stereotypes. However, this point does not detract from the harm done when human beings are treated simplistically. There is, for example, a powerful argument to be made that blood screening techniques can reduce or eliminate the need to prevent blood donations by MSM, or a to have a holding period delay separating time from sex act to time eligible to give blood (Sturrock & Mucklow, 2018). The idea of technology as a panacea that makes choices easier is not a new one--the idea of science solving all problems is at least as old as the start of the scientific revolution in the sixteenth century (Hudson-Rodd, 1995). The fact that technology can be seen as a panacea does not make technology's utility untrue. Rather, tools like blood screens are just one more element that humans must consider, and a particularly powerful one, as we determine what mental shortcuts to make. As a powerful example of the promise and peril of modern techniques, it is important to point out that their parameters tend to be set by humans--with bad inputs and bad rules put in place for machines to follow, even extremely precise outputs by machines can have little meaning (Shi, 2003).

LEPROSY

It may be useful at this point to take a step back, and consider an older example of an infectious disease carrying much stigma, to better understand the features of how stigma functions. This disease in this case will be leprosy. Here is an excerpt from a translation of William of Tyre's "A History of Deeds Done Beyond the Sea," a contemporary history of the part of the world surrounding the crusader kingdoms (Chadwick, 2016). The protagonist, who will become King Baldwin IV of Jerusalem, also has an affliction:

The other boys gave evidence of pain by their outcries, but Baldwin, although his comrades did not spare him, endured it altogether too patiently, as if he felt nothing. After this had occurred several times it was reported to me. At first I supposed that it proceeded from his capacity for endurance and not from lack of sensitiveness. But when I called him and began to inquire what it meant, I discovered that his right arm and hand were partially numb so that he did not feel pinching or even biting in the least. (Chadwick, 2016)

Baldwin's disease progressed in the time that followed, despite the efforts of those who wished to help him (Chadwick, 2016). While the point of view of this excerpt is sympathetic, presenting the lack of feeling in an almost saintly way, the sense of Baldwin's otherness seems palpable. William of Tyre seems to have nothing against Baldwin, quite the opposite, and yet half the stigma is present. There is not clear condemnation, but condemnation is not necessary to present separation. And, of course, not every person with leprosy in the medieval period had anywhere near the resources of a future king. Throughout history and locations, leprosy has had an association with sin, probably even more than contagion, since it was reasonably well known that leprosy is limited in its ability to be infectious (Sermrittirong & Van Brakel, 2014). There was, nevertheless, a substantial outbreak centered in Western Europe from 1000 to 1300, and this helped shape the complicated cultural context of the Christendom that Baldwin inhabited (Miller & Smith-Savage, 2006).

To put the culture in comparison with the disease itself, leprosy is a condition created by the pathogen *Mycobacterium leprae*, which requires the pathogen to be extensively in the presence of a susceptible individual (Lastória & Abreu, 2014). The susceptible aspect is very important--genetic predisposition is important to catching the disease, even though *M. leprae* passes through nasal mucosa. This interaction between the pathogen and genetics, to create disease, has a meaningful connection to the interaction between disease and social or personal context to create illness, or effect. As much as 95% of the population has resistance to catching leprosy (Bennett et al., 2008), and thanks to modern science, we know that genetic risk to leprosy comes from variations in the PARK2 and PACRG genes (MIra et al., 2004) but out of the remaining group, the experience is still very real.

ILLNESS AND VULNERABILITY

Thinking about leprosy in a modern sense lends itself also to thinking about precise terminology. How does leprosy specifically relate to stigma? As to another related question--what is illness? In other words, what does it mean to be sick at all? The desire of the scientific aspects of modernity to place specific definitions on concepts runs into some difficulties when it comes to the idea of illness. Illness has a vague definition, but is tied to perception (Emerson, 1987). That is, how someone feels as a result of acquiring a condition, such as the presence of a pathogen. The idea that what one person considers "sick" might not be considered "sick" to another person opens up a number of interesting questions about what the experience of infectious disease actually is, questions that appear to be so essential that the nature of what we consider as "illness" seems to be passed down generationally, through conversations like that of a parent to a child (Campbell, 1975).

The value of bringing up illness here is because it is a way of thinking about "deep stigma." That is, the way in which stigma is more than merely a phenomenon that exists on a macrosocial level, but is also something that has specific implications for individuals who are trying to navigate a world with stigma. Stigma can be considered a secret burden of illness that reduces access to resources for those who may need resources most (Weiss et al., 2006). Those who are homeless and those who are mentally ill are two categories of individuals whose stigma seems fundamentally associated with their need for resources. The concept of "penalty for vulnerability" is certainly a social phenomenon, but it is also a personal one. Consider, as an example that may be particularly familiar to those who have lived in certain cities, the ways in which many passerby are socialized to ignore individuals who are homeless (Artz, 2001). Being ignored is necessarily personal to the person who is being ignored, while, as a method of alienation, being an embodiment of stigma. Engaging with the range of ways stigma impacts the everyday life of many people likely goes beyond the scope of this chapter, but what does not go beyond the scope is the idea that stigma exacerbates illness. Stigma causes stress (Rüsch et al., 2014). Stress leads to illness, and even can be linked to pathology, or specific disease progression (Cohen & Williamson, 1991). When the role of institutions are factored in, the role stigma can play on progression of infectious disease is even more extreme. Stigma can lead institutions to deny services (Brown et al., 2017). For example, Martins (2008) raises a term called "social triage" in the context of homeless experience in emergency rooms. While the theory behind triage is that everyone will be seen eventually, the fact that priority decisions may be made based on factors unrelated to need is enough to reinforce the idea of disparity. Informal tendencies towards stigma-based decisions appear to have created a contest with the prerogatives of public health starting as early as the field of public health could be articulated (Hatzenbuehler et al., 2013). Nineteenth century asylums for the mentally ill are a clear example of a real need for services--and real capacity to provide them--in complicated interaction with the stigma-driven tendency to put the "other" out of sight.

By making the connection between stigma and individual experience, and outcomes, it is possible to broaden the discussion of stigma more systematically, and consider how individual vulnerabilities lead to concrete categories of social need. One clear example of specific group stigma has already been presented--that of stigma to homeless people. Homeless people are particularly vulnerable to infectious disease (Raoult et al., 2001). Individuals who are refugees are also particularly vulnerable to infectious disease (Mockenhaupt et al., 2016). There appears to be a reciprocal link between having a status associated with stigma, and having increased burden of infectious disease, because of the way stigma increases stress and decreases access to services.

So far, the discussion in this chapter has broadly covered the concept of stigma, covered some ways stigma can relate to HIV and leprosy, and then broadened again and engaged with the linkages between the concepts of stigma, illness, infectious disease, stress, and vulnerable populations. As the chapter progresses, additional emphasis will be placed on personal testimonies. In the illness concept, the personal experience of the patient is critical, and it is particularly valuable in the context of this chapter's topic to show how the personal experience of individuals with infectious diseases can have their experiences substantively shaped by stigma, and their social context. However, before the section with personal testimonies begins in earnest, there is value in putting some emphasis on the mechanism by which stigma can interact with infectious disease, and society, and produce these outcomes. Smith (2012) finds that stigma can be generated from something as potentially contrived as an infectious disease alert (consider numbers of cases on a television screen or website, linking the disease implicitly or explicitly to specific regions or groups of peoples). Tenuous geographic association mediated by externally imposed racial identifications can spread social penalties of disease to noninfected persons--the coronavirus outbreak that began in 2019 has led to increases in anti-Asian stigma and discrimination, in part surrounding assumptions of who does and does not have the diesease (Misra et al., 2020). Smith and Huges (2014) press the idea that stigma from infectious disease is not helpful in our modern society, which has more sophisticated tools to deal with strange experiences that are potential threats.

PERSONAL EXPERIENCE: LEPROSY

With certain abstractions and specifics about stigma settled, the chapter can move on to direct experiences. The first direct experience involves an individual who acquired leprosy, and goes like this:

In 2003, a doctor in Phnom Penh told me that I had leprosy. "What is leprosy?" I asked him.

As he explained the disease, he told me that I could be cured. But he also said leprosy stigmatizes those who have it, and many people are afraid of it.

When I heard this, it made me very sad. I didn't want to live in this world anymore. I wanted to die.

I didn't tell my family about leprosy. I kept my condition to myself and lived alone with my worries, which were so big. I stayed in my room in the pagoda for one year. I didn't want to go out and meet people.

Between 2003 and 2004 I was treated with MDT at a health center in Kandal Province. At the end of 2004, I had reconstructive surgery on my hands and feet.

After that, I got a job with CIOMAL at the Kien Khleang national leprosy rehabiliation unit. I now work as a Khmer language teacher and support worker. I stopped being a monk in 2005. (Sophea, 2006)

The mechanism by which stigma acts is extremely visible here. First the author of the passage is diagnosed. Then they seek clarification about their condition, including social clarification. The doctor, in response, lets the author know that leprosy is the subject of stigma, and there may well be social sanctions associated with having the condition, whether or not they are deserved. This clarification then seems to overwhelm the author. The fact that in the author's age, leprosy can be cured, does not seem to be as significant as the fact that leprosy is associated with social consequences. The author's description of subsequent behavior suggests that they act accordingly. They hide their condition from family. They live alone. However, as they do so, they obtain treatment, and get a job at a group associated with leprosy rehabilitation. Then they ultimately obtain further work. What is striking about this passage is how the bulk of the difficulty surrounding the condition seems to be social. To state that the condition itself was not burdensome seems to be going much too far. However, the fact remains that the difficulties actually presented in the above passage are social in nature, not physical, and, insofar as they are true to the author's recollection, emphasize a disease burden that is very different from a list of physical symptoms.

PERSONAL EXPERIENCE: HIV

With this presentation of leprosy stigma presented in approximately contemporary words, the chapter will turn to a pathogen that for many has more contemporary associations, including association with stigma--HIV. The nature of HIV was discussed to some degree earlier in this chapter, but for the present purposes, one aspect of the related pathology that is worth mentioning is how HIV spends a great deal of time hiding in the body. Ruelas and Green (2013) go so far as to state that HIV is incurable because of the way HIV integrates into host DNA, and while technology and research and time are working to overcome this, the 34 million infected at the time of their writing as of yet have a disease not known to be curable. (As of 2022, there is major hope and mounting evidence around a procedure involving transplantation of HIV-resistant stem cells (Weill Cornell Medicine, 2022).) The following set of passages comes from a speaker known as Boris, a gay man who was diagnosed with HIV at the age of nineteen (Boris, 2019).

I was very scared and realised that I wasn't really aware of what was happening to me. The very next day I went back to my doctors and told them that I wanted to postpone starting the treatment. I was devastated and couldn't really see myself taking treatment for the rest of my life or at least until they invent cure [sic] for it.

...

After almost three years of not taking treatment, and a lot of sleepless nights and sadness, I finally decided to stop allowing this thing to defeat me. I don't even know how but I found strength in me and went to the doctors again. They put me on antiretroviral treatment which I've been taking for two years now. (Boris, 2019)

One detail that is interesting about these paragraphs is the way in which the experience of HIV was mediated through the author's perceptions. That is–"I wasn't really aware of what was happening to me." This shock then leads to a decision that also seems tied to being overwhelmed--the decision not to take treatment. The author then goes through a series of personal experiences that allow them to confront their condition, and, after three years, begin antiretroviral treatment. The experience in this story seems, in terms of the author's personal experience, almost purely mental and social. With the nature of HIV, someone with the virus can go for years with minimal to no symptoms, before a particular threshold is hit and the condition presents with symptoms that are very apparent. In the three years in which the author was coming to terms, the physical symptoms appear to have been mild, but, tellingly, not the mental or social ones. The experience of these three years is defined as "sleepless nights and sadness." These may not be "expected" symptoms directly caused by a serious virus, but as indirect effects, they make a lot of sense. The perceptions of the author matter, and even seem to describe the bulk of their experience with HIV to the time period mentioned in the writing.

To reframe, the personal aspect of stigma is critical. Human beings are emotional creatures, and part of our emotions are tied to the way in which we relate to presented facts. The strength the author describes as needing to present is the strength to get treatment. From a perspective that purely focuses on physical symptoms, the idea of "strength to get treatment" may make no sense. Treatment is what fixes problems. Fixing problems prior to getting treatment seems to miss the idea of treatment. However, the supplement to this logic is that the nature of illness places the social problems that arise from a disease as part of the disease experience--phenomena that may need to be treated in their own right.

The next passage is from an HIV-positive heterosexual male who was diagnosed in the late 1980s (Mooney, 2005):

R: You never considered telling your family?

J: No no no chance it's just that on the list of people to tell your family would be the lowest on the list you were gonna tell one one one of the reasons was and still is to a certain extent was that the family might think you're gay and I mean I I I mean that's still an issue now but it was certainly a big issue back when it was a gay plague I mean now it's not quite so bad because there's a lot more heteros whoare positive and and a lot more black and no one's gonna think of you're black because I'm not but being gay is nothing to do with the colour of your skin so again from a hetero guy's point of view it's like [inaudible] if you're down the pub or whatever and you want to insult someone you call them a poof and particularly in the early 90s it was because there weren't that many black Africans coming to the UK with it it was very much a it was gay plague. And the last thing on earth on top of all the other insults would be people thinking I was gay (Mooney, 2005, p.76)

From this passage, it is apparent just how much the social dimension of HIV contributed to the speaker's experience. The speaker thinks of HIV in terms of how it connects to "insults," and minority groups in his UK home. In his eyes, Blacks and gay people are the ones to get HIV, and understanding that shows awareness of historically high-risk groups (Eaton et al., 1999). However, the way in which the speaker engages with thought about these groups shows problems with stigma. In the passage, being seen as gay is seen as inherently problematic, and being African, or Black, is associated with having HIV too. The nuance of a risk group is missing from this analysis. The bad condition, HIV, is associated with groups that have been historically disadvantaged in the UK, and that is where the analysis rests--on the idea that one marker of difference, having HIV, hints at another marker of difference, being gay, and association with either is socially dangerous. This sort of thinking creates obvious barriers for treatment and quality of life for all groups involved. The phrase "gay plague" is a clear example of the confusion between two categories, and, aside from not being accurate--the speaker in the passage is heterosexual--actively contributes to lack of awareness in anyone who hears it. The barriers to treatment and quality of life associated with stigma seem to come from two different sources. First, internal belief. Second, efforts to protect oneself from the label. In the passage, the speaker doesn't explicitly say how HIV makes him feel, though later in the article he does ("it is summed up I feel dirty" (Mooney, 2005, p.77)). However, what he does emphasize is the way the social confusion of the concepts of HIV and being gay, as well as the stigma he sensed surrounding both, put up real barriers to him being able to communicate openly, even with people very important in his life. This has an element of practicality in a context of danger--in the social world we live in, the attitudes others have towards you matter, for work, life, and even physical safety. In the world in which the speaker was diagnosed, even someone who does not see any credence in thinking of HIV as a generic negative has to navigate the attitudes others have towards the disease.

In other words, one of the key problems with stigma is the way in which it is simplistic. Stigma identifies outgroups, and conveys a sense of exclusion, which would be useful for the extremely limited purpose of encouraging an individual to not have unprotected sex with another individual who has HIV. However, once one adds in the miasma of everything associated with HIV being bad, including the person, and including other conditions the sensitive individual finds unusual, the targeting becomes overbroad and inefficient in a society where people must live with each other in a broad community, and cannot simply run from things they do not understand.

PERSONAL EXPERIENCE: SEXUALLY-TRANSMITTED INFECTIOUS DISEASE

Now that multiple narratives have been provided, there should be new value in going through more patterns associated with stigma of infectious disease, including sexually-transmitted disease. The possibility of moral sigma leads to underplaying of the risks of sexually-transmitted infectious diseases (Young et al., 2007). College students avoid testing because of stigma (Barth et al., 2002). Stigma is a barrier to treatment in the Deep South of the United States (Lichtenstein, 2003). Stigma is a barrier in similar ways in China (Liu et al., 2002). Environments where particular stigma is present seem to affect rates of condom usage in Sierra Leone (Kelly et al., 2017). Stigma is a barrier to seeking care in sexually-transmitted diseases ranging from HIV to gonorrhea (Fortenberry et al., 2002). Stigma can interfere with health-promoting behaviors during disease outbreaks (Fischer et al., 2019). Finally fear and stigma generally delay detection and treatment efforts (Barrett & Brown, 2008).

To begin to close out this chapter, the last narrative presented will focus on human papillomavirus (HPV). HPV is thought to be the main factor in cervical carcinoma (Durson et al., 2009) even though it is sometimes perceived as a less-threatening sexually-transmitted infection (Gillis et al., 2020). The narrative that follows is uniquely human but shares common patterns to those seen above:

At the time, I was in denial about it. I told myself that that wasn't what it was because my sister had a similar thing happen, the displasia. So, I just kind of told myself that it was hereditary. That was kinda funny because I asked the nurse that called if it could be hereditary, and she said "No, this is completely sexually transmitted"--I really didn't accept it until a few months after my cryosurgery. (Nack, 2000, p. 102)

The idea of sexual transmission as being a particular source of shame is common between this source and the source interviewed by Mooney (2005, p. 77). The theme of lack of knowledge presented in some of the earlier passages is continued here, and, in this instance, there is specific denial. The speaker in the passage is not the sort of person who can get HPV, so goes the denial, because her sister--a social comparison--had a condition that seemed similar and was not as stigmatized. The speaker gets treatment regardless, and it is this treatment that gives the speaker the space to accept their condition--after it is no longer a part of them. It seems they are better able to accept an apparent source of stigma after the stigma was removed.

CONCLUSION

Infectious disease is experienced by humans, and acts through a wide variety of biological and social mechanisms. Big history, belief, science, and stigma are among the ways in which infectious disease can be examined, and from a given perspective, any one of these might be the easiest to explore, while others might struggle to seem relevant. However, all of the analysis paths may always exist together, highlighting both human strength and human vulnerability, as well as the strengths and vulnerabilities of pathogens.

It is the hope of the author that the reader comes away from this text with increased interest in the interplay of the different factors that contextualize infectious disease, as well as the ways any perspective might affect or influence any other. Medical pathology threads with sociology–science must necessarily be interpreted by all people who wish to use it to contribute to population health. With the coronavirus pandemic that originated in 2019, infectious disease has become a more mainstream topic, perhaps helping to remove some stigma surrounding a range of different associations with the subject. Infectious disease is one of many important issues, and will likely stay that way, as it is deeply embedded into the world humans live in.

REFERENCES

Artz, L. (2001). Critical ethnography for communication studies: Dialogue and social justice in service-learning. *Southern Journal of Communication*, *66*(3), 239–250. doi:10.1080/10417940109373202

Barrett, R., & Brown, P. J. (2008). Stigma in the time of influenza: Social and institutional responses to pandemic emergencies. *The Journal of Infectious Diseases*, *197*(s1), S34–S37. doi:10.1086/524986 PMID:18269326

Barth, K. R., Cook, R. L., Downs, J. S., Switzer, G. E., & Fischhoff, B. (2002). Social stigma and negative consequences: Factors that influence college students' decisions to seek testing for sexually transmitted infections. *Journal of American College Health, 50*(4), 153–159. doi:10.1080/07448480209596021 PMID:11910948

Bennett, B. H., Parker, D. L., & Robson, M. (2008). Leprosy: Steps along the journey of eradication. *Public Health Reports, 123*(2), 198–205. doi:10.1177/003335490812300212 PMID:18457072

Boris. (2019, September 26). *Boris - Go and get tested for HIV*. https://www.avert.org/living-with-hiv/stories/boris

Boyer, P. (1996). What makes anthropomorphism natural: Intuitive ontology and cultural representations. *Journal of the Royal Anthropological Institute, 2*(1), 83–97. doi:10.2307/3034634

Brown, G., Leonard, W., Lyons, A., Power, J., Sander, D., McColl, W., Johnson, R., James, C., Hodson, M., & Carman, M. (2017). Stigma, gay men and biomedical prevention: The challenges and opportunities of a rapidly changing HIV prevention landscape. *Sexual Health, 14*(1), 111–118. doi:10.1071/SH16052 PMID:27977386

Campbell, J. D. (1975). Illness is a point of view: The development of children's concepts of illness. *Child Development, 46*(1), 92–100. doi:10.2307/1128837

Carmona-Gutierrez, D., Kainz, K., & Madeo, F. (2016). Sexually transmitted infections: Old foes on the rise. *Microbial Cell, 3*(9), 361–362. doi:10.15698/mic2016.09.522 PMID:28357374

Chadwick, E. (2016, February 6). *Primary source Saturday: Baldwin IV The leper king*. Elizabeth Chadwick: The official website. https://elizabethchadwick.com/blog/primary-source-saturday-baldwin-iv-the-leper-king/

Coffey, E. J. (1992). The anthropomorphic fallacy. *Journal of the British Interplanetary Society, 45*(1), 23–29.

Cohen, S., & Williamson, G. M. (1991). Stress and infectious disease in humans. *Psychological Bulletin, 109*(1), 5–24. doi:10.1037/0033-2909.109.1.5 PMID:2006229

Colvin, C. J. (2014). Evidence and AIDS activism: HIV scale-up and the contemporary politics of knowledge in global public health. *Global Public Health: An International Journal for Research, Policy and Practice*, *9*(1-2), 57–72. doi:10.1080/17441692.2014.881519 PMID:24498918

De Waal, F. B. (1999). Anthropomorphism and anthropodenial: Consistency in our thinking about humans and other animals. *Philosophical Topics*, *27*(1), 255–280. doi:10.5840/philtopics199927122

Duffy, B. R. (2003). Anthropomorphism and the social robot. *Robotics and Autonomous Systems*, *42*(3-4), 177–190. doi:10.1016/S0921-8890(02)00374-3

Dursun, P., Senger, S. S., Arslan, H., Kuşçu, E., & Ayhan, A. (2009). Human papillomavirus (HPV) prevalence and types among Turkish women at a gynecology outpatient unit. *BMC Infectious Diseases*, *9*(1), 1–6. doi:10.1186/1471-2334-9-191 PMID:19948015

Eaton, L. A., Matthews, D. D., Bukowski, L. A., Friedman, M. R., Chandler, C. J., Whitfield, D. L., Sang, J. M., & Stall, R. D. (1999). Elevated HIV Prevalence and Correlates of PrEP Use Among a Community Sample of Black Men Who Have Sex With Men. *Journal of Acquired Immune Deficiency Syndromes*, *79*(3), 339–346. doi:10.1097/QAI.0000000000001822 PMID:30063650

Emson, H. E. (1987). Health, disease and illness: Matters for definition. *Canadian Medical Association Journal*, *136*(8), 811–813. PMID:3567788

Finzi, D., Blankson, J., Siliciano, J. D., Margolick, J. B., Chadwick, K., Pierson, T., Smith, K., Lisziewicz, J., Lori, F., Flexner, C., Quinn, T. C., Chaisson, R. E., Rosenberg, E., Walker, B., Gange, S., Gallant, J., & Siliciano, R. F. (1999). Latent infection of CD4+ T cells provides a mechanism for lifelong persistence of HIV-1, even in patients on effective combination therapy. *Nature Medicine*, *5*(5), 512–517. doi:10.1038/8394 PMID:10229227

Fischer, L. S., Mansergh, G., Lynch, J., & Santibanez, S. (2019). Addressing disease-related stigma during infectious disease outbreaks. *Disaster Medicine and Public Health Preparedness*, *13*(5-6), 989–994. doi:10.1017/dmp.2018.157 PMID:31156079

Fortenberry, J. D., McFarlane, M., Bleakley, A., Bull, S., Fishbein, M., Grimley, D. M., Malotte, C. K., & Stoner, B. P. (2002). Relationships of stigma and shame to gonorrhea and HIV screening. *American Journal of Public Health*, *92*(3), 378–381. doi:10.2105/AJPH.92.3.378 PMID:11867314

Galarneau, C. (2010). Blood donation, deferral, and discrimination: FDA donor deferral policy for men who have sex with men. *The American Journal of Bioethics*, *10*(2), 29–39. doi:10.1080/15265160903487619 PMID:20131170

Gigerenzer, G., & Gaissmaier, W. (2011). Heuristic decision making. *Annual Review of Psychology*, *62*(1), 451–482. doi:10.1146/annurev-psych-120709-145346 PMID:21126183

Gillis, J. L., Grennan, T., Grewal, R., Ogilvie, G., Gaspar, M., Grace, D., Lofters, A., Raboud, J. M., Saarela, O., MacPherson, P., Rosenes, R., Salit, I. E., & Burchell, A. N. (2020). Low human papillomavirus (HPV) knowledge related to low risk perception among men living with HIV: Implications for HPV-associated disease prevention. *Preventive Medicine*, *9*, 191. doi:10.1016/j.ypmed.2020.106274 PMID:33022315

Hatzenbuehler, M. L., Phelan, J. C., & Link, B. G. (2013). Stigma as a fundamental cause of population health inequalities. *American Journal of Public Health*, *103*(5), 813–821. doi:10.2105/AJPH.2012.301069 PMID:23488505

Hudson-Rodd, N. (1995). Hygeia or panacea? Ethnogeography and health in Canada: Seventeenth to eighteenth century. *History of European Ideas*, *21*(2), 235–246. doi:10.1016/0191-6599(94)00262-E

Jeffries, W. L. IV, Townsend, E. S., Gelaude, D. J., Torrone, E. A., Gasiorowicz, M., & Bertolli, J. (2015). HIV stigma experienced by young men who have sex with men (MSM) living with HIV infection. *AIDS Education and Prevention*, *27*(1), 58–71. doi:10.1521/aeap.2015.27.1.58 PMID:25646730

Kelly, J. D., Reid, M. J., Lahiff, M., Tsai, A. C., & Weiser, S. D. (2017). Community-level HIV stigma as a driver for HIV transmission risk behaviors and sexually transmitted diseases in Sierra Leone: A population-based study. *Journal of Acquired Immune Deficiency Syndromes*, *75*(4), 399–407. doi:10.1097/QAI.0000000000001418 PMID:28406807

Kretzschmar, M. E., Rozhnova, G., & van Boven, M. (2021). Isolation and contact tracing can tip the scale to containment of COVID-19 in populations with social distancing. *Frontiers in Physics*, *8*, 677. doi:10.3389/fphy.2020.622485

Lastória, J. C., & Abreu, M. A. (2014). Leprosy: Review of the epidemiological, clinical, and etiopathogenic aspects - part 1. *Anais Brasileiros de Dermatologia*, *89*(2), 205–218. doi:10.1590/abd1806-4841.20142450 PMID:24770495

Lichtenstein, B. (2003). Stigma as a barrier to treatment of sexually transmitted infection in the American deep south: Issues of race, gender and poverty. *Social Science & Medicine*, *57*(12), 2435–2445. doi:10.1016/j.socscimed.2003.08.002 PMID:14572849

Link, B. G., & Phelan, J. C. (2001). Conceptualizing stigma. *Annual Review of Sociology*, *27*(1), 363–385. doi:10.1146/annurev.soc.27.1.363

Liu, H., Detels, R., Li, X., Ma, E., & Yin, Y. (2002). Stigma, delayed treatment, and spousal notification among male patients with sexually transmitted disease in China. *Sexually Transmitted Diseases*, *29*(6), 335–343. doi:10.1097/00007435-200206000-00005 PMID:12035023

Marcus, J. L., Chao, C. R., Leyden, W. A., Xu, L., Quesenberry, C. P. Jr, Klein, D. B., Towner, W. J., Horberg, M. A., & Silverberg, M. J. (2016). Narrowing the Gap in Life Expectancy Between HIV-Infected and HIV-Uninfected Individuals With Access to Care. *Journal of Acquired Immune Deficiency Syndromes*, *73*(1), 39–46. doi:10.1097/QAI.0000000000001014 PMID:27028501

Martins, D. C. (2008). Experiences of homeless people in the health care delivery system: A descriptive phenomenological study. *Public Health Nursing (Boston, Mass.)*, *25*(5), 420–430. doi:10.1111/j.1525-1446.2008.00726.x PMID:18816359

Meehan, T. C. (2012). Spirituality and spiritual care from a careful nursing perspective. *Journal of Nursing Management*, *20*(8), 990–1001. doi:10.1111/j.1365-2834.2012.01462.x PMID:23151101

Miller, T. S., & Smith-Savage, R. (2006). Medieval leprosy reconsidered. *International Social Science Review*, *81*(1/2), 16–28. https://www.jstor.org/stable/41887256

Mira, M. T., Alcais, A., Van Thuc, N., Moraes, M. O., Di Flumeri, C., Thai, V. H., ... Schurr, E. (2004). Susceptibility to leprosy is associated with PARK2 and PACRG. *Nature*, *427*(6975), 636–640. doi:10.1038/nature02326 PMID:14737177

Misra, S., Le, P. D., Goldmann, E., & Yang, L. H. (2020). Psychological impact of anti-Asian stigma due to the COVID-19 pandemic: A call for research, practice, and policy responses. *Psychological Trauma: Theory, Research, Practice, and Policy*, *12*(5), 461–464. doi:10.1037/tra0000821 PMID:32525390

Mockenhaupt, F. P., Barbre, K. A., Jensenius, M., Larsen, C. S., Barnett, E. D., Stauffer, W., Rothe, C., Asgeirsson, H., Hamer, D. H., Esposito, D. H., Gautret, P., & Schlagenhauf, P. (2016). Profile of illness in Syrian refugees: A GeoSentinel analysis, 2013 to 2015. *Eurosurveillance*, *21*(10), 30160. doi:10.2807/1560-7917.ES.2016.21.10.30160 PMID:26987893

Mooney, A. (2005). Some body wants to be normal: An account of an HIV narrative. *Medical Humanities*, *31*(2), 72–80. doi:10.1136/jmh.2005.000198 PMID:23674664

Nack, A. (2000). Damaged goods: Women managing the stigma of STDs. *Deviant Behavior*, *21*(2), 95–121. doi:10.1080/016396200266298

Nelson, T. E., Acker, M., & Manis, M. (1996). Irrepressible stereotypes. *Journal of Experimental Social Psychology*, *32*(1), 13–38. doi:10.1006/jesp.1996.0002

Parsons, S. (2019). Fear of punishment in another world: A follow-up examination of the religious beliefs about HIV/AIDS—a decade of progress? *Journal of Religion and Health*, •••, 1–13. doi:10.100710943-019-00962-z PMID:31863262

Porter, K., Johnson, A. M., Phillips, A. N., & Darbyshire, J. H. (1999). The practical significance of potential biases in estimates of the AIDS incubation period distribution in the UK Register of HIV seroconverters. *AIDS (London, England)*, *13*(14), 1943–1951. doi:10.1097/00002030-199910010-00018 PMID:10513654

Raoult, D., Foucault, C., & Brouqui, P. (2001). Infections in the homeless. *The Lancet. Infectious Diseases*, *1*(2), 77–84. doi:10.1016/S1473-3099(01)00062-7 PMID:11871479

Ruelas, D. S., & Greene, W. C. (2013). An integrated overview of HIV-1 latency. *Cell*, *155*(3), 519–529. doi:10.1016/j.cell.2013.09.044 PMID:24243012

Rüsch, N., Müller, M., Lay, B., Corrigan, P. W., Zahn, R., Schönenberger, T., Bleiker, M., Lengler, S., Blank, C., & Rössler, W. (2014). Emotional reactions to involuntary psychiatric hospitalization and stigma-related stress among people with mental illness. *European Archives of Psychiatry and Clinical Neuroscience*, *264*(1), 35–43. doi:10.100700406-013-0412-5 PMID:23689838

Sabin, C. A. (2013). Do people with HIV infection have a normal life expectancy in the era of combination antiretroviral therapy? *BMC Medicine*, *11*(1), 1–7. doi:10.1186/1741-7015-11-251 PMID:24283830

Sermrittirong, S., & Van Brakel, W. H. (2014). Stigma in leprosy: Concepts, causes and determinants. *Leprosy Review*, *85*(1), 36–47. doi:10.47276/lr.85.1.36 PMID:24974441

Shaw, G. M., & Hunter, E. (2012). HIV transmission. *Cold Spring Harbor Perspectives in Medicine*, *2*(11), a006965. doi:10.1101/cshperspect.a006965 PMID:23043157

Shi, Y. (2003). Stochastic dynamic model of SARS spreading. *Chinese Science Bulletin*, *48*(13), 1287–1292. doi:10.1007/BF03184164 PMID:32214705

Smith, R. A. (2012). An experimental test of stigma communication content with a hypothetical infectious disease alert. *Communication Monographs*, *79*(4), 522–538. doi:10.1080/03637751.2012.723811

Smith, R. A., & Hughes, D. (2014). Infectious disease stigmas: Maladaptive in modern society. *Communication Studies*, *65*(2), 132–138. doi:10.1080/10510974.2013.851096 PMID:25477728

Sophea, L. (2006, December). *Overcoming Stigma*. https://leprosyhistory.org/testimonies/overcoming-stigma

Sturrock, B. R., & Mucklow, S. (2018). What is the evidence for the change in the blood donation deferral period for high-risk groups and does it go far enough? *Clinical Medicine*, *18*(4), 304–307. doi:10.7861/clinmedicine.18-4-304 PMID:30072554

Weill Cornell Medicine. (2022, February 18). *Patient Possibly Cured of HIV Infection by Special Stem-Cell Transplant*. https://news.weill.cornell.edu/news/2022/02/patient-possibly-cured-of-hiv-infection-by-special-stem-cell-transplant

Weiss, M. G., Ramakrishna, J., & Somma, D. (2006). Health-related stigma: Rethinking concepts and interventions. *Psychology Health and Medicine*, *11*(3), 277–287. doi:10.1080/13548500600595053 PMID:17130065

Yang, L. H., Kleinman, A., Link, B. G., Phelan, J. C., Lee, S., & Good, B. (2007). Culture and stigma: Adding moral experience to stigma theory. *Social Science & Medicine*, *64*(7), 1524–1535. doi:10.1016/j.socscimed.2006.11.013 PMID:17188411

Young, S. D., Nussbaum, A. D., & Monin, B. (2007). Potential moral stigma and reactions to sexually transmitted diseases: Evidence for a disjunction fallacy. *Personality and Social Psychology Bulletin*, *33*(6), 789–799. doi:10.1177/0146167207301027 PMID:17488871

Zhang, B. C., & Chu, Q. S. (2005). Msm and HIV/AIDS in China. *Cell Research*, *15*(11), 858–864. doi:10.1038j.cr.7290359 PMID:16354560

Zolopa, A. R., Andersen, J., Komarow, L., Sanne, I., Sanchez, A., Hogg, E., Suckow, C., & Powderly, W. (2009). Early antiretroviral therapy reduces AIDS progression/death in individuals with acute opportunistic infections: A multicenter randomized strategy trial. *PLoS One*, *4*(5), e5575. doi:10.1371/journal.pone.0005575 PMID:19440326

About the Author

Edward Greenberg is a social science researcher and technology professional with a PhD in criminology from the University of Massachusetts Lowell and an MA in history from the University of Rochester. His healthcare-field experience includes specialized studies in the life sciences at Brandeis University, research at the National Center for Adaptive Neurotechnology as well as volunteer work at Brigham and Women's Hospital. He also has experience as a software engineer for the health services company Cigna.

Index

O

P

Q

R

S

T

V

W

Z

www.ingramcontent.com/pod-product-compliance
Lightning Source LLC
LaVergne TN
LVHW081520300926
849161LV00006B/1238